INTRODUCTION TO COMMUNITY-BASED NURSING

INTRODUCTION TO COMMUNITY-BASED NURSING

SECOND EDITION

Roberta Hunt, RN, MSPH
Assistant Professor, Nursing
The College of Saint Catherine
St. Paul, Minnesota

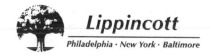
Lippincott
Philadelphia · New York · Baltimore

Acquisitions Editor: Margaret Zuccarini
Managing Editor: Barclay Cunningham
Editorial Assistant: Helen Kogut
Project Editor: Nicole Walz
Senior Production Manager: Helen Ewan
Production Coordinator: Nannette Winski
Senior Art Director: Carolyn O'Brien
Interior Design: Joan Wendt
Manufacturing Manager: William Alberti
Indexer: Michael Ferreira
Compositor: Peirce Graphic Services
Printer: R. R. Donnelley & Sons—Crawfordsville

2nd Edition

9 8 7 6 5 4 3 2 1

Library of Congress Cataloging-in-Publication Data

Hunt, Roberta.
    Introduction to community-based nursing / Roberta Hunt.—2nd ed.
        p. ; cm.
    Includes bibliographical references and index.
    ISBN 0-7817-2814-2 (alk. paper)
    1. Community health nursing.   I. Title: Community-based nursing.   II. Title.
    [DNLM: 1. Community Health Nursing. WY 106 H946i 2001]
    RT98.H86 2001
    610.73'43—dc21   00-050682

DEDICATION

To my husband, Tim Heaney, with love.

RJH

Contributor

Paula Swiggum, MS, RN
Assistant Professor of Nursing
Gustavus Adolphus College
Saint Peter, Minnesota

Reviewers

Christine Brosnan, RNC, DrPH
Assistant Professor and Lead Faculty for Community Health
  Nursing
University of Texas—Houston Health Science Center
Houston, Texas

Mary Emily Cameron, RN, PhD
Assistant Professor of Nursing
Rutgers, the State University of New Jersey
Camden, New Jersey

Karen Cassidy, RN, EdD
Associate Professor of Nursing
Bellarmine College
Louisville, Kentucky

Katherine A. Conroy, RNC, MS
Assistant Professor of Nursing
West Chester University
West Chester, Pennsylvania

Grace P. Erickson, RNC, MPH, MSN, EdD
Assistant Professor of Nursing
University of South Florida
Tampa, Florida

Lucille C. Gambardella, RN, CS, APN, PhD,
Chair and Professor, Division of Nursing
Wesley College
Dover, Delaware

Ruth N. Knollmueller, RN, PhD
Clinical Associate, School of Nursing
University of Connecticut
Hamden, Connecticut

Carol M. Patton, CRNP, DrPH
Director, RN to BSN and Second Degree Programs
Director, Family Nurse Practitioner Program
Assistant Professor of Nursing
Duquesne University
Pittsburgh, Pennsylvania

Preface

The changing health care delivery system presents new challenges for contemporary nurses. Schools of nursing are struggling with the best way to restructure curriculum to meet current needs and to give students experiences in a variety of clinical situations and settings that will prepare them for their careers in the diversified field of nursing. This textbook is designed to fill such a need. *Introduction to Community-Based Nursing*, second edition, is a textbook about community-based nursing. The foundational concepts in this text spring from my experience of more than 20 years of teaching community health nursing and working in community settings. These concepts are articulated with careful attention to the National League for Nursing competencies.

Purpose of the Text

As *Introduction to Community Based Nursing*, second edition, was developed, four major goals were considered:

1. *To give an informative and experiential introduction to nursing care in the community.*

   Before now, most schools of nursing have focused on preparing students to provide care in the hospital. Under the new health care delivery system, much of nursing care has moved out of these acute care settings into a variety of settings and specialties throughout the community. This book presents fundamental aspects of community-based care and builds a knowledge base that the nurse can use in any community setting.

2. *To illustrate the variety of settings and situations in which the community-based nurse gives care.*

   Because of the variety of settings in which a nurse may practice and the limitation of time in the curriculum of schools of nursing, it is often difficult to schedule sufficient diversified clinical experiences. One of the purposes of this text is to address this problem by using a variety of clinical applications. This is accomplished in several ways. First, representative examples of different settings and situations are scattered throughout the body of the text. Second, one of the features of the text, *Example of a Client Situation,* integrates and synthesizes chapter concepts, showing the student step-by-step how the theory in the chapter relates to the reality of clinical practice. Third, additional *Client Care Studies* appear in *Learning Activities* at the end of each chapter and in the Instructor's Manual. Such client care situations give the student an opportunity to practice skills while applying chapter concepts. Last, *Questions for Reflection* for use with a clinical journal or individual assignments are found in the *Learning Activities* at the end of each chapter.

3. *To clarify the cultural diversification of the community in which nurses provide quality care.*

Another important emphasis of *Introduction to Community-Based Nursing*, second edition, is its cross-cultural approach. Our society is diversified with many racial, ethnic, and minority groups. The community-based nurse will care for clients from many diverse cultures and must be prepared to give quality and culturally competent care. Chapter 3, Culture Care, is written by Paula Swiggum, who has extensive experience in cross-cultural nursing in both recruiting and providing academic support for students from diverse cultural backgrounds, as well as in curriculum development. As a member of the Transcultural Nursing Society, she will complete the process of becoming a Certified Transcultural Nurse in 2001. Consideration of cross-cultural issues is woven throughout the text.

4. *To integrate the importance of the individual to the family and the family to the individual throughout the text.*

Most clients will be part of a family. The client's health and the client's care during illness are influenced by the family. At the same time, the client's health status and outlook will influence the continuous growth and development of the family. This symbiotic relationship plays a prominent role in *Introduction to Community-Based Nursing*, Special attention is given to nursing support of the lay caregiver.

Organization of the Text

Introduction to Community-Based Nursing is divided into five units: basic concepts, nursing skills, application, settings, and implications for future practice.

▶ *Unit I, Basic Concepts in Community-Based Nursing*, includes essential elements of community-based nursing. An introductory chapter discusses definitions of a community and a healthy community, components of community-based nursing, and nursing skills and competencies needed to give quality care in the community. The unit also includes information on health promotion and disease prevention, cultural considerations, and family implications.

▶ *Unit II, Skills for Community-Based Nursing Practice*, reviews basics of assessment, teaching, case management, and continuity of care, and addresses those skills specific to community-based settings.

▶ *Unit III, Community-Based Nursing Across the Life Span*, provides assessment guides, teaching materials, and strategies for addressing health promotion and disease prevention across the life span.

▶ *Unit IV, Settings for Practice*, discusses a wide sampling of practice settings and opportunities and practice specialties. A second chapter discusses home health care in depth.

▶ *Unit V, Implications for Future Practice*, discusses trends in health care and implications on community-based nursing.

Consistency of approach was one of the goals in the development of the text. Many chapters include a short section giving a historical perspective on the chapter subject. Most chapters address nursing skills and competencies. These sections may include information on the nursing process or on such things as communication, teaching, and management. Seeming repetition of any information is for the purpose of reinforcing knowledge or skills in light of the chapter's subject. Documentation is covered in many chapters because of its importance to community-based nursing. All chapters end with *Learning Activities*.

Key Features of the Text

The following features of the book were developed as pedagogical aids for the student. They help clarify text information, give the student guidelines for actions, or require the student to use critical thinking.

- ▶ Learning Activities: three to five activities at the end of every chapter. These contain the following exercises:
  - ▶ Questions for Reflection: to be used for a clinical journal or as individual assignments to assist the student in applying theoretical content to clinical situations to become a reflective practitioner.
  - ▶ Client Care Study: at least one in most chapters. A client situation is given with critical thinking exercises.
  - ▶ Critical Thinking Exercises: at least one in every chapter. A problem is presented in a sentence or two with directions for critical thinking.
  - ▶ Practical Application: appear in many chapters. Not related to a specific client, these include activities to prepare the student for clinical application.
- ▶ Community-Based Nursing Care Guidelines: boxed information that includes specific interventions for the community-based nurse.
- ▶ Community-Based Teaching: boxed lists of information to give clients and their families.
- ▶ Research Related to Community-Based Nursing Care: boxed information that includes short paragraphs of descriptive research.
- ▶ Assessment guides: many chapters provide sample assessment forms to be used in community-based nursing care.
- ▶ Health promotion and disease prevention teaching material: plentiful materials in Chapters 9, 10, and 11 for health teaching, and addresses of Web sites from which numerous additional materials can be downloaded.
- ▶ Glossary: helps the student review terminology or understand new terminology used in the book.
- ▶ Other pedagogical aids: Objectives, Key Terms, Chapter Outlines, References and Bibliography.
- ▶ What's on the Web. Found in most chapters, these features contain addresses and descriptions of Web sites related to the chapter material and providing additional resources. Chapter 14 includes a list of general Web sites helpful in community-based nursing.

We have tried to avoid sexist terms for the nurse and clients. Throughout the text we have used the term "family" for consistency. However, the term refers to anyone who is concerned about and supportive of the client and can signify a relative or significant other.

Instructor's Manual

The Instructor's Manual was prepared with an ongoing emphasis on practical application of the student's knowledge base. More than 50 assignments, test questions, and additional client care studies are designed to develop skills and knowledge essential for the unique role of the associate-degree nurse in

community-based nursing. Suggestions of how to identify, develop, and structure community-based clinical experiences are also found in the manual. Many
of the assignments have been used and improved over the years of teaching
community health nursing.

Roberta Hunt, RN, MSPH
hunthean@pro-ns.net

Acknowledgments

I am grateful to many individuals, especially family, friends, and colleagues, for their encouragement and assistance in the development of this textbook. It is impossible to acknowledge everyone, given the limitations of memory and space.

To all my colleagues who have given encouragement and validation and who have made the teaching of nursing an exciting and stimulating profession—you have contributed to this project. The more than 2,000 students whom I have had the pleasure of working with in the classroom and in clinical settings in the community, who have provided feedback and suggestions about my teaching and assignments, have each made an invaluable contribution to this book.

There are several people in the Nursing Education department of Lippincott Williams & Wilkins who have provided invaluable expertise and assistance. If it weren't for Donna Hilton, who contacted me with enthusiastic encouragement to consider using my course manual as the basis for a textbook, this project never would have gotten off the ground. Margaret Zuccarini, Senior Acquisitions Editor, has given professional guidance to craft and redefine the focus of this text. Hilarie Surrena has been terrific with her quick, competent assistance. Jackie Smith made important contributions with her valuable editorial assistance. Most of all, thanks to Barclay Cunningham, Managing Editor, whose congenial personality coupled with elegant editorial suggestions has made the last leg of this journey pleasant and painless. Thanks to Nicole Walz, Project Editor, for her quick response time and her kind and sweet temperament. She made the last of the "dirty details" quick and easy.

To my dear friend of many years, Paula Swiggum, I owe an enormous thanks for writing Chapter 3, Culture Care. This expertly crafted and beautifully written chapter adds a great deal to the overall message of the importance of respectful care, which is the central premise of *Introduction to Community-Based Nursing*.

Finally, I am grateful to my family and friends who provide day-to-day support and encouragement. To all of my colleagues, at the College of St. Catherine: Susan, Linda, Marva, Barbara, Romana, Pam, Vicki, Pat, Sara, Kathleen, Mary, Alice, Carol, JoAnne, Brenda, Suellen, Maggie, and Deb, the most professional and supportive faculty group an educator could ever hope to work with—thanks for the daily sustenance. I especially want to thank Joann O'Leary,

Sue Larson, and Meg Carolan, for their ongoing friendship and listening ear. Thanks to my family, especially Becky Hunt Carmody, Ila and John Harris, and Steve Hunt, for your continuing encouragement. To Andrew and Mark, you guys are the most terrific young men, you make your Dad and me so proud of you. To my wonderful daughters—Jackie, for your cheerful attitude plus valuable editorial assistance prodding me forward, and Megan, for your thoughtful advice and balanced view of the world—a heartfelt thank-you. Most of all, I am grateful to my loving husband, Tim Heaney—your committed attitude towards me and all that I do has helped me become more than I ever imagined.

Roberta Hunt

Contents

Basic Concepts in Community-Based Nursing

Before you practice nursing in a community-based setting, you must understand the basic concepts behind community-based health care. Unit I introduces these concepts as a knowledge base for further exploration as you begin to apply what you have learned.

Chapter 1 gives an overview of community-based nursing, beginning with a brief historical perspective. Health care reform and health care funding, which have taken health care out of the hospital and into the community, are discussed, along with the definition of a community, especially a healthy community. Components of community-based care and nursing skills and competencies round out the introductory chapter.

Health promotion and disease prevention, as outlined by the federal government's *Healthy People 2010,* is the focus of Chapter 2.

Chapter 3 discusses the ever-changing makeup of our society and asks you to look at your own cultural background and your attitudes about diversity. The chapter promotes culturally competent care.

Chapter 4 discusses family involvement, an important consideration in community-based care.

The remainder of the book will use these concepts to build your knowledge base and relate it to practical experiences.

Overview of
Community-Based Nursing

R O B E R T A   H U N T

▶LEARNING OBJECTIVES◀

- Identify major issues leading to the development of community-based nursing.

- Discuss the current reimbursement system for health care services and its impact on nursing.

- Describe the factors that define community.

- Indicate the relationship between health and community.

- Compare acute care nursing, community-based nursing, and community health nursing.

- Discuss components of community-based care.

- Examine the skills with which you perform necessary competencies.

▶KEY TERMS◀

acute care
advance directives
community
community-based nursing
continuity
demographics
diagnosis-related groups (DRGs)
extended family

health maintenance organizations
living will
nuclear family
preferred provider
   organizations
prospective payment
self-care
vital statistics

Historical Perspectives

Health Care Reform

Health Care Funding

The Community

Community Nursing Versus Community-Based Nursing

Focus of Nursing

Components of Community-Based Care

Nursing Skills and Competencies

Conclusions

Changes in settings for nursing practice have occurred since the early 1980s as a result of public concern regarding our health care system. Concerns center on quality, access, and cost of health care as well as fragmentation of health care. These concerns and the resultant changes give nurses an opportunity to help shape health care at the beginning of the millennium. In 1999, the National League for Nursing (NLN) predicted 10 trends in health care that will affect nursing education and practice (Box 1–1).

These trends and the implications for nursing educational preparation and quality nursing practice are the focus of this book. This chapter provides an overview of nursing care by first giving historical background and introducing the reader to the community and community-based nursing. Components of community-based nursing practice, skills, and competencies are covered.

 HISTORICAL PERSPECTIVES

During most of the 20th century, nursing care was associated primarily with hospital settings (Bellack & O'Neil, 1999). However, historically, the setting for nursing care was in the home. The first written reference to care of the ill in the home

---

► **Box 1–1.** The Future of Nursing Education: 10 Trends to Watch ◄

1. Changing demographics and increasing diversity
2. The technologic explosion
3. Globalization of the world's economy and society
4. The era of the educated consumer, alternative therapies and genomics and palliative care
5. Shift to population-based care and the increasing complexity of patient care
6. The cost of health care and the challenge of managed care
7. Impact of health policy and regulation
8. The growing need for interdisciplinary education for collaborative practice
9. The current nursing shortage/opportunities for lifelong learning and workforce development
10. Significant advances in nursing science and research

Source: National League for Nursing. (1999). *The future of nursing education: Ten trends to watch*. New York: Author. (http://www.nln.org/infotrends.htm)

is found in the New Testament, in which mention is made of visiting the sick at home to aid in their care.

Florence Nightingale is credited as the mother of modern nursing. Typically her contribution of developing a model for educating nurses in hospital-based programs is cited. Nightingale's curriculum also included the first training programs to educate district nurses, with 1 year of training devoted to promoting self-care and the health of communities (Monteiro, 1991).

William Rathbone, a resident of Liverpool, England in the 1850s, is credited with establishing the modern concept of the visiting nurse (Kalish & Kalish, 1995). Lillian Wald and Mary Brewster began a program for visiting nurses in the United States in the early 1900s (Frachel, 1988). Wald, the founder of public health nursing, drew on contemporary ideas that linked nursing, motherhood, social welfare, and the public. Her work was designed to respond to the needs of those populations at greatest risk through nursing the sick in their homes and providing preventive instructions to reduce illness. Wald argued that the nurse, through her "peculiar introduction to the patient and her organic relationship with the neighborhood," could be the "starting point" for wider service in the community. Wald believed that nurses could reach and educate their clients in the broadest sense, drawing on diversity of cultural beliefs and societal demands of the populace (Reverby, 1993).

Shift From Community to Hospital

In 1910, 90% of all nursing care was provided in the home. After World War I, care of the sick began the move to the hospital. Early in the 1950s, the growing complexity in health care technology resulted in an increase in the need for hospital care. During the 1960s and 1970s, it was not uncommon for a person to stay in the hospital for 7 to 10 days for uncomplicated conditions or surgery (Craven & Hirnle, 1996).

This trend continued until the early 1980s, when escalating health care costs prompted changes in the health care delivery system and its financing. In summary, the nursing care provided in the home in the 1800s migrated to the acute care hospital in the middle of the 20th century and then back to the home in the 1980s. This move is depicted in Figure 1-1.

An Era of Cost Containment

President Reagan signed the Tax Equity and Fiscal Responsibility Act (TEFRA) in 1982 and the Social Security Amendments of 1983. This legislation changed the way Medicare and Medicaid services were reimbursed, initiating a service called the **prospective payment system**. The prospective payment system calculates reimbursement to hospitals based on the client's diagnosis according to federally mandated **diagnosis-related groups (DRGs)**. The client's diagnosis is categorized according to the federal DRG coding system and payment is bundled into one fee, which is then paid to the hospital. Payment by client diagnosis, therefore, was an attempt to contain Medicare and Medicaid costs.

Gradually, many insurance companies, health maintenance organizations, and other third-party payers adopted the DRG method of payment. As the reimbursement system for health care changed, the average length of stay for a hospitalized client decreased substantially. In fact, it became financially advantageous for the hospital if clients had shorter stays. As a result, a scenario was created in which clients were discharged "quicker and sicker." With this transition, it became evident that it was more cost-effective to provide services outside the hospital.

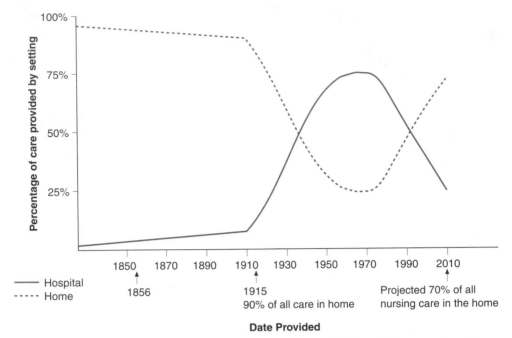

Figure 1–1. ▶ Settings for nursing care as changed from 1850 until the present and as projected into the future.

Shift From Hospital to Community

Acute Care Setting

Acute care became the term used for people who were receiving intensive hospital care. The term is used today for the setting in which this care is provided. An acute care setting contrasts with the hospital setting, which also can be used as an ambulatory clinic or day surgery unit. In general, individuals in acute care settings are very sick. Many are postsurgical clients or need highly technical care. Many of these clients have life-threatening conditions and require close monitoring and constant care. The care given these clients is specialized and requires considerable expertise in physical caregiving. Acute nursing care is very different from community-based nursing care, as evidenced by differences between hospital and home environments shown in Table 1–1.

Community Setting

Clients affected by the transition into community-based health care were not in need of fewer services. Rather, the focus of services simply shifted from the hospital to the community. Care that once was considered safe only within the hospital became routine in outpatient settings such as ambulatory care centers, surgical centers, dialysis centers, rehabilitation centers, walk-in clinics, physicians' offices, and the home.

   The change in health care services resulted in changes in nursing care as well. Settings changed to the community, and especially the home. It is projected that by 2010, as shown in Figure 1–1, 70% of all nursing care will be provided in the home, with an adjunct increase in the availability of care in the community, including more technically complicated and "hi-tech" services and procedures

TABLE 1–1 • Differences Between Hospital and Home

Factors	Hospital	Home
Practice		
Resources	Predetermined	Variable
Environment	Predictable	Highly variable
Locating client	Simple	Requires planning
Access to client	Routine	Determined by client's family
Focus	Individual	Client in family system
Family support	Helpful	Critical
Client role	Relatively dependent	Highly autonomous
Instruction		
Student safety	Awareness	Central concern
Supervision of practice	Mostly direct	Mostly indirect
Teaching style	Often teacher-directed	Collaborative problem-solving

Source: Reed, F. C., & Wuyscik, M. A. (1998). Community health strategies: Teach what? Reflections on the transition from hospital teaching to teaching in the community. *Nurse Educator, 23*(3), 11–13.

(Clarke & Cody, 1994). In the past decade, the number of nurses working in every employment setting has increased. However, the rate of increase in hospitals is less than in previous years. The greatest increase occurred in community-based settings (NLN, 1997).

The Bureau of Labor Statistics predicts that health care services will increase by 30% by the year 2006, accounting for 3.1 million jobs. Nursing is one of the five occupations projected to have the largest number of jobs in the next decade. However, it is anticipated that the size of the registered nurse workforce will be nearly 20% below projected requirements by 2020. Unlike nursing shortages in the past, this shortage will be driven by a permanent shift in the labor market which is unlikely to reverse in the next few years (Buerhaus, Staiger, & Auerbach, 2000).

With these changes it becomes imperative for nursing educators to prepare graduates for positions outside the walls of the acute care setting and for roles in the community. The NLN (2000a) recommends that there be a shift in emphasis for all nursing education to continue to ensure that all nurses from all education levels are prepared to function in a community-based, community-focused health care system. This means that nurses must be competent to practice in varied settings across the continuum of care (American Organization of Nurse Executives [AONE], 2000).

Nursing care also has changed from a medical view of healing the sick to an orientation that focuses on disease prevention and health promotion. As the health care system is evolving and changing, there will be an increased need for nurses. Nurses are also developing relationships with the communities, in which they work and are becoming active in policy-making and client advocacy.

 HEALTH CARE REFORM

Health care in general is in transition. The United States is in the midst of reviewing and revising its health care system, and few people deny that some changes must occur. Legislation on state and national levels may result in the most dramatic changes of all. *Healthy People 2010* (U.S. Department of Health and Human

Services, 2000), which lists government goals (discussed further in Chapter 2), has stirred our imagination in meeting the needs of all Americans. Particular populations have been targeted for care. The question has been raised: Is health care a right or a privilege? Who gets health care and who pays for this health care will be at the center of the debate for some time. These issues present challenges and opportunities for the nurse in the first decade of the new century.

How do nurses fit into health care reform? Huston and Fox (1998) answer this by saying that (1) all nurses must be prepared for practice in community settings, (2) nurses must understand the business aspects of health care, and (3) nurses in community settings need highly developed skills in assessment, communication, interdisciplinary collaboration, and working with culturally diverse populations.

 HEALTH CARE FUNDING

Health care is extremely expensive, and costs continue to rise. Increasing health care costs have affected many health care agencies and organizations. They must now find funds, in addition to fee-for-service charges, in the form of voluntary donations and state and federal programs.

Few individuals can afford to pay their health care costs out of their own pockets. Many individuals belong to health maintenance organizations or rely on government-funded health care such as Medicare and Medicaid. Insurance plans, health maintenance organizations, and government programs provide a variety of coverage plans. Many, however, do not cover preventive care, psychiatric treatment, outpatient support services, or medications. Many limit the amount of service paid for a particular type of care, such as home health care visits.

Federally Funded Health Care

Primary government funding comes through Medicare and Medicaid. Under Medicare, home health care is an important service for the elderly and will be of growing concern as the elderly population increases in the United States. Medicare covers nursing, physical, speech, and occupational therapies; home care aids; medical social services; and some medical supplies. With the Balanced Budget Act in 1997, changes were made to Medicare's payment system to contain cost. These changes have affected and will continue to affect the role of the nurse in the delivery of home care services (Jitramontree, 2000).

Group Plans

Group plans include health maintenance organizations (HMOs), preferred provider organizations (PPOs), and private insurance. **Health maintenance organizations** are prepaid, structured, managed systems in which providers deliver a comprehensive range of health care services to enrollees. **Preferred provider organizations** allow a network of providers to provide services at a lower fee in return for prompt payment at prenegotiated rates. Private insurance may be obtained through large, nonprofit, tax-exempt organizations or through small, private, for-profit insurance companies. This type of insurance is called third-party payment. Long-term care insurance may also be obtained through private insurance companies.

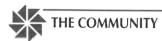 THE COMMUNITY

Nurses who practice community-based nursing need to understand the community within which they practice. Knowledge of the community helps nurses maintain quality of care.

Defining Community

Community can be defined in numerous ways, depending on the application. This text uses the definition of community as "a people, location, and social system" (Josten, 1989).

People: Families, Culture, and Community

The variety of individuals, families, and cultural groups represented in a community contributes to the overall character of that community. The simplest way to understand a community is through **vital statistics** and **demographics.** These data may be thought of as the community's vital statistics, similar to an individual's vital signs. A community consisting primarily of senior citizens has a totally different personality from a community of young, unmarried adults.

The characteristics of the families living in a community contribute to the overall complexion of that community and in turn the community health care needs. In communities where families are strong and nurturing, there is an opportunity for a strong and caring community. In communities where families are nonexistent or fail to provide an adequate basis for individual growth, problems with physical abuse, neglect, substance abuse, and violence may arise. A strong family unit is the basic building block for strong communities.

Culture contributes to the overall character of a community and, in turn, its health needs. In most of the world, a scarcity of resources necessitates **extended family** residences. Included in the extended family are grandparents, aunts, uncles, and other relatives. When living together in one household, many members may be involved with child care and care of the sick or injured. In these communities, there are different needs related to child and health care than in communities such as those in the United States and Western Europe, where the **nuclear family** is the norm. In the 6% of the world where nuclear family structures prevail, isolation and self-reliance affect the design and delivery of services. A client, then, who has a nuclear family and no extended family often has different needs from the client with numerous extended family members living in the same household or close by.

The role of individuals according to their age is often dictated by culture. In some cultures, the older people are retired from leadership and governing responsibilities, whereas in other cultures these members are considered essential to the governing structure of the community. In this situation, the more prestigious positions of authority and responsibility are assigned to the older members of the community.

Health is affected by culture. Madeleine Leininger (1970) observed that "health and illness states are strongly influenced and often primarily determined by the cultural background of an individual." The culture of the individual and his or her family has an impact on the community's definition of health and on the service needs of that community.

Location: Community Boundaries

A community usually is defined by boundaries. Boundaries may be geographic, such as those defined as a city, county, state, or nation. Boundaries may be political; precincts and wards may determine them. Boundaries to a community may also emerge as the result of identifying or solving a problem. Consequently, a community may establish a boundary within which a problem can be defined and solved. Figure 1–2 depicts this variety of community boundaries.

Community boundaries are important because they often determine what services are available to individuals living within a particular geographic area. Eligibility for services may be limited, or not allowed, depending on whether or not one resides within a certain geographic area. It is important for the nurse to realize that community boundaries limit availability of, and eligibility for, services. For example, you are a nurse working at Ramsey County Hospital. Your patient is from Hennepin County. You will refer the client to services in Hennepin County. The client, however, may also be eligible for services with a home health care agency that serves multiple counties but is not located in Hennepin County. It is helpful for you to be familiar with eligibility requirements of a variety of community organizations.

It is important to have a working knowledge of service restrictions for agencies in a geographic area. In some counties, the first assessment visit by the county nurse is free; in some areas this may not be the case. Not only should the nurse be familiar with boundaries and basic eligibility criteria and restriction, the nurse also needs to know about the available resources within the area.

A community defined by its problems and solutions has a fluid boundary. The problems and those who are affected by those problems determine this

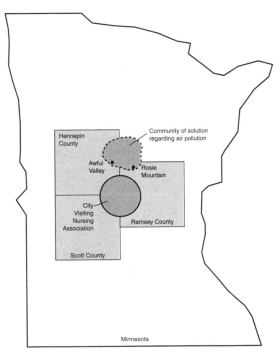

Figure 1–2. ▶ A community's boundaries may be many things: geographic, political, problematic. These boundaries are used in the example in this chapter.

boundary. This allows all those who may be affected by the problems to partic- ipate in the solutions and the resulting outcome. Thus, a more fluid boundary may allow for greater eligibility or opportunity for service.

The problem of air pollution in one community provides us with an exam- ple of a community solution where the boundary is fluid. In the suburbs of Rosie Mountain and Awful Valley (see Fig. 1–2), two school nurses in different ele- mentary schools notice that the percentage of children they are seeing with symptoms of asthma is on the increase. The school nurses talk to each other and note that most of the children with asthma in both school districts live west of a large oil refinery. The school nurses contact the Department of Health. The parents of the children from both schools are invited to a public meeting to dis- cuss the issue of air pollution and the incidence of asthma. After several meet- ings, a group of parents from both schools forms a constituency devoted to the identification of the problem and potential solutions. The theoretical boundaries of this community are shown in Figure 1–2. Established school boundaries be- come fluid in this scenario when a problem arises.

Social Systems

Social systems have an impact on a community and, consequently, the health of that community. Social systems include a community's economy, education, re- ligion, welfare, politics, recreation, legal system, health care, safety and trans- portation, and communication systems. Depending on the infrastructure, these systems may have a beneficial or detrimental impact on the health of individu- als living in a given community. Where recreational facilities provide opportu- nities for health promotion activities, for instance, the health of the citizens will be enhanced.

It is a documented fact that the infant mortality rate is lower in communi- ties where prenatal care is available and readily accessible to all pregnant women. Here is a social system at work within a community; it has a profound impact on the quality of health of its individual members.

A Healthy Community

Just as there are characteristics of healthy individuals, so are there character- istics of healthy communities. These include:

- ▶ Awareness that "we are community"
- ▶ Conservation of natural resources
- ▶ Recognition of, and respect for, the existence of subgroups
- ▶ Participation of subgroups in community affairs
- ▶ Preparation to meet crises
- ▶ Ability to solve problems
- ▶ Communication through open channels
- ▶ Resources available to all
- ▶ Settling of disputes through legitimate mechanisms
- ▶ Participation by citizens in decision-making
- ▶ Wellness of a high degree among its members

A dynamic relationship exists between health and community. In this rela- tionship, health is considered in the context of the community's people, its lo- cation, and its social system (Fig. 1–3). Healthy citizens can contribute to the overall health, vitality, and economy of the community. Similarly, if a large pro- portion of individuals in a community is not healthy, not productive, or poorly

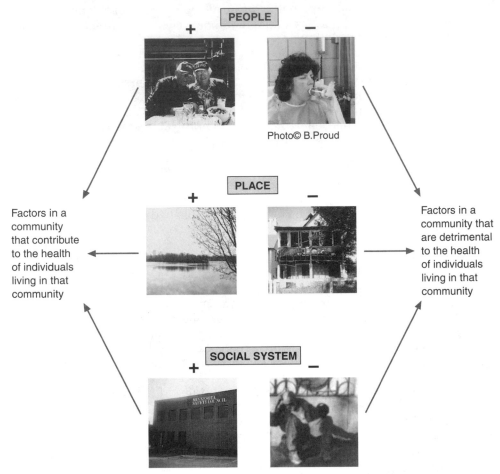

Figure 1–3. ▶ A community's health is considered in the context of its people, its location, and its social system.

nourished, the community can suffer from a lack of vitality and productivity (Fig. 1–4).

Location also influences the health of a community. If a toxic landfill or refinery contaminates the earth, water, or air, the health of the people in the area will obviously be detrimentally affected. Figure 1–5 illustrates the relationship between the location and the level of health in a given community.

Social systems and public policy also affect health. Figure 1–6 shows how a community's social systems affect its health. For example, there will be fewer smokers in communities where smoking is not allowed in public buildings or the sale of cigarettes to minors is restricted and strictly enforced. In a community where all pregnant women receive prenatal care, the infant mortality rate will be lower. In a community where immunizations are available and accessible to all children, the immunization rate will be higher and the communicable disease rates low. The array of social systems that affect health is pictured in Figure 1–6.

The public sees lowering crime rates, strengthening families and their lifestyles, improving environmental quality, and providing behavioral or mental

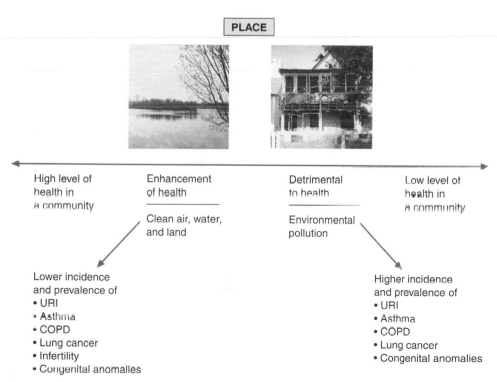

PEOPLE		
Functional		Nonfunctional

High level of health in a community → Productive / Able to: • Work • Care for self or others • Volunteer • Pay taxes → Nonproductive / Unable to: • Work • Care for self or others • Volunteer • Pay taxes → Low level of health in a community

Figure 1–4. ▶ Functional and dysfunctional individuals affect the health of the community.

PLACE

High level of health in a community

Enhancement of health
————
Clean air, water, and land

Detrimental to health
————
Environmental pollution

Low level of health in a community

Lower incidence and prevalence of
• URI
• Asthma
• COPD
• Lung cancer
• Infertility
• Congenital anomalies

Higher incidence and prevalence of
• URI
• Asthma
• COPD
• Lung cancer
• Congenital anomalies

Figure 1–5. ▶ Location affects the health of the community.

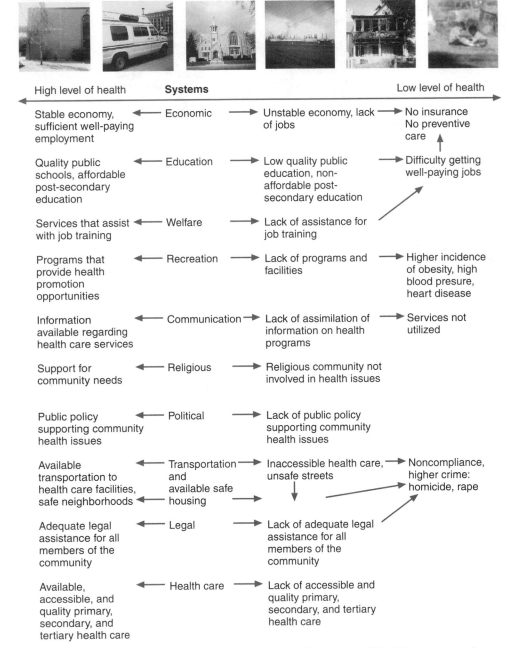

Figure 1–6. ▶ Social system and public policy affect the health of the community.

health care as critical elements to creating healthy communities. A Healthcare Forum survey in 1993 points out " . . . the emergence of public recognition that one's health is somehow related to the health of one's neighbors; suggesting that perhaps, the most practical approach to pursuing a healthier life is the pursuit of a healthier community."

 ## COMMUNITY NURSING VERSUS COMMUNITY-BASED NURSING

More opportunities are created for nurses in the community as the setting for nursing care moves outside the acute care setting. (Many of these settings, positions, and opportunities are discussed in Chapter 12.) The prominent nursing role in the community in the past was that of public health or community health nurse, but this has changed with the current health care delivery system. Although a monumental need for provision of nursing care in the community has resulted from the changes in the health care delivery system, this increase for nurses has been not for community health nurses but for community-based nurses.

The American Nurses Association (1986) stated, "While community health nursing practice includes nursing directed to individuals, families and groups, the dominant responsibility is to the population as the whole." Thus, community, or public, health nursing is defined by its role in promoting the public's health. Community health nursing is a subset of community-based nursing. Community health nursing has a definitive philosophy of practice and requires specific knowledge and skill.

Community-based nursing is not defined by the setting or by the level of academic preparation but by a philosophy of practice (Hunt, 1998). It is about how the nurse practices, not where the nurse practices. Community-based nursing is based on the following concepts (NLN, 2000a):

► The individual and the family have primary responsibility for health care decisions.
► Health and social issues are acknowledged as interactive.
► Treatment effectiveness, rather than the technologic imperative, drives decisions.

Community-based nursing care can be defined as nursing care directed toward specific individuals and families within a community. It is designed to meet needs of people as they move between and among health care settings. The emphasis is on a "flowing" kind of care that does not necessarily occur in one setting (Craven & Hirnle, 1996).

High-technology care that previously was available only in acute care settings is now provided in the home. The community-based nurse must teach clients and families how to manage highly technical equipment and to be responsible for complex self-care.

 ## FOCUS OF NURSING

Nursing, in any setting and with any nursing theory, involves a focus of four components: the client, the environment, health, and nursing (Fawcett, 1984). Each area is approached differently depending on whether the care is provided in the acute care setting or in the community-based setting (Table 1–1).

In the acute care setting, the client is typically identified by the medical diagnosis and is separated from the family. The environment is controlled by the facility with restriction of the family's access to the client and a limitation on the client's freedom. Health and illness are seen as separate and apart from one another. If the client is discharged, the goals of acute care are met. Nursing functions are largely delegated medical functions that center on treatment of illness.

In community-based nursing, the client is in his or her natural environment, in the context of the family and community. Illness is seen as merely an aspect of life, and the goals of care are focused around maximizing the client's quality of life. Nursing in the community is an autonomous practice, for the most part, with nursing interventions decided on by both the client and family and the health care team and based on the values of the client or family and the community. The community model of care reflects the principles of community-based nursing where the goal of care is to encourage self-care in the context of the family and community with a focus on prevention and continuity of care.

 ## COMPONENTS OF COMMUNITY-BASED CARE

Transitions in health care settings and consumer participation have brought about some changes in the directions of health care. Several components make up community-based care: self-care, preventive health care, care within the context of the community, continuity of care, and collaborative care. These are described here and expanded on throughout the text.

Self-Care: Client and Family Responsibility

The consumer movement within the past several decades has led to self-care awareness. Consumers are becoming aware that it is better to take care of themselves and remain healthy than to neglect their health and have to treat an illness or injury. Programs on stress management, nutrition, exercise and fitness, antismoking and antidrug use are examples of this health-seeking behavior on the part of consumers. As a further result, political and government factions have promoted such things as seatbelt use, motorcycle and bicycle safety, pollution control, and handgun control.

The first component of community-based nursing is self-care. **Self-care** charges the individual client and the family with primary responsibility for health care decisions and actions. Because more and more health care is provided outside the acute care setting, by design this care must be provided by the client, family, or other caregiver such as a friend or neighbor rather than a health care professional. It has become too expensive to do otherwise.

Empowering the individual to make informed health care decisions is an essential component of self-care. One example is the recently introduced federal mandate for advance directives. **Advance directives** allow clients to participate in decisions about their care, including the right to refuse treatment. One type of advance directive is the **living will,** which is the client's statement regarding the medical treatment he or she chooses to omit or refuses in the event the client is unable to make those decisions for himself or herself.

Although community-based nursing affords the opportunity for direct intervention, it also requires self-care teaching for the client and caregiver. The nurse's participation in self-care requires use of the nursing process. In other words, assessment, planning, implementation, and evaluation revolve around this question: How much care can the client and other caregivers safely provide themselves?

Preventive Care

Treatment efficacy rather than technologic imperative promotes nursing care that emphasizes prevention. Community-based nursing considers all three levels of prevention (discussed in Chapter 2). Unlike community health nursing, community-based nursing focuses primarily on tertiary prevention. This emphasis is evident in all settings of community-based nursing.

For example, a nurse in the emergency room considers not only the impact of the child's poisoning, but also what preventive nursing interventions will maximize recovery and prevent a repeat of the incident. Careful teaching about wound care to avoid infection is an important preventive intervention for the client who is having a laceration sutured. Likewise, referral of a client for substance abuse assessment is an appropriate preventive nursing intervention for an intoxicated person who presents at the urgent care center after a fall.

Care Within the Context of the Community

Another component of community-based nursing recognizes that health and social issues are interactive. Nursing care is provided while considering the culture, values, and resources of the client, the family, and the community. If the client requests a particular religious or social ceremony before tube feeding, then the nurse attempts, within the constraints of safety, to comply with the client's request. In situations where family members want to participate in the client's care but their psychomotor skills restrict their ability to do so, the nurse will accommodate the desire within the constraints of time and safe care. If the client lives in a community where older individuals enjoy the social functions of religious services every week, the visiting nurse honors that community value by careful scheduling of visits.

Care in the context of the client, family, and community is affected by the location and social systems of each community. Location often defines eligibility for health care services. Consequently, access and availability of services affect the health of the community. For instance, access to care is impeded by location when an adolescent who does not drive lives in the suburbs where there is no public transportation and seeks information about family planning services offered only in the nearby metropolitan area. In such a case, the social systems of the community affect access to care.

Continuity of Care

Fragmentation of care has long been a concern of health care professionals. For instance, a client with a variety of problems may be seen by several physicians: the family physician, cardiologist, endocrinologist, consultants, and surgeon. A variety of other health care providers may be involved in the care also. This fragmentation of care can result in conflicting directions for care, overmedication or undermedication, and a confused client. **Continuity** of care is a bridge to quality care.

Community-based care becomes essential when clients are seen by several health care practitioners and move from one health care setting to another. Continuity allows for quality of care to be preserved in a changing health care delivery system. If all providers follow the basic principles of continuity of care, then the possibility of a detrimental impact from a decreased length of stay in the acute care setting, where care is coordinated, to a community setting where care is provided through a variety of individuals, can be minimized. Continuity is the glue that holds community-based nursing care together and is one of the philosophies behind the writing of this book. Continuity of care is discussed in Chapter 8.

Collaborative Care

Closely related to continuity of care is collaborative care. Collaborative care among health care professionals is an essential part of holistic care because the primary goal of each practitioner should be to promote wellness and restore health. Regardless of the setting, the community-based nurse works with a variety of professionals as care for the client is assessed, planned, implemented, and evaluated.

The physician is responsible primarily for the diagnosis of the illness and medical or surgical treatment required. Some physicians may specialize. Physicians have the authority to admit clients into a specific health care setting and to discharge them from that setting into another setting. The orders they write are followed by other professionals and the client, who report to the physician on outcomes. The pharmacist dispenses medications as directed by the physician.

Various therapists may be involved in the client's care. They specialize in such fields as physical therapy, occupational therapy, respiratory therapy, and speech therapy. They may provide therapy in the acute care setting, a rehabilitation setting, a residential care setting, or in the home. The client may visit the facility or the therapist may visit the home.

A dietitian may be asked to adapt a specialized diet to a specific individual and family or to counsel and educate clients and their families. The social worker helps clients and families make decisions related to use of community resources, life-sustaining treatments, and long-term care. A chaplain or the client's spiritual advisor will also counsel the client and family and give spiritual support.

Although each professional is responsible for a specialized concern, each is also responsible for sharing that information with others or for evaluating how care is proceeding. If one person in the chain fails to communicate, the bridge of continuity is weakened. Usually one person is designated as coordinator of these communications. In many cases this coordinator is the nurse. The nurse who coordinates collaborative care is discussed in Chapter 7.

NURSING SKILLS AND COMPETENCIES

Although transitions have been made in health care in the past two decades, models of community-based care continue to develop. The Pew Health Professions Commission (1998) identified 21 competencies that health care professionals will need in the 21st century. These competencies, listed in Box 1–2, emphasize community-based nursing care principles. Although these competencies apply to all

▶ Box 1–2. Pew Commission: 21 Competencies for the 21st Century ◀

1. Embrace a personal ethic of social responsibility and service.
2. Exhibit ethical behavior in all professional activities.
3. Provide evidence-based, clinically competent care.
4. Incorporate the multiple determinants of health in clinical care.
5. Apply knowledge of the new sciences.
6. Demonstrate critical thinking reflection, and problem-solving skills.
7. Understand the role of primary care.
8. Rigorously practice preventive health care.
9. Integrate population-based care and services into practice.
10. Improve access to health care for those with unmet health needs
11. Practice relationship-centered care with individuals and families.
12. Provide culturally sensitive care to a diverse society.
13. Partner with communities in health care decisions.
14. Use communication and information technology effectively and appropriately.
15. Work in interdisciplinary teams.
16. Ensure care that balance individual, professional, system and societal needs.
17. Practice leadership.
18. Take responsibility for quality of care and health outcomes at all levels.
19. Contribute to continuous improvement of the health care system.
20. Advocate for public policy that promotes and protects the health of the public.
21. Continue to learn and help others learn.

Source: Bellack, J., & O'Neil, E. (2000). Recreating nursing practice for a new century. *Nursing and Healthcare Perspectives, 21*(1), 14–18.

health care professionals, the term "nurse" can be substituted in place of the term "practitioners" in the statements.

Nursing care in the acute care setting and the community differ greatly. Consequently, the nursing roles in each setting require different practice skills. Nursing roles differ in acute care, community-based health care, and home care. In the acute care setting, nurses spend the majority of their time in direct patient care and have little time for administrative, supervisory, or consultant roles, as shown in Table 1–2.

The home care and community-based health nurses spend almost three times as many hours as the acute care nurse in the consultant roles (teacher,

TABLE 1–2 • Care Performed by Setting

	Percentage of Time Spent		
	Home Care Nurse	Hospital Nurse	Community-Based Health Nurse
Physical caregiver	61%	84%	63%
Manager (administration)	10%	2%	10%
Manager (supervisor)	12%	6%	9%
Communicator/Teacher (consultant)	14%	5%	15%

Source: Hughes, K., & Marcantonio, R. (1992). Practice patterns among home health, public health, and hospital nurses. *Nursing and Health Care, 13*(10), 532–536.

communicator). The community-based and home care nurses also spend five times as many hours in the administrator/manager role as the acute care nurse. In acute care, nurses spend 84% of their time doing direct client care; in community-based and home care nursing it is about 60%.

The home care nurse spends more time in the supervision/management role than in the teaching or physical caregiver role. Home care incorporates critical aspects of both the hospital and community health nurse role. Nurses in home care express more job satisfaction than those working in acute care or community health and are less likely to work weekends or nights.

Professional roles for the nurses in community-based care require competency in both knowledge and skills in communication, teaching, management, and direct physical caregiving (Box 1–3).

Communication and Teaching

A competent nurse knows the principles and techniques of interpersonal communication and applies these in interactions with clients, caregivers, and other health care providers. In practice, the nurse identifies and interprets verbal and nonverbal communications. It is essential to recognize all recurring variables that influence the communication process. The nurse consistently and effectively uses interpersonal communication to establish, maintain, and terminate a therapeutic relationship. The interaction must effectively support the goals that are mutually established by the multidisciplinary team.

The nurse in the community-based setting must have a working knowledge of the principles of teaching and learning as they relate to the scope of practice. The nurse collects and interprets information to assess the learner's need to learn or readiness to learn. Individualized learning outcomes are developed and implemented in the teaching plan. Learning outcomes are evaluated and modifications are made as indicated. Teaching is further developed in Chapter 6.

▶ Box 1–3. Community-Based Nursing Competencies ◀

Communication

The nurse applies principles of interpersonal communication to interactions with clients, families, and other caregivers in all settings in the community.

Teaching

The nurse applies principles of teaching and learning to all learners, including the client, family member or caregiver, coworkers, and other care providers or community member.

Management

The nurse applies knowledge of leadership by performing the management functions of planning, organizing, coordinating, delegating, and evaluating care for a group of clients.

Physical Caregiving

The nurse applies knowledge of principles and procedures for providing safe and effective physical care.

Management

As a manager of care in the community, the nurse uses his or her leadership ability and carries out the management functions of planning, organizing, coordinating, delegating, and evaluating care for one client or a group of clients. This involves collecting and interpreting relevant data that leads to meeting priority needs of the client. The nurse assesses resources, capabilities of other providers, and the client's or family's ability to provide ongoing care. This assessment and the established care plan goals provide the foundation used to develop a management plan geared toward the client's recovery.

The manager of care oversees the care of a group of clients, delegates nursing activities to coworkers, and assumes responsibility for care given under his or her direction. The manager may also work to maintain and improve the work environment by identifying opportunities for improvement and implementing change.

The nurse as manager is responsible for evaluation of every aspect of care. Evaluation of the client's ability to assess his or her own situation and condition and to plan and implement care is an essential component of the recovery process. The manager role extends not only to clients but also to other nursing personnel who are providing care under the direction and leadership of the registered nurse.

Assessment and Physical Caregiving

The nurse must have knowledge about the principles and procedures required for safe and effective physical care. Some of these procedures are ordered by the physician. The nurse either performs these procedures or observes the client or caregiver in performing the tasks. The community-based nurse performs less physical care than does the nurse in the acute care setting.

Assessment is key to quality nursing care in all settings. Because the nurse in the community often functions in a more autonomous role than the nurse in the acute care setting, sound assessment skills are even more essential. After systematically collecting and interpreting data related to the client's condition, the nurse initiates, continues, alters, or terminates physical nursing care. He or she identifies environmental variables in the home that may affect physical nursing care. Assessment also includes identification of the variables in the community that may influence physical nursing care.

The client, caregiver, and nurse set expected outcomes and outcome criteria and then develop a plan of care for providing the necessary physical care that will meet these goals. The plan is then implemented. The nurse removes hazards from the environment that threaten the safety of the client or others.

Effectiveness of the physical care, expected outcomes, and outcome criteria are modified according to need. The nurse also evaluates the ability of other caregivers to provide adequate physical care for the client.

Critical Thinking

Although thinking is a normal human skill, critical thinking is a skill that requires development. Critical thinking helps the nurse find options for solving client care problems. The home care nurse will find many problems to solve. He or she will need to identify signals that indicate an emergency situation or merely a need to call the physician. The nurse may have to think of adaptations that can be made with tools or facilities in the house or how to address situations that present a cultural or religious problem. The nurse may also help the client, caregiver, or family develop critical thinking skills to help them work through their own problems.

The critical thinking process is similar to the nursing process. There are many definitions of critical thinking, but the American Association of Colleges of Nursing (AACN) determined that an ideal critical thinker has the following abilities: questioning, analysis, synthesis, interpretation, inference, inductive and deductive reasoning, intuition, application, and creativity. Several models have been suggested for developing critical thinking skills (AACN, 1998). Box 1–4 will help the student or nurse to strengthen and build natural skills.

Application of Nursing Process

Critical thinking is part of the nursing process. The nurse uses skillful thinking in knowing what assessments to make for each client and picking up on the cues of those assessments. Those assessments help the nurse determine the strengths and weaknesses of the client, family, and caregiver. Together they develop a problem statement, the nursing diagnosis. They plan expected outcomes and outcome criteria. Interventions are identified that are reasonable and acceptable to all parties. The person who will carry out those interventions is designated. The nurse may teach a procedure. The client may be able to do the procedure, but a caregiver may need to buy the supplies or help set up the equipment for the procedure each time it is used. Thinking is used in making evaluations.

Many community-based nurses follow a managed care plan or are given physician's orders to follow. But the community-based nurse also uses the nursing process in therapeutic relationships with clients and caregivers. Nursing process is used in many of the chapters that follow.

Documentation

Complete, accurate documentation is an essential element of nursing care in any setting but it is of particular importance in community-based settings. Cre-

---

▶ Box 1–4. Developing Self-Growth in Thinking Skills ◀

1. Make a list of your current thinking skills.
2. Keep a log (diary) of how you use thinking skills on a regular basis.
3. Share your log with a classmate. Learn from and applaud each other.
4. Read an article or book on thinking in nursing and discuss it with a classmate.
5. Draw a picture or write a paragraph that describes how you would like to enhance your thinking and the factors that hinder your thinking. Share it with a classmate.
6. Promise yourself always to consider at least three possible answers (hunches/conclusions) for every question.
7. Remind yourself that the path to responsible nursing care is along the path of critical thinking.
8. Give yourself a reward for your development of thinking skills.
9. Set goals for further development of your thinking skills.

Source: R. F. Craven, & C. J. Hirnle (Eds.) (2000) *Fundamentals of nursing: Human health and function* (3rd ed., p. 135). Philadelphia: Lippincott Williams & Wilkins.

ating a clear account of what the nurse saw and did not only provides a record of care but also creates a log of client progress. Unlike the acute care setting where several caregivers may be documenting care simultaneously, in some community settings such as the home, only the nurses may be documenting care.

Charting is used to determine eligibility for reimbursement for care provided. If services rendered by the nurse fall within the requirements of Medicaid/Medicare or other third-party payers, then the agency will be paid for the care rendered.

Charting is a legal document. In cases in which an agency and nurse are sued, charting of the incident in question will be used as the record of care provided and client response to that care. Litigation is often avoided or readily resolved if care is accurately and completely documented.

Ethical–Legal Concerns

In community-based nursing, ethical dilemmas present challenges that differ from those in the acute care setting. There may be lack of formal institutional support such as an ethics committee or ethics rounds in community-based care. In the acute setting, the nurse has 24-hour contact with the client and family, whereas care is intermittent and brief in the community setting. Problem identification and problem-solving are troublesome when communication is fragmented over several weeks or months.

When care is provided in the home, respecting the client's and family's desire to self-determination is foremost. This may limit the nurse's influence in the decision-making process. In contrast, the acute care setting is often thought of as "the turf" of the nursing and medical staff.

When family and nurse values collide, frustrating dilemmas may result. Some clients have limited resources and support systems. This may profoundly affect whether caregivers are accessible, available, and affordable. Interdisciplinary communication is difficult in community-based care; this fact may intensify difficulties with ethical issues.

The nurse may facilitate the discussion of ethical concerns as they arise, using an ethical framework and encouraging open dialogue between the client and appropriate family and friends. It is important to know one's own values. If conflicts arise when the nurse and family do not agree, the nurse may have to recommend the family identify another party to facilitate discussions.

 CONCLUSIONS

Community-based nursing is not defined by a setting but by a philosophy of practice. Increasingly, health care is provided in community settings and not in acute care facilities. As a result, the client, family, friend, or neighbors provide care, rather than professional providers. The community-based nurse helps clients and families adapt to providing self-care.

Focusing on prevention, community-based nursing averts the initial occurrence of disease or injury and provides early identification and treatment or a comprehensive rehabilitation of a disease or injury. Continuity and collaborative care allow for quality care to be preserved in a changing health care delivery system. Community-based nurses use special skills and competencies to provide care within the context of the client's culture, family, and community.

References and Bibliography

American Association of Colleges of Nursing. (1998). *Essentials of baccalaureate education and professional nursing practice.* Washington, DC: Author.

American Nurses Association. (1986). Community Health Nursing Division. *Standards of community health nursing practice.* (Publication No. CH-10). Kansas City, MO: Author.

American Organization of Nurse Executives. (2000). *The evolving role of the registered nurse.* Chicago: Author. Available at: http://www.aone.org/practiceresearch/evolving_role_registered_nurse.htm.

Baldwin, J., O'Neill, C., Abegglen, J., & Hill, E. (1998). Population-focused and community-based nursing-moving toward clarification of concepts. *Public Health Nursing, 13*(1), 12–18.

Bellack, J., & O'Niel, E. (2000). Recreating nursing practice for a new century: Recommendations and implications of the Pew Health Commission's final report. *Nursing and Health Care Perspective, 21*(1), 14–18.

Bryan, Y., Babley, E., Grindel, C., Kingston, M., Tuck, M., & Wood, L. (1997). Preparing to change from acute to community-based care: Learning needs of hospital-based nurses. *JONA, 27*(5), 35–44.

Buerhaus, P., Staiger, D., & Auerbach, D. (2000). Implications of an aging registered nurse workforce. *JAMA, 283*(22), 2948–2952.

Bureau of Labor Statistics, United States Department of Labor. (1998). *Occupational Outlook Handbook 1998–1999* (pp. 202–203). Washington, DC: Superintendent of Documents, U.S. Government Printing Office.

Cahill, M., Devlin, M., LeBlanc, P., Lowe, B., Norgon, V., Tassin, K., & Vallette, E. (1998). Reexamining the associate degree curriculum: Assessing the need for community concepts. *Nursing and Health Care Perspectives, 19*(4), 158–161, 165.

Chafey, K. (1996). Caring is not enough: Ethical paradigms for community-based care. *Nursing and Health Care: Perspectives on Community, 17*(1), 10–15.

Chalmers, K., Bramadat, I., & Andrusyszyn, M. (1998). The changing environment of community health practice and education: Perceptions of staff nurses, administrators, and educators. *Journal of Nursing Education, 37*(3), 109–117.

Chiu, L., Shyu W. C., & Chen, T. R. (1997). A cost-effectiveness analysis of home care and community-based nursing homes for stroke patients and their families. *Journal of Advanced Nursing, 26,* 872–879.

Clarke, H., Beddome, G., & Whyte, N. (1993). Public health nurses' vision of their future reflects changing paradigms. *Image: Journal of Nursing Scholarship, 25,* 305–309.

Clarke, P., & Cody, W. (1994). Nursing theory based practice in the home and community: The crux of professional nursing education. *Advances in Nursing Science, 17*(2), 41–53.

Craven, R. C., & Hirnle, C. J. (2000). *Fundamentals of nursing: Human health and function* (3rd ed.). Philadelphia: Lippincott Williams & Wilkins.

David, A. (1999). New ideas, strangely familiar. *Nursing Times, 95*(35), 24.

Documentation Tips. (1998). *Home Healthcare Nurse, 17*(3), 193–194.

Fawcett, J. (1984). *Analysis and evaluation of conceptual models of nursing.* Philadelphia: F.A. Davis.

Frachel, R. (1988). A new profession: The evolution of public health nursing. *Public Health Nursing, 51*(12), 84–91.

Green, P., & Adderley-Kelly, B. (1999). Partnership for health promotions in an urban community. *Nursing and Health Care Perspectives 20*(2), 76–81.

Hahn, E. J., Bryant, R., Peden, A., Robinson, K. L., & Williams, C. A. (1998). Entry into community-based nursing practice: Perceptions of perspective employers. *Journal of Professional Nursing, 14,* 305–313.

Healthcare Forum. (1994). *What creates health?* San Francisco.

Heller, B. R., Oros, M. T., & Durney-Crowley, J. (1999). *The future of nursing education: Ten trends to watch.* New York: National League for Nursing. Available at: http://www.nln.org/infotrends.htm.

Hunt, R. (1998). Community based nursing: Philosophy or setting. *American Journal of Nursing, 98*(10), 44–47.

Huston, C. J., & Fox, S. (1998). The changing healthcare market: Implications for nursing education in the coming decade. *Nursing Outlook, 46*(3), 109–114.

Jitramontree, N. (2000). The impact of medicare reimbursement changes on home healthcare: A nursing perspective. *Home Healthcare Nurse, 18*(2), 116–121.

Johnson, A. (1998). The revitalization of community practice: Characteristics, competencies, and curricula for community-based services. *Journal of Community Practice, 5*(3), 37–62.

Josten, L. (1989). Wanted: Leaders for public health. *Nursing Outlook, 37*, 230–232.

Kalish, P., & Kalisch, B. (1995). *The advance of American nursing* (3rd ed.). Philadelphia: Lippincott.

Kirk, S., & Glendinning, C. (1998). Trend in community care and patient participation: Implications for the roles of informal careers and community nurses in the United Kingdom. *Journal of Advanced Nursing, 28*, 370–381.

Kulbok, P., Gates, M., Vicenzi, A., & Schultz, P. (1999). Focus on community: Directions for nursing knowledge development. *Journal of Advanced Nursing, 29*, 1188–1196.

Leininger, M. (1970). *Nursing and anthropology: Two worlds to blend.* New York: Wiley.

Moneyham, L., & Hodgson, N. (1997). A model emerges for community-based nurse care management of older adults. *Nursing and Health Care: Perspectives on Community, 18*(2), 68–73.

Monteiro, L. (1991). Florence Nightingale on public health nursing. In B. Spradley (Ed.), *Readings in community health nursing.* Philadelphia: Lippincott.

National League for Nursing. (1997). *Final report: Commission on a workforce for a restructured health care system.* New York. Author. Available at: http://www.nln.org/infrest3.htm.

National League for Nursing. (2000a). *A vision for nursing education.* New York: Author. Available at http://www.nln.org/info-vision.htm.

National League for Nursing. (2000b). *Educational competencies for graduates of associate degree nursing programs.* Council of Associate Degree Nursing Competencies Task Force. Boston: Jones & Bartlett Publisher.

Naylor, M., & Buhler-Wilderson, K. (1999). Creating community-based care for the new millennium. *Nursing Outlook, 47*(3), 120–127.

News from NLN Research. (1998). *Nursing and Health Care Perspectives, 19*(1), 54–55.

Pew Health Professions Commission. (1998). *Health America: Practitioners for 2005.* Durham, NC: Author.

Pinch, W. J. (1996). Research and nursing: Ethical reflections. *Nursing and Health Care: Perspectives on Community, 17*(1), 26–31.

Rafael, A. (1999). From rhetoric to reality: The changing face of public health nursing in southern Ontario. *Public Health Nursing, 16*(1), 50–59.

Reed, F. C., & Wuyscik, M. A. (1998). Community health strategies: Teach what? Reflections on the transition from hospital teaching to teaching in the community. *Nurse Educator, 23*(3), 11–13.

Reverby, S. M. (1993). From Lillian Wald to Hillary Rodham Clinton: What will happen to public health nursing? [Editorial]. *American Journal of Public Health, 83*, 1662–1663.

Sanderson, C. (1998). The new challenge in community based nursing education. *Tennessee Nurse, 61*(2), 15–17.

Shoultz, J., Kiiker B., & Sloat, A. (1998). Community-based nursing education research study from the NLN Vision for nursing education Hawaii/phase. *Nursing and Health Care Perspectives, 19*(6), 278–282.

Smith-Stoner, M. (1999). Another 10 tips to think more critically. *Home Healthcare Nurse, 17*(3), 144–145.

Taylor, C., Lillis, C., & LeMone, P. (1997). *Fundamentals of nursing: The art and science of nursing care.* Philadelphia: Lippincott-Raven.

Trnobranski, P. H. (1994). Nurse practitioner: Redefining the role of the community nurse. *Journal of Advanced Nursing, 19*, 134–139.

U.S. Department of Health and Human Services. (2000). *Healthy people 2010: National health promotion and disease prevention objectives, full report, with commentary.* Washington, DC: U.S. Government Printing Office.

Zotti, M., Brown, P., & Stotts, R. (1996). Community-based nursing versus community health nursing: What does it all mean? *Nursing Outlook, 44*, 211–217.

LEARNING ACTIVITIES

LEARNING ACTIVITY 1-1

▶ **Client Care Study:** Community-Based Nursing Care

How can the nurse encourage self-care in the following client situations?

Jane is the 31-year-old mother of Jackie, a 4-month-old baby who has frequent apnea spells. Jane states, "I am afraid she will stop breathing at home. I can't figure out the monitor."

Stephan is a 60-year-old widower whose wife died 3 years ago. There is an increasing possibility that he will have to have his leg amputated below the knee as a result of a very large leg ulcer. Stephan has been hospitalized three times in the past 6 months because of uncontrolled diabetes. The last time there were maggots in his leg ulcer.

LEARNING ACTIVITY 1-2

▶ **Critical Thinking Exercise:** Self-Evaluation and Reflection

1. In your clinical journal, discuss a community you are familiar with and describe what defines that community.
2. Identify some of the health needs of that community.
3. Where do members of this community receive health care?

CHAPTER 2

Health Promotion and Disease Prevention

ROBERTA HUNT

The U.S. health care system is the most expensive in the world, using 14% of the U.S. gross national product (GNP), at a cost of nearly $4,000 per person. The next most expensive health care system is in Canada, where 9% of the GNP is used for health care, at a per capita cost of $2,000. Most industrialized nations spend 8% to 10% of their GNP on health care. Every industrialized nation except the United States has a national health plan in place that covers all citizens (Anderson & Poullier, 1999).

Despite having the most expensive health care in the world, the United States lags behind other nations in key health indicators. The United States ranks 24th among nations in its infant mortality rate at 7.8/1,000 births. This average does not show the higher rates for certain minority groups. Life expectancy in the United States ranks behind Sweden, Germany, Italy, France, and Canada. Twenty-five percent of the nation's 1 1/2- to 3-year-old children are inadequately immunized against diphtheria, tetanus, pertussis, polio, measles, mumps, or rubella. Disadvantaged populations rank significantly worse than average in these and other health indicators (Federal Interagency Forum on Child and Family Statistics, 1999).

Nursing is a reflection of society's needs. Although a great deal of money is spent on health care in the United States, the level of health of U.S. citizens is disappointing. The consumer movement toward increased participation in wellness, weight loss, smoking cessation, and exercising has resulted in the preventive health movement. Settings for practice have evolved naturally as nurses focus on health rather than illness. Nursing has taken on a new look as it assumes the role of health promotion and illness prevention.

This chapter begins with a discussion of health and its place on the health–illness continuum. The goals and priorities in the federal government's program—*Healthy People 2010*—are presented. A large part of the chapter is devoted to illustrating the difference between health promotion and disease prevention, the major strategies nurses will use to meet the goals of *Healthy People 2010*, with emphasis on the preventive focus. Levels of prevention and nursing roles are outlined. The chapter ends with a brief section on advocacy.

 HEALTH AND ILLNESS

Rather than focus on curing illness and injury, community-based care focuses on promoting health and preventing illness. **Health** is defined by the World Health Organization (1986) as a "state of physical, mental and social well being and not merely absence of disease or infirmity." This holistic philosophy differs greatly from that of the acute care setting.

Considering health—rather than illness—as the essence of care requires a shift in thinking. The **health–illness continuum** illustrates this model of care (Fig. 2–1). Health is conceptualized as a resource for everyday living. It is a pos-

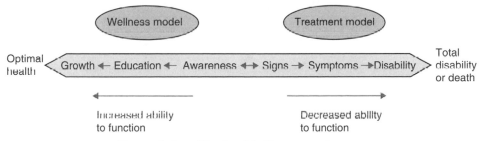

Figure 2–1. ▶ The health–illness continuum.

itive idea that emphasizes social and personal resources and physical capabilities. Wellness is a lifestyle aimed at achieving physical, emotional, intellectual, spiritual, and environmental well-being. The use of wellness measures can increase stamina, energy, and self-esteem. These then enhance quality of life.

Improvement of health is not seen as an outcome of the amount and type of medical services or the size of the hospital. Treatment efficacy, rather than technology, drives care in this model. Here health is viewed as a function of collaborative efforts at the community level.

Care provided in acute care settings usually is directed at resolving immediate health problems. In the community, care focuses on maximizing individual potential for self-care regardless of any illness or injury. The client assumes responsibility for health care decisions and care provision. Where health is the essence of care, the client's ability to function becomes the primary concern. The intent of care is not to "fix" with treatment but to enhance the quality of life and support actions that make the client's life as comfortable as possible.

Function is defined by subjective and objective measurements. Both the client's abilities to perform activities of daily living (ADL) and the client's perception of how well he or she is functioning are considered. Clients may state that they are satisfied with their ability to care for themselves; however, objective data from laboratory reports, diagnostic tests, and caregivers' observations reveal that this may not be the case (Fig. 2–2). On the other hand, clients may that they are concerned about their ability to perform ADL, yet contrasting reports indicate that they are functioning quite well. In the Example of a Client Situation accompanying Figure 2–2, Mary's situation reflects this dichotomy.

A person's lifestyle is a dynamic process that involves needs, beliefs, and values. Choices in life then are seen as opportunities for moving toward optimal health or wellness.

Carroll and Miller (1991) have defined wellness as "involving good physical self-care, using one's mind constructively, expressing one's emotions effectively, interacting creatively with others, and being concerned about one's physical and psychological environment." Regardless of the setting for health care, wherever nurses practice, their concern is for the whole person and they provide holistic care (Fig. 2–3).

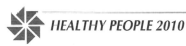 *HEALTHY PEOPLE 2010*

Healthy People 2010 offers a simple but powerful idea: provide the information and knowledge about how to improve health in a format that enables diverse

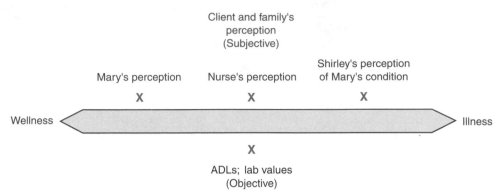

Figure 2–2. ▶ Subjective perceptions of health and function may differ from each other and from objective data.

EXAMPLE OF A CLIENT SITUATION

▶ Perceptions of Health and Illness

Mary had a myocardial infarction 3 days ago. After two episodes of crushing chest pain, she reluctantly went to the emergency room. Laboratory values showed moderate heart damage. She is a 46-year-old single parent and sole provider for three adolescents. Mary is a physical therapist and works at an ambulatory clinic during the week and a nursing home on weekends. She says she feels fine and asks to go home so she can go back to work.

Mary's mother, Shirley, is extremely distraught about her daughter's condition and believes Mary is dying. Figure 2–2 illustrates the objective data versus Mary's subjective communication. The dissonance between subjective perceptions and objective data can interrupt and delay recovery.

groups to combine their efforts and work as a team. It is a road map to better health for all, which can be used by many different people, communities, professional organizations, and groups whose concern is a particular threat to health or a particular population group (U.S. Department of Health and Human Services [DHHS], 2000). Publication of this vision was the result of a national consortium of health care professionals, citizens, and private and public agencies from across the United States.

Healthy People 2010 states that its purpose is to commit the nation to the attainment of two broad goals:

1. To increase quality and years of healthy life
2. To eliminate health disparities

Measurable targets or objectives to be achieved are organized into 28 priority areas (Box 2–1).

The fact that individual health is closely linked to community health was discussed in Chapter 1. Likewise, community health is affected by the collective behaviors, attitudes, and beliefs of everyone who lives in the community. The underlying premise of *Healthy People 2010* is that the health of the individual is almost inseparable from the health of the larger community.

This road map for improving health provided by *Healthy People 2010* is based

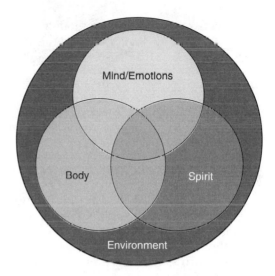

Figure 2–3. ► Schematic representation of holism. The system is greater than and different from the sum of the parts. Wherever the setting, the nurse's concern is for the whole person.

► Box 2–1. *Healthy People 2010* Focus Areas ◄

1. Access to quality health services
2. Arthritis, osteoporosis, and chronic back conditions
3. Cancer
4. Chronic kidney disease
5. Diabetes
6. Disability and secondary conditions
7. Education and community-based programs
8. Environmental health
9. Family planning
10. Food safety
11. Health communication
12. Heart disease and stroke
13. Human immunodeficiency virus (HIV)
14. Immunization and infectious diseases
15. Injury and violence prevention
16. Maternal, infant, and child health
17. Medical product safety
18. Mental health
19. Nutrition and obesity
20. Occupational safety and health
21. Oral health
22. Physical activity and fitness
23. Public health infrastructure
24. Respiratory diseases
25. Sexually transmitted diseases
26. Substance abuse
27. Tobacco use
28. Vision and hearing

on the concepts of health promotion, disease prevention, and health protection. **Health promotion** strategies relate to individual lifestyles having a powerful influence over one's health prospects. Educational and community-based programs can be designed to address lifestyle. **Health protection** strategies relate to environmental or regulatory measures that confer protection on large population groups. Rather than an individual focus, health protection involves a community-wide focus. **Preventive services** include counseling, screening, immunization, or chemoprophylactic interventions for individuals in clinical settings.

HEALTH PROMOTION VERSUS DISEASE PREVENTION

Sometimes people confuse health promotion and disease prevention. It is easy to do so because some approaches or interventions are the same or overlap. For instance, consider exercise. Jill jogs every morning before work. She enjoys jogging, and she likes to start her day that way. She finds it stimulates her for the day's activities. She feels tired when she has not been able to jog. Jill jogs to promote wellness, so Jill is participating in a health promotion activity. On the other hand, Nancy jogs because her physician has told her to do so. She is overweight and has a family history of heart problems. Her physician tells her she needs exercise to help prevent future cardiovascular problems. Nancy jogs to prevent illness, so Nancy is participating in a disease prevention activity.

Health promotion activities are used to make a person who already feels well feel better, and disease prevention activities are used to make a person who feels well prevent possible future illness. Many health promotion practices are also directed toward raising the health of the general community.

THE PREVENTION FOCUS

The prevention focus is a key concept of community-based nursing. Prevention is conceptualized on three levels: primary prevention, secondary prevention, and tertiary prevention. An overview of these levels of prevention appears in Table 2–1. Health promotion activities may be included also at the level of primary prevention. Health protection activities, conducted by nurses in community-based settings, usually occur at the primary level, although they may occur at secondary and tertiary levels also.

Different preventive strategies are found at each level of prevention. These strategies fall into a continuum of essential activities that prevent disease or injury, prolong life, and promote health. The following services are categorized as preventive strategies: counseling, screening, immunization, and chemoprophylactic interventions for clients in clinical settings.

Some of the preventive activities listed in Table 2–1 are further developed in Table 2–2, which shows the goals of these selected activities.

There are numerous reasons for adopting preventive steps; cost benefit is one. For example, the direct and indirect costs of infectious diseases are significant. Every hospital-acquired infection adds an average of $2,100 to a hospital or home care bill. Bloodstream infections result in an average of $3,517 in additional hospital charges per infected individual because the client stay averages an additional 7 days (DHHS, 2000). These costs are realized in every setting where health care is provided. A typical case of Lyme disease diagnosed in the early stages incurs about $174 in direct medical treatment costs. Delayed diag-

TABLE 2–1 • Levels of Disease Prevention and Examples of Activities

Level	Description	Activities
Primary	Prevention of the initial occurrence of disease or injury	Immunization, family planning, retirement planning, well-child care, smoking cessation, hygiene teaching, fluoride supplements, fitness classes, alcohol and drug prevention, seatbelts and child car restraints, environmental protection
Secondary	Early identification of disease or disability with prompt intervention to prevent or limit disability	Physical assessments, hypertension screening, developmental screening, breast and testicular self-examinations, hearing and vision screening, mammography, pregnancy testing
Tertiary	Assistance (after disease or disability has occurred) to halt further disease progress and to meet one's potential and maximize quality of life despite illness or injury	Teaching and counseling regarding lifestyle changes such as diet and exercise, stress management and home management after diagnosis of chronic illness, support groups, support for caretaker, Meals On Wheels for homebound, physical therapy after stroke or accident, mental health counseling for rape victims

Some prevention activities listed above overlap into health promotion or health protection.

nosis and treatment can result in complications that cost from $2,228 to $6,724 per client in direct medical costs in the first year alone.

As medicine develops more technology and treatment choices, these costs (and, therefore, potential cost savings) increase. The lifetime costs of health care associated with HIV, in light of recent advances in diagnostics and therapeutics, have grown from $55,000 to $155,000 or more per person (DHHS, 2000). These costs mean that HIV prevention efforts may be even more cost effective and even cost saving to society.

In addition to being cost effective, appropriate prevention interventions result in enhanced client satisfaction and faster recovery. Historically, the major portions of primary and tertiary prevention services have been delivered from community-based settings. This is still appropriate in the current health care system.

Primary Prevention

Primary prevention is commonly defined as prevention of the initial occurrence of disease or injury. Primary prevention activities include such things as immunizations, family planning services, classes to prepare people for retirement, and counseling and education on injury prevention. These are categorized as primary prevention because they prevent the initial occurrence of a disease or injury. Table 2–1 lists examples of specific primary prevention activities.

Also included in primary prevention are health promotion and health pro-

TABLE 2–2 • Activities at Each Level of Prevention

Level	Activities	Goal of the Activity
Primary	Immunization clinics	Prevention of communicable diseases such as polio, pertussis, rubella
	Smoking cessation	Prevention of lung and heart disease, cancer
	Tobacco chewing prevention	Prevention of cancer of the mouth, tongue, and throat
	Sex education, including emphasis on the use of condoms	Prevention of acquired immunodeficiency syndrome (AIDS) and other sexually transmitted diseases (STDs)
Secondary	Programs to teach and motivate men to do self-exam for testicular masses	Early identification and treatment of testicular cancer
	Blood pressure screening	Early identification and treatment of hypertension to prevent strokes and heart disease
	Programs to teach and motivate women to do self-exam of breasts	Early identification and treatment of breast cancer
Tertiary	Counseling, low-sodium diet, exercise for management of hypertension	Minimize the effects of hypertension
	Exercises and speech therapy after a cerebrovascular accident	Restore function and limit disability

tection activities. Health promotion focuses on activities related to lifestyle choices in a social context for individuals who are already essentially healthy. Examples of health promotion include exercise and nutrition classes and prevention programs for alcohol and other drug abuse. Smoking cessation programs are often targeted at healthy individuals, offering a lifestyle choice for already healthy individuals.

Prevention is also accomplished through health protection. Health protection focuses on activities related to environmental or regulatory measures that provide protection for large population groups. This category would include activities directed at preventing unintentional injuries through motor vehicle accidents, occupational safety and health, environmental health, and food and drug safety. Other examples of health protection include seatbelt and child car seat restraint laws and laws prohibiting smoking in public places. Implementation of child car seat restraint laws have prevented a significant number of deaths and disabilities among children in the United States over the past 15 years. It has been effective as a health protection activity. Environmental protection and pollution control are other primary levels of prevention that are also health protection factors.

Secondary Prevention

The intent of **secondary prevention** is the early identification and treatment of disease or injury to limit disability. Identification of health needs, health problems, and clients at risk are inherent components of secondary prevention. Activities of secondary prevention include screening programs for blood pressure, breast cancer, scoliosis, hearing, and vision. Intervention does not prevent scoliosis, but it does provide early identification and subsequent treatment of a condition that already exists in school-age children. Likewise, mammography does not prevent breast cancer, but it provides an opportunity for early identification and treatment. Typically, screening efforts should address conditions that cause significant morbidity and mortality in the target age group. Table 2–1 lists other examples of specific secondary prevention activities.

Tertiary Prevention

Tertiary prevention maximizes recovery after an injury or illness. Most care provided in acute care facilities, clinics, and skilled nursing facilities focuses on tertiary care. Rehabilitation is the major focus in this level of prevention. Rehabilitation activities assist clients to reach their maximum potential despite the presence of chronic conditions. Teaching a client who has had a hip replacement how to create a safe home environment that prevents falls is an example of tertiary prevention.

Shelters for battered women and counseling and therapy for abused children are further examples of tertiary prevention. Other examples are listed in Table 2–1.

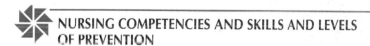

NURSING COMPETENCIES AND SKILLS AND LEVELS OF PREVENTION

As early as Florence Nightingale, the role of nurses as health promoters has been valued. Despite an increasing emphasis on disease prevention and health promotion, and ample evidence demonstrating the effectiveness of preventive services, such services are underutilized (Amonkar, Madhavan, Rosenbluth, & Simon, 1999). This emphasis has generated numerous opportunities for nurses to participate in health promotion and disease prevention activities in all levels of prevention (Dixon, 1999). Now that you understand the levels of prevention, this section discusses the role of the nurse at each level of prevention in two types of community-based care: the ambulatory and home care settings. Typically, the prominent nursing competencies in these settings are those of communicator and teacher. Competencies as manager and physical care provider also are essential in the home setting. This can be true of ambulatory care as well, depending on the setting.

The role responsibilities for each level of prevention differ in each setting. Levels of prevention and the role of the nurse in community-based care may be affected by the particular position and the educational preparation of the nurse. Table 2–3 illustrates this relationship. Table 2–1 provides additional examples of preventive strategies in community-based settings.

Primary Prevention

Ambulatory Health Care

Nurses communicate information about primary prevention in the ambulatory setting. For example, a nurse may provide information on the importance of infant seats, child restraints, and helmets to all the mothers at a well-child clinic. School nurses may communicate with families through written flyers sent home

TABLE 2–3 • Educational Preparation Needed to Provide Community-Based Nursing at Three Levels of Prevention

Client Served	Levels of Prevention		
	Primary	Secondary	Tertiary
Individual client	Sexuality; teaching about use of condoms Family planning Dietary teaching and exercise programs to assist clients with obesity	Counseling and HIV testing Early prenatal care Screening for early identification of diabetes	Nutrition teaching to the client with AIDS to maximize health Support groups for parents of low-birth-weight infants Teaching newly diagnosed diabetic about diet and how to administer insulin
Family	Education about infection control in the home of a family member at home on a respirator	Tuberculosis screening for a family at risk	Teaching a family caregiver how to follow sterile procedure for a dressing change
Group	Prenatal classes for pregnant adolescents Sexuality teaching about AIDS and other STDs	Vision screening for first graders Hearing screening at a senior center	Support groups for children with asthma Swim therapy for physically disabled
Communities	Fluoride water supplementation Environmental cleanup of paint and other substances containing lead	Organized screening programs such as health fairs Lead screening of children in a community	Shelter or relocation for victims of natural disasters Development of programs to assist children with developmental delays caused by lead exposure

Key:
.... Associate Degree Nurse
----- Baccalaureate Nurse
——— Master of Science in Public Health

with the children. Subjects may include the communicability and the methods of transmission of high-risk diseases, and prevention for conditions such as chickenpox, influenza, or head lice.

Teaching in clinics, schools, and occupational settings may be directed to individuals or groups. Topics cover a wide range and include such things as immunizations, family planning, and prenatal care. At adult clinics, nurses can provide current information to clients about health promotion, diet, exercise, stress management, and weight reduction. Women of childbearing age may attend classes on family planning and prenatal teaching, an essential primary prevention strategy. Parents of preschool children can obtain vital information and clarification from school nurses about when, where, and why their children can receive periodic check-ups and immunizations. Teaching is one of the main responsibilities of the nurse working in the school.

In the occupational setting, nurses may provide information about injury prevention, repetitive motion injuries, and sensory losses secondary to job tasks. They disseminate information about shift work, offer strategies to avoid sleep disturbances, and provide information about the importance of health promotion activities such as exercise. Many companies provide recreational programs and physical activities at work or in the community through their occupational health programs.

The manager of care in these settings applies knowledge about the principles of leadership by performing management functions for a group of clients. This includes managing all aspects of care and involves communication, teaching, and physical care.

The physical caregiver role in the clinic, school, occupational health setting, and home is usually provided at the tertiary level of prevention. Evaluation of the physical care provided to a client, however, is a function of the manager of care and may take place in all of the above settings. The manager evaluates the teaching, physical care, and communication skills of the home health aide, for instance, or the care manager teaches a licensed practical nurse in the clinic and school.

Home Health Care

Clients in the home frequently require episodic care for acute health care conditions. Opportunities for primary prevention are limited. Home care nurses communicate information to the client and family regarding primary prevention strategies because in community-based care the nurse considers the client in the context of the family. The nurse influences the family's health behaviors in many areas that are not directly related to the client's condition. For example, if the client's spouse asks about immunizations for their children, the nurse has the opportunity to teach about the immunization schedule and where to get affordable care.

Secondary Prevention

Ambulatory Health Care

Secondary prevention can involve alerting clients about the time frames for health screening (eg, mammography, Pap smears, glaucoma screening, breast examinations, lipid levels). The clinic nurse may see clients who are at risk for certain conditions, alert them to their condition, and provide information about community services that may be able to assist them.

Preschool screening, vision and hearing testing, and scoliosis screening are secondary prevention strategies provided in the school. In addition, school nurses teach secondary prevention by educating parents about these screening programs available for their children.

Often the workplace is the site where screening is done for hypertension, hearing loss, exposure to hazardous substances, or breast cancer. The nurse disperses information about these services and gives the educational programs.

Client need determines in which setting information may be presented. For example, as a manager of care in the clinic, the nurse may not have the opportunity to assess the family caregiver's abilities in assisting a client with insulin injections. However, the nurse in the home can better assess how well the family can assist and support the client. The nurse, as the manager of care in the home, may decide that the family caregiver needs additional teaching to administer the insulin because he or she could not accurately draw up the insulin during an early morning nursing visit.

Home Health Care

Care in the home usually involves short visits. Thus, opportunities for communicating secondary prevention information are limited. However, home health care nurses do inform the client and family about services in the community that may help them with the client's care and with early identification and treatment of conditions revolving around the client's diagnosis.

Tertiary Prevention

Ambulatory Health Care

Clinic nurses often give their clients information about community resources. Parents of children with a chronic disease, for instance, may receive a list of organizations that provide emotional support, respite care, or information and referral. Clients with chronic conditions benefit from teaching that is directed at successful rehabilitation and prevention of related complications. Physical care in the clinic may include changing a dressing, wrapping a sprained ankle, or giving an intravenous infusion.

Through the schools, parents can learn about community services available for children with chronic conditions. In some states, children with disabilities are mainstreamed into the public schools. These children and their families need tertiary prevention education. In all states, children with less severe chronic conditions attend school and benefit from health care instructions.

Some schools provide a significant amount of physical caregiving through school-based clinics. Services may include physical examinations, routine screenings, venipuncture for laboratory studies, family planning, and even prenatal care. Nurses may also provide direct nursing care to some children on an ongoing basis (eg, children on a mechanical ventilator or children with conditions that result in frequent urinary catheterization). The school nurse also dispenses prescription medications and provides first aid in emergencies.

In the occupational setting, physical care is primarily first aid. The nurse may tell personnel with chronic conditions, or recent acute conditions, about opportunities and advantages of returning to work. Return-to-work programs assist personnel with chronic injuries or illnesses and illustrate the tertiary prevention approach of maximizing individual potential for health through teaching.

Home Health Care

A primary role of the home health care nurses is to provide health instruction to clients and family members. Because home health care clients generally require only episodic care and usually have a chronic condition, most teaching is directed toward tertiary prevention. Teaching may focus on rehabilitation or restoration for those with a recent stroke, head injury, fractured hip, diagnosis of a chronic condition, surgery, and so forth.

Physical care in the home is usually at the tertiary level of prevention. To receive payment for services, most home health care has a physical care component such as completing dressing changes while teaching and implementing good infection control techniques with the client and the family.

Although the client is the main concern, a holistic nursing style means that nurses also provide care for family and other support persons. Chapter 13 covers this topic in more detail.

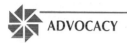

ADVOCACY

An advocate is a person who pleads or defends the cause of another. Advocates work to change the system by revealing injustices and inadequacies. **Advocacy** involves teaching, changing the system, guidance, role modeling, professional collaboration, prevention, and community resources. Steps in advocacy, listed in Box 2–2, represent power that is inherent in knowledge. The expertise and competence of nurses can also be used in supporting the needs and views of their clients and their clients' families. Nurses can be advocates for clients who feel they have been excluded from participation in health care decisions or who have little trust in health care or political representatives.

Community-based nurses who have rapport with their clients know the problems their clients face: the mother who lacks child care, the older adult who lacks transportation, the school child who is afraid to use the restrooms in the school, the adolescent who is afraid of the violence on the street, the wife who faces abuse from her husband, the poor who struggle to make

---

▶ **Box 2–2.** Steps of Advocacy ◀

Understanding and Knowledge of Self Personally and Professionally

- Knowing oneself: Awareness of personal goals and how these goals may affect relationships with clients
- Realistic self-concept: Awareness of one's own limitations and abilities that will affect what one can and cannot support
- Self-knowledge about values clarification: Awareness of one's biases and prejudices, moral and ethical values. This gives one a good knowledge and understanding of personal views of what is fair and acceptable and how that may affect one's approach to a relationship with the client

Knowledge of Treatment and Intervention Options

- Development of knowledge base of procedures and actions
- Awareness of rationale for specific therapies

Knowledge of Health Care System

- Awareness of how systems relate to each other, the client, and the community
- Awareness of relationship of outside influences such as politics and economics

Knowledge of How to Put Advocacy Into Action

- Assessment—contextual approach
    What does the client feel the most important problem is?
    What support or resources does the client already have in place?
    What does the client know or not know? (eg, health services, treatment options)
    In what areas does the client feel a need for personal control to be established in his or her life?
- Planning—mobilize resources, consultations, collaboration with other disciplines
- Implementation—education, empowerment of client (Nurse assists the client in asserting control over the variables affecting the client's life. The nurse must role model assertiveness to make this important step effective.)

ends meet. One nurse characterized her home visits as mutual disclosure: "It's you and that person listening to each other" (Zerwekh, 1992). Together the client and the nurse have power and use it to improve the client's health status.

Who is better situated as an advocate for the individual and families than the community-based nurse who knows clients' needs? From trusting relationships such as the nurse experiences, he or she has a knowledgeable understanding of both local needs and services.

 ## CONCLUSIONS

Settings for nursing practice have evolved as a reflection of society's need to focus on health rather than illness. State and local health departments are using *Healthy People 2010* as a framework to put disease prevention into action. The prevention focus is a key concept of community-based nursing. Different preventive strategies are found at three levels of prevention. Advocacy is another form of community-based nursing in which the nurse supports the needs and views of the people he or she serves. The nurse and client working together have power.

References and Bibliography

Amonkar, M., Madhavan, S., Rosenbluth, S., & Simon, K. (1999). Barriers and facilitators to providing common preventive screening services in managed care settings. *Journal of Community Health, 24*(3), 229–247.

Anderson, G. F., & Poullier, J. P. (1999). Health spending, access, and outcomes: Trends in industrialized countries. *Health Affairs, 18*(3), 178–192.

Bownson, R., Riley, P., & Bruce, T. (1998). Demonstration projects in community-based prevention. *Journal of Public Health Management Practice, 4*(2), 66–77.

Breslow, L. (1999). From disease prevention to health promotion. *Journal of the American Medical Association, 281*(11), 1030–1031.

Carroll, C., & Miller, D. (1991). *Health: The science of human adaptation* (5th ed.). Madison, WI: Brown & Benchmark.

Craven, R. C., & Hirnle, C. J. (1996). *Fundamentals of nursing: Human health and function* (2nd ed.). Philadelphia: Lippincott-Raven.

Cutler, L. (1999). The contribution of nursing to cancer prevention. *Journal of Advanced Nursing, 29*(1), 169–177.

Dahl, R. W. (1995). The development of a community-based nursing practice: Shifting the focus to health promotion. *Advanced Practice Nursing Quarterly, 1*(3), 1–6.

Dille, J. (1999). Worksite influenza immunization: Successful program. *AAOHN Journal, 47*(7), 293–299.

Dixon, E. (1999). Community health nursing practice and the Roy Adaptation Model. *Public Health Nursing, 16*(4), 290–300.

Federal Interagency Forum on Child and family Statistics. *American's children: Key national indicators of well being, 1999.* Federal interagency Forum on Child and Family Statistics. Washington, DC: U.S. Government Printing Office.

Healthcare Forum. (1994). *What creates health?* San Francisco: Author.

Hughes, K., Kostbade, K., & Marcantonio, R. (1994). Practice patterns among home health, public health and hospital nurses. *Nursing & Health Care, 13*(10), 532–536.

Mouton, C., & Espino, D. (1999). Health screening in older women. *American Family Physician, 59*(7), 1835–1837.

Murashima, S., Hatono, Y., Whyte, N., & Asahara, K. (1999). Public health nursing in Japan: New opportunities for health promotion. *Public Health Nursing, 16*(2), 133–139.

National League for Nursing. (1997). *National League for Nursing final report commission on a workforce for a restructured health care system.* New York: Author.

Norton, L. (1998). Health promotion and health education: What role should the nurse adopt in practice? *Journal of Advanced Nursing, 28*(6), 1269–1275.

Poss, J. (1999). Providing culturally competent care: Is there a role for health promoters? *Nursing Outlook, 47*(1), 30–36.

Ruppert, R. A. (1996). Caring for the lay caregiver. *American Journal of Nursing, 96*(3), 40–45.

Tsouros, A. O. (1990). *World Health Organization healthy citizens project: A project becomes a movement.* Copenhagen, Denmark: FADL Publishers.

U.S. Department of Health and Human Services. (2000). *Healthy people 2010* (Conference edition, in two volumes). Washington, DC: Author.

Whitehead, D. (1999). The application: Health promoting practice within the orthopaedic setting. *Journal of Orthopaedic Nursing, 3*(2), 101–107.

World Health Organization. (1986). *Basic documents* (36th ed.). Geneva, Switzerland: Author.

Wisewoman Workgroup. (1999). Cardiovascular disease prevention for women attending breast and cervical cancer screening programs: The WISEWOMAN project. *Preventive Medicine, 28*(5), 496–502.

Zerwekh, J. (1992). Laying the groundwork for family self-help: Locating families, building trust, and building strength. *Public Health Nursing, 9*(1), 15–21.

LEARNING ACTIVITIES

LEARNING ACTIVITY 2-1

▶ **Client Care Study:** Primary Nursing Roles and Levels of Prevention

Determine the primary nursing role(s) and level of prevention for each of the following clients.

▶ **Client:** Jack

Jack is a 43-year-old man with a colostomy. He has evidence of early skin breakdown around the stoma site despite the fact that he has followed the established protocol. The clinic nurse notes the problem at Jack's first visit to the clinic after his surgery. She teaches him about a new product that may interrupt the skin breakdown.

1. Determine the primary nursing role.
2. Identify the level of prevention the nurse is using.

▶ **Client:** Stephen

Stephen is 12-years-old and has a neurologic condition that requires self-catheterization every 2 hours. He has had three bladder infections in the past 2 months. The school nurse has taught Stephen about the infectious cycle and the importance of handwashing and has watched Stephen self-catheterize in an attempt to identify the reason for the frequent infections.

3. Determine the primary nursing role.
4. Identify the level of prevention the nurse is using.

LEARNING ACTIVITY 2-2

▶ **Practical Application:** Community Support Group

You have been asked to start a support and education group for people in your community who have had strokes.

1. Describe how you will decide who in the community should participate in the group. You have identified those who will be attending your group. Now you must write objectives for the group.
2. Discuss how the components of community-based nursing apply to this problem:
   a. Self-care
   b. Preventive care
   c. Care within the context of the community
   d. Continuity of care
   e. Collaborative care
3. Identify levels of prevention on which you will focus. Determine if there are levels you will not include.
4. State two likely basic or physical needs at each level of prevention for your group.
5. List two goals for the basic or physical needs you have chosen in number 4.
6. State two likely psychosocial needs at each level of prevention for your group.
7. List two objectives for the psychosocial needs for group members at each level of prevention.

LEARNING ACTIVITY 2-3

▶ **Critical Thinking Exercise:** Levels of Prevention

You work in an Emergency Department. An older woman and her husband enter. The woman is loud and combative, and her blood alcohol level is well above normal.

Identify the level of prevention on which you will focus.
Determine if any level of prevention will not be included at all.

LEARNING ACTIVITY 2-4

▶ **Critical Thinking Exercise:** Home Health Care and Tertiary Prevention

List the reasons for focusing on tertiary prevention in home health care.

LEARNING ACTIVITY 2-5

▶ **Critical Thinking Exercise:** Self-Evaluation and Reflection

1. In your clinical journal, identify issues you have observed in your clinical experiences that relate to health rather than to illness.
2. Discuss how this differs from what you previously thought of as health.
3. How does this affect your impression of the role of the nurse in the community?
4. In your clinical journal, identify issues you have observed in your clinical experiences that relate to *Healthy People 2010* goals.
5. What can you do as a nurse to affect these health issues?

Culture Care

PAULA SWIGGUM

▶ L E A R N I N G   O B J E C T I V E S ◀

- Define the following: culture, cultural care, transcultural nursing, ethnocentrism, cultural blindness, acculturation, assimilation, lifeway, emic care, and etic care.

- Describe the history of transcultural care in nursing.

- Describe how culture influences worldview, communication, time orientation, family, society, and health.

- Describe the components of a cultural assessment.

- Discuss transcultural nursing skills and competencies in community settings.

- Describe the nursing role as advocate for those clients from diverse cultures.

- Identify transcultural nursing resources.

▶ K E Y   T E R M S ◀

acculturation	culture
assimilation	culturologic assessment
cultural awareness	emic care
cultural blindness	ethnocentrism
cultural care	etic care
cultural encounter	lifeway
cultural knowledge	transcultural nursing
cultural skill	

Historical Perspectives

Cultural Awareness

The increasing diversity of people in the United States is becoming more evident each day. One needs only to walk the streets of urban areas and farming communities to notice the changing face of America. Recent immigrants have come from the far reaches of the world, primarily southeast Asia, east Africa, and Latin American countries. New groups bring with them a variety of languages, customs, modes of dress and other cultural practices. Nurses in the 21st century are challenged to provide care to persons whose customs are unfamiliar. Culture influences health and well-being in myriad ways, so the professional nurse must understand what that means for each client encountered.

Nurses have always been concerned with the whole person, including the physical, emotional, psychological, spiritual, and developmental dimensions. With the increasing numbers of immigrants coming to the United States, especially in the past 30 years, the new challenge is to understand the cultural dimension. **Culture** incorporates not only customs, but beliefs, values, and attitudes shared by a group of people and passed down through generations.

Healthy People 2010 (U.S. Department of Health and Human Services [DHHS], 2000) calls for the elimination of disparity among groups in access to quality health care services and an increase in community-based programs that are culturally and linguistically appropriate. Transcultural nursing knowledge is essential to attain those goals.

This chapter will discuss transcultural nursing and its historical beginnings. In addition, key concepts relating to cultural care, including cultural awareness, and culturally appropriate nursing competencies related to assessment and intervention, will be explored. Because such a multitude of cultural groups and practices exists, nurses cannot have knowledge of each and every one. Therefore, a culturally sensitive approach that incorporates knowing how to discover important cultural beliefs affecting health and wellness will be discussed, along with available resources.

 ## HISTORICAL PERSPECTIVES

Discussions of cultural competence in nursing are not new. In fact, the field of transcultural nursing has its roots in the early 1900s, when public health nurses cared for immigrants from Europe who came from a wide range of cultural backgrounds and had diverse health care practices (Poss, 1999). In the late 1940s, Dr. Madeleine Leininger held the belief that "care is the essence of nursing, and the central, dominant and unifying focus of nursing" (Leininger, 1991, p. 3). She then began to see the importance of nursing care that was based on the client's culture, that is, the unique values, beliefs, practices, and **lifeways** (beliefs about dress, diet, and other activities of daily living) passed down from one generation to the next. The idea that culture and care are inextricably linked led her to study other cultures, and she became the first nurse to obtain a doctorate in anthropology. **Transcultural nursing** (a term coined by Leininger) is a body of knowledge and practice for caring for people from other cultures.

Since those early days, the theory of Cultural Care Diversity and Universality has been developed by Leininger to "generate substantive knowledge for the discipline of nursing" (Leininger, 1991, p. 15). The world was on a fast track to multiculturalism, and nurses did not have the knowledge to provide care that was culturally appropriate. Having this knowledge is a moral and ethical obligation for nurses as they strive to provide the best care possible to all their clients. Community nurses have been among those most interested in this field, because they work directly with individuals and families in their own settings and see the need firsthand.

Although the first large groups of immigrants came to America primarily from Europe in the early 1900s, the recent wave of immigrants to the United States has come from all over the world including Africa, Asia, and Central and South America. Table 3–1 depicts the country of origin for immigrants in 1900 and 1990. Today, both urban and rural communities have significant numbers of members whose country of origin is other than the United States. Many Native Americans live off the reservation and contribute to the multicultural composition of cities and towns.

Many nurse leaders and educators have embraced the need for culture-specific care, and various approaches to gaining this knowledge have been developed. One such model was developed by Dr. Josepha Campinha-Bacote, a Cape Verdean native who now lives and works in the United States. Her model involves the components of cultural awareness, cultural knowledge, cultural skill, and cultural encounter (Campinha-Bacote, 1995). It will be used here as a framework to help nurses learn the concepts necessary to gain cultural competence in working within the community setting.

 ## CULTURAL AWARENESS

Before nurses can intervene appropriately with clients from another culture, they must first understand their own—that is, they must have self-awareness of their own cultural background, influences, and biases. Only with this **cultural awareness** can they appreciate and be sensitive to the values, beliefs, lifeways, practices, and problem-solving methods of a client's culture.

One exercise that can be illuminating for nurses is to respond to a "cultural tree" in which one's own cultural heritage is evaluated in terms of the various elements that make up a culture. The components of the cultural tree are depicted in Figure 3–1. By considering specific examples and anecdotes about family traditions and beliefs, one becomes aware of beliefs and practices that are highly

Year	Europe	Asia	Africa	Oceania	Latin America	North America
TABLE 3–1 • Region of Birth of the Foreign-Born Population: 1900 and 1999						
Number						
1900	8,881,548	120,248	2,538	8,820	137,458	1,179,922
1990	4,350,403	4,979,037	363,819	104,145	8,407,837	753,917
Percent Distribution						
1900	86.0%	1.2%	—	0.1%	1.3%	11.4%
1990	22.9%	26.3%	1.9%	0.5%	44.3%	4.0%

U.S. Bureau of the Census, 1999.

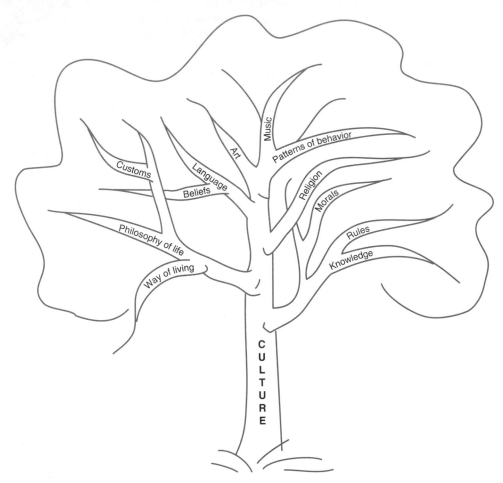

Figure 3–1. ▶ The cultural tree.

influenced by one's cultural background. There can be amazing diversity even within a group that outwardly appears very much alike.

This new awareness of one's own cultural influences helps the nurse avoid attitudes that can be detrimental to the nurse–client relationship. **Cultural blindness** occurs when the nurse does not recognize his or her own beliefs and practices or the beliefs and practices of others. **Ethnocentrism** refers to the idea that one's own ways are the only way or the best way to behave, believe, or do things. For example, a dominant cultural value in the United States is planning for the future. Calendars are kept religiously, goals are set, events are planned weeks and months in advance, and money is saved for retirement. In other cultures, value is placed on the present and there is a belief that because life is pre-ordained, there is no point in planning for or trying to change the future. Future-oriented individuals may feel that this is the only correct way to live and may be disdainful of those with another orientation to time. This is ethnocentrism.

Another concept in mainstream American culture that is taken for granted as normal is the concept of time. Americans live by the clock, make time, waste time, kill time, want to know what time, and worry about having enough time. In many cultures, one's daily activities take place as the need arises, without regard to a prescribed time of day. For members of these cultures, "being on time" for an appointment may have a range of several hours. The community nurse must be aware of these views and accommodate them accordingly.

The reliance on self is another dominant cultural value in the United States. More than 100 words in the English language begin with the word self. In many other languages, there is no translation for the word self. In these cultures, the individual needs are secondary to the needs of the group. This has strong implications for the concept of self-care.

Mainstream American culture places high value on taking care of one's self. People are reluctant to have someone do for them what they think they can do for themselves. This is not so for all cultures. For example, when a Mexican woman gives birth there is a period of time called *Quarentena* or *LaDieta* during which specific rules apply regarding the postpartum woman's activity and diet (Andrews & Boyle, 1999). During this time, she is not to do heavy lifting, exercise, or housework. Family and community members take over the chores of the household, including child care and meal preparation. A community nurse visiting during this postpartum period who is not aware of this cultural practice may provide teaching according to his or her own values that may dictate a more active approach to the mother's recovery from childbirth. Because nurses working in the community frequently visit postpartum mothers and their newborns, it is essential that they understand how strongly culture influences postpartal self-care and how much it may vary from Western practices (Horn, 1981).

Health decision-making is culturally based. For some people, these decisions are very private and individual, whereas others wouldn't think of making a treatment decision without first consulting their extended families. Some people come from backgrounds where stoicism is the norm and pain is not expressed, whereas others have the view that openly verbalizing pain is expected. In each situation, cultural self-awareness is essential to help the nurse recognize and value the right of others to follow their cultural beliefs and practices. Awareness of one's own cultural values opens the nurse's mind to the possibility that the client's values, beliefs, and practices may vary in ways that significantly affect the provision of care.

The effective nurse will recognize other cultural beliefs and practices as valid and accommodate the client's ways in providing care. The nurse should ask, "How will knowing these things about my patient influence my care?"

 ## CULTURAL KNOWLEDGE

Once nurses are more sensitive to and aware of their own cultures and biases, they are ready to discover the culture and lifeways of the community(ies) within which they work. "The goal of **cultural knowledge** is to become familiar with a culturally or ethnically diverse group's world view, beliefs, values, practices, lifestyles, and problem-solving strategies." (Campinha-Bacote, 1997, p. 81).

Community-based nursing practice requires that the nurse have cultural knowledge of the community. This knowledge allows the nurse to use a preventive approach and facilitate self-care according to the client's particular culture. Collaboration and continuity are also enhanced when the nurse knows the cultural community in which he or she is working with the client. Having cultural knowledge about the community will influence what is seen, leading to more thorough and appropriate assessment and intervention (Fig. 3–2).

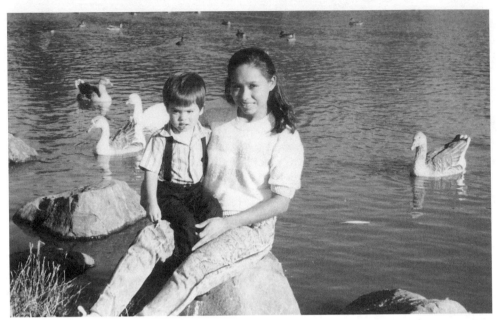

Figure 3–2. ▶ Family relationships and child care are strongly influenced by cultural traditions.

Lack of cultural knowledge stands in the way of cultural competence. Nurses can have wonderful intentions, and be sensitive and caring, but if there is a lack of specific knowledge about the patient's culture, then mistakes are bound to be made.

For example, a public health nurse visits a family in a Hmong community in the Midwest. As he walks in the door, he sees a young boy standing there, and he reaches out to touch the boy's head in greeting and as an expression of caring. Lacking cultural knowledge of the Hmong, the nurse is unaware of a strong taboo against touching the head, which is considered the most sacred part of the body, being the location of the brain and thinking processes. This unintentional affront compromises the nurse's ability to provide care to the family.

As a new immigrant to the United States, a young Guatemalan woman takes her 2-week-old infant in for a check-up. Because the umbilical cord had dried and was ready to fall off, the physician plucks it away and tosses it into the trash as the mother looks on in horror. An American mother would probably think nothing of this, but in Guatemalan culture, the umbilical cord is precious and is saved by the mother. The physician was not being cruel, but was ignorant of cultural knowledge related to postpartum practices in Guatemalan culture. A simple question asked by the doctor or nurse, such as, "What cultural practices are important to you in the care of your newborn?" would have alleviated the trauma to this young woman.

Generic and Professional Knowledge

Dr. Madeleine Leininger uses the terms emic and etic to describe types of care (Leininger, 1991). **Emic** refers to the local or insider's views and values about a phenomenon. **Etic** refers to the professional or outsider's views and values about a phenomenon. The community nurse uses both these types of care knowledge and verifies with the client and family which areas are meaningful and acceptable to them. Discovering how generic (emic) and professional (etic) systems are alike or different assists the nurse to provide culturally congruent care to individuals or groups.

In Mexican American culture there are several levels of healers within the *curanderismo* folklore system. At one level is a *curendero*, or folk healer, who is believed to have God-given gifts of healing. This folk healer may treat people with a wide range of physical and psychological problems ranging from back pain and gastrointestingal distress to irritability or fatigue. After a diagnosis is made, the *curandero* may use treatments such as massage, diet, rest, indigenous herbs, prayers, magic, or supernatural rituals (Giger & Davidhizer, 1995). The nurse working in a Mexican American community should have knowledge of the levels of folk healers used by her clients and should inquire as to the consultation and treatment already rendered.

Using this emic understanding of the client's beliefs about the health issue, the community nurse can coordinate that care with professional (etic) care that will be acceptable to the client. If massage or a specific diet treatment has been successful, then those interventions can be incorporated into a plan of care. When cultural practices are acknowledged, respected, and given value by the professional nurse, clients are more willing to incorporate Western medicine that may augment and enhance the response to treatment.

Components of Cultural Assessment

Six phenomena related to a cultural assessment are discussed in this section. These are summarized in Box 3–1.

Communication

Because the community based nurse spends much time in teaching and communicating roles, knowledge of communication styles and meanings is essential. Verbal and nonverbal behavior, eye contact, salutations, and intergender communication patterns vary significantly among cultures. For example, in Western cultures, lack of eye contact is seen as impolite and may indicate indifference or noninterest. In Native American and Southeast Asian cultures, on the other hand, lack of eye contact is a gesture of respect. In conversation, Americans tend to answer quickly, often before the person speaking has finished; however, Native Americans use silence before answering to carefully absorb what the other has said and to formulate their own response. A nurse working within this community must be aware of this and allow time for these interactions.

In many Eastern cultures, agreeing by nodding or saying yes is considered polite, whether the individual in reality agrees or understands what has been asked. For a Hmong person, responding "yes" to a medical explanation may simply mean that the person is politely listening, not that he or she agrees or even understands what was said. The Hmong appear passively obedient to protect their own dignity by not appearing ignorant and also to protect the doctor's dignity by acting deferential (Fadiman, 1997).

A nurse teaching about medication regimens or wound care in a community setting, for example, should use other means of ensuring understanding rather than simply asking, "Do you understand?" Return demonstrations or verbal explanations back to the nurse help to ensure that teaching is effective. For exam-

> ▶ Box 3–1. Six Phenomena of Cultural Assessment ◀

- *Communication.* A continuous process by which one person may affect another through written or oral language, gestures, facial expressions, body language, space, or other symbols.
- *Space.* The area around a person's body that includes the individual, body, surrounding environment, and objects within that environment.
- *Social organization.* Includes the family and other groups within a society that dictate culturally accepted role behaviors of different members of the society and rules for behavior. Behaviors are prescribed for significant life events, such as birth, death, childbearing, childrearing, and illness.
- *Time.* Refers to the meaning and influence of time from a cultural perspective. Time orientation refers to an individual's focus on the past, the present, or the future. Most cultures combine all three time orientations, but one orientation is more likely to dominate.
- *Environmental control.* Refers to the ability or perceived ability to an individual or persons from a particular cultural group to plan activities that control nature, such as illness causation and treatment.
- *Biologic variations.* Refers to the biologic differences among racial and ethnic groups; can include physical characteristics, such as skin color; physiologic variations, such as lactose intolerance; or susceptibility to specific disease processes.

Giger J. N., & Davidhizar R. E. (1991). *Transcultural nursing: Assessment and intervention.* St. Louis: Mosby–Year Book.

ple, a nurse may say, "To be sure that your mother will get her medication in the best way to help her, tell me the times you will give her this pill." Or, "Give me some examples of the kinds of foods that you can prepare for your father so that he will minimize the amount of grease in his diet." A respectful and caring approach is a universal dimension of care.

Space and Physical Contact

The concept of space is another important dimension of cultural knowledge. How close people stand to each other in conversation, overt expressions of affection and caring with touch, and rules relating to personal space and privacy vary greatly among cultures. For example, in Italian and Mexican cultures, physical presence and touching are valued and expected. Family members of both sexes embrace, kiss, and link arms when walking. In Middle Eastern cultures, close face-to-face conversations in which one can almost feel the breath of the other is the norm, whereas in the United States the normal amount of space between people in conversation is an arm's length. In Muslim cultures, it is inappropriate for men and women to even shake hands before marriage. It would be highly improper and distressing for a female Somalian patient to be assessed by a male nurse.

The nurse learns about these cultural traditions and beliefs by reading, observing, and asking questions. When in doubt, it is always appropriate to ask, "In your culture, what is considered proper relating to touching and physical space?"

Time

The Western orientation to time and its value was discussed previously. Because the concept of time has such different meanings in various cultures, it is important for the nurse to have knowledge of this dimension within the cultural group receiving care. Implications for making appointments, follow-up care, and proper medication administration need to be considered. For example, a medication may be prescribed to be taken three times a day with meals. Three meals a day is the norm for most Americans, but not so in all other cultures. The nurse should find out when the family has a meal and how much time there is between meals to determine how to explain the regimen within this patient's normal patterns of eating.

When scheduling a home visit, 2:00 PM is an exact time to a nurse accustomed to Western orientation to time, but may mean "sometime in the afternoon" to a person who doesn't share that value of exactness to clock time. Clarifying with the patient and family what is meant by a designation of an appointment time saves frustration for both parties.

Another aspect of time orientation is that of past, present, or future orientation. Traditional American culture is very future oriented. Calendars and plans for the future are a part of everyday American life. In contrast, Native American cultures tend to be past oriented, with a focus on ancestors and traditions. African American culture tends to focus on the present with an emphasis on "now" and day-to-day activities. People without a future orientation need a different approach when discussing preventive care, for example. The nurse may involve the patient by saying, "Because of the strong tendency toward developing diabetes that exists in your family, in what ways can we work together to help you avoid this disease in the future?"

Social Organization

The community-based nurse must understand the social organization of the groups within the community being served. This "includes the family and other groups within a society that dictate culturally accepted role behaviors of different members of the society and rules for behavior" (Kozier, Erb, Blais, & Wilkinson, 1995, p. 298). Things to consider, learn, and assess for include:

What is the definition of family in this cultural group? Does it include primarily the nuclear family, or is the extended family considered the basic unit?

Are there gender or age roles that affect the choice of whom the nurse should address when entering the home or in consultation about a client's health?

What are the traditional roles within the family that affect caregiving?

What value is placed on children and the elderly, and how does that affect health care decision-making within the family?

What is the status of females within the culture, and how does that affect who is considered an acceptable health care provider?

What is the expected family involvement in health care decisions, and who is the primary decision-maker within the family?

How is information regarding the health of a family member shared with others in the community?

What role does religion play in health care practices and decision-making within the culture and the family unit?

Biologic Variations

To perform a thorough assessment and provide culturally congruent care, the community-based nurse who knows the biologic variations specific to his or

TABLE 3–2 • Biocultural Aspects of Disease

Disease	Remarks
Alcoholism	Native Americans have double the rate of whites; lower tolerance to alcohol among Chinese and Japanese Americans
Anemia	High incidence among Vietnamese due to presence of infestations among immigrants and low-iron diets; low hemoglobin and malnutrition found among 18.2% of Native Americans, 32.7% of blacks, 14.6% of Hispanics, and 10.4% of white children under 5 years of age
Arthritis	Increased incidence among Native Americans Blackfoot 1.4% Pima 1.8% Chippewa 6.8%
Asthma	Six times greater for Native American infants < 1 year; same as general population for Native Americans ages 1–44 years
Bronchitis	Six times greater for Native American infants < year; same as general population for Native Americans ages 1–44 years
Cancer	Nasopharyngeal: High among Chinese Americans and Native Americans Breast: Black women 1½ times more likely than white Esophageal: No. 2 cause of death for black males ages 35–54 years *Incidence:* White males 3.5/100,000 Black males 13.3/100,000 Liver: Highest among all ethnic groups are Filipino Hawaiians Stomach: black males twice as likely as white males; low among Filipinos Cervical: 120% higher in black females than in white females Uterine: 53% lower in black females than white females Prostate: Black males have highest incidence of all groups Most prevalent cancer among Native Americans: biliary, nasopharyngeal, testicular, cervical, renal, and thyroid (females) cancer Lung cancer among Navajo uranium miners 85 times higher than among white miners Most prevalent cancer among Japanese Americans: esophageal, stomach, liver, and biliary cancer Among Chinese Americans, there is a higher incidence of nasopharyngeal and liver cancer than among the general population
Cholecystitis	*Incidence:* Whites 0.3% Puerto Ricans 2.1% Native Americans 2.2% Chinese 2.6%
Colitis	High incidence among Japanese Americans
Diabetes mellitus	Three times as prevalent among Filipino Americans as whites; higher among Hispanics than blacks or whites Death rate is 3–4 times as high among Native Americans ages 25–34 years, especially those in the West such as Utes, Pimas, and Papagos *Complications* Amputations: Twice as high among Native Americans versus general U.S. population Renal failure: 20 times as high as general U.S. population, with tribal variation, (eg, Utes have 43 times higher incidence)
G6PD	Present among 30% of black males
Influenza	Increased death rate among Native Americans ages 45+
Ischemic heart disease	Responsible for 32% of heart-related causes of death among Native Americans; blacks have higher mortality rates than all other groups

(continued)

TABLE 3–2 • Biocultural Aspects of Disease (*Continued*)

Disease	Remarks
Lactose intolerance	Present among 66% of Hispanic women; increased incidence among blacks and Chinese
Myocardial infarction	Leading cause of heart disease in Native Americans, accounting for 43% of death from heart disease; low incidence among Japanese Americans
Otitis media	7.9% incidence among school-aged Navajo children versus 0.5% in whites Up to ⅓ of Eskimo children < 2 years have chronic otitis media Increased incidence among bottle-fed Native Americans and Eskimo infants
Pneumonia	Increased death rate among Native Americans ages 45+
Psoriasis	Affects 2–5% of whites, but < 1% of blacks; high among Japanese Americans
Renal disease	Lower incidence among Japanese Americans
Sickle cell anemia	Increased incidence among blacks
Trachoma	Increased incidence among Native Americans and Eskimo children (3–8 times greater than general population)
Tuberculosis	Increased incidence among Native Americans Apache 2.0% Sioux 3.2% Navajo 4.6%
Ulcers	Decreased incidence among Japanese Americans

Based on data reported in Overfield, T. (1995). *Biologic variation in health and illness: Race, age, and sex differences.* New York: CRC Press; and Office of Minority Health. (1995). Cancer In minority communities. *Closing the gap.* Washington, DC: U.S. Government Printing Office. Andrews, M., & Boye J. (1999). *Transcultural concepts in nursing care* (pp. 46–47). Philadelphia: Lippincott Williams & Wilkins.

her clients will be most effective. Although some biologic variations are more obvious (eg, skin color, hair texture, facial features, stature, and body markings), others require familiarity with medical knowledge and research. For example, Africans and African American persons have a much higher incidence of sickle cell disease than other groups. Much of the world's population (many Asians, Africans, Hispanics, and Native Americans) is lactose intolerant, or unable to digest milk sugars. To provide health teaching related to a diet that includes milk and milk products to people in these groups is ethnocentric. Native Americans have a very high incidence of diabetes mellitus. Health assessment by community-based nurses working with this population should include screening for high blood sugar levels and culturally appropriate preventive teaching.

The action, absorption, excretion, and dose parameters of many pharmacologic agents also vary among ethnic groups. Genetic differences, structural variation in binding receptor sites, and environmental conditions may affect the drug action in different groups of people. Blood pressure medications, analgesics, and psychotropic drug doses may be significantly different depending on the ethnic group (Kudzma, 1992). Adult doses for many medications are not determined by weight as for pediatric doses, but body mass should be considered for groups of small stature, such as people of Japanese or Korean descent. The nurse should also ask about herbal remedies the client might be taking that could affect the action or metabolism of certain medications (Andrews & Boyle, 1999). Table 3–2 lists some common diseases and their effect on different populations.

Environmental Control

There are three predominant views on the relationship between the environment and health: magicoreligious, biomedical, and humoral. The magicoreligious view sees illness as a having a supernatural force; that is, malevolent or evil spirits cause disease or illness as a punishment from God. People from Hispanic and Caribbean cultures may have this health belief system. Because the belief is that a supernatural influence (rather than organic) caused the health problem, people with this perspective will look for a supernatural counterforce to rid themselves of the problem. People with this belief will seek out a voodoo priestess or spiritualist who has the powers to remove "spells" from a variety of sources. Although Western medicine has classified voodoo illness as a psychiatric disorder (Campinha-Bacote, 1992), nurses who practice cultural care will understand this view of illness and intervene accordingly.

In the biomedical view, disease and illness are believed to be caused by microorganisms or a malfunction of the body. People with this health belief view look to medicines, medical treatment, or surgery to cure their illness.

The humoral health belief view looks for a balance or harmony with nature (Kozier et al., 1995). Many Eastern cultures ascribe to the theory of yin and yang being opposite forces that must be kept in balance. Imbalance results in illness or disease. The hot and cold theory of many Latino and Asian cultures is similar. "Central to humoral theory is the belief that the healthy body is characterized by evenly distributed warmth and that illness results when the body is attacked by an increase of either hot or cold" (Horn, 1990). For example, childbirth is seen as an experience where the body loses heat balance, which must be restored. A postpartum Chinese woman will refuse ice water served in the hospital and will accept only foods that are seen as "warm," such as chicken and rice. Bathing would contribute to the loss of body warmth and would be refused for a period of time after childbirth. The nurse visiting a client in a community setting with this health belief should be sensitive to these practices and provide care accordingly.

Many variations exist among cultural groups as to how health care is managed and decisions are made. It is important to also keep in mind that individual families may have their own roles, beliefs, and practices that differ from those of the larger cultural group. This may be a result of the degree to which the family has been acculturated to Western cultural patterns and beliefs, or it may be a regional or familial variation. Professional nurses who desire to provide effective care that is culturally congruent to the beliefs of the client are aware of the potential for variations and know what questions to ask. Although it is very helpful to have a holding knowledge (ie, knowledge of a group learned from transcultural nursing texts, literature, and previous encounters) of cultural groups encountered, the nurse must always verify with each client which beliefs and practices are personally relevant. In this way, cultural sensitivity and respect are conveyed even when the nurse is not well versed in the lifeways of a particular group.

Acculturation and Assimilation

Two other concepts are important for nurses to keep in mind as they learn about the culture of particular groups. Individuals within a group may adhere to the traditional culture to varying degrees; this variation may be a result of acculturation or assimilation.

As new groups enter a new society, **acculturation** may occur as they learn the ways to exist in a new culture. These include learning to drive, going to school, negotiating public transportation, getting a job, and living in an environment very unlike that in the home country. As these activities become more comfortable, individuals become more acculturated to the dominant society yet may retain much of their own cultural traditions within their communities. For example, a young Somalian girl may continue to wear her traditional Muslim attire (hajib) and retain traditional gender roles while going to an American high school and working at a fast food restaurant on weekends.

Assimilation occurs when individuals or groups identify more strongly with the dominant culture in values, activities, and daily living. This usually occurs over longer periods of time, sometimes generations. The nurse must keep in mind that there may be a wide variation in how cultural traditions are carried out even within the same family when the parents have immigrated from another country but the children have been raised surrounded by the dominant culture.

CULTURAL SKILL

Campinha-Bacote defines **cultural skill** as the ability to collect relevant cultural data regarding the client's health history, which "involves the process of learning how to conduct a culturologic assessment" (Campinha-Bacote, 1997, p. 83). Up to this point we have discussed the need for nurses to examine their own cultural traditions, beliefs, values, and practices to increase awareness of how influential their culture is on their view of the world and to open their minds to the valid variations in worldviews of varying cultures. This helps to avoid cultural blindness, cultural imposition, and ethnocentrism. It is then the nurse's responsibility to learn as much as possible about the ethnic or cultural groups encountered in the community where the nursing care is being delivered. A holding knowledge of the emic or folk care practices along with the etic or professional care practices gives the community nurse a basis from which to individualize care that is culturally sensitive to the client as an individual or as a family. Practices within cultural groups or families may vary significantly from general descriptions; therefore, knowing the questions to ask for culturally specific care is essential to avoid stereotyping. Having cultural skill is essential to that process.

Leininger defines a **culturologic assessment** as a "systematic appraisal or examination of individuals, groups and communities as to their cultural beliefs, values, and practices to determine explicit needs and intervention practices within the cultural context of the people being evaluated" (Leininger, 1994, pp. 85–86). Community-based nurses focus on preventive care. These nurses assess the health risks of a particular group and consider cultural practices and beliefs to plan teaching and activities to prevent diseases or health risks (primary prevention). Using culturally based knowledge of generic or folk health care practices in the group, community-based nurses then incorporate their **etic** and **emic** care knowledge to diagnose and treat threats to health and wellness (secondary prevention). Tertiary prevention in the community seeks to rehabilitate or prevent recurrence of health problems. Through a skillful culturologic assessment, the community nurse has listened to the clients' perception of the health problem and compared it with his or her own, explaining and acknowledging the similarities and differences. Involving members of the community, the nurse then negotiates a treatment plan that will be seen as beneficial to the community.

Numerous models for culturologic assessment have been developed by various authors in the field of transcultural nursing (Andrews & Boyle, 1999; Giger

& Davidhizer, 1995; Leininger, 1994; Purnell & Paulanka, 1998; Tripp-Reimer, Brink, & Saunders, 1984). Each organizes assessment data in a different manner, and individual nurses will determine which model works best within their scope of practice and the communities they serve. Pfifferling (1980) developed a cultural assessment tool (Box 3–2) to be used in the mental health field, which can be used with any client. The six questions are open ended and allow the client to describe his or her perception of the health problem. For example, in response to the first question, "How would you describe your problem?" the parents of a Hmong child with epilepsy might respond, "The spirit catches you and you fall down" (Fadiman, 1997).

The culturologic assessment gives the nurse good information with cultural implications to use as a basis for planning teaching and treatment plans. "The basic premise of the culturologic assessment is that clients have a right to their cultural beliefs, values, and practices and that these factors should be understood, respected and considered when rendering culturally competent nursing care" (Campinha-Bacote, 1994, p. 10).

 CULTURAL ENCOUNTER

The **cultural encounter** is the opportunity for the nurse to engage in direct contact with the members of cultural communities. Through frequent contact with numerous members of a cultural group, the nurse stays aware that variations will exist within the community and that stereotypical expectations are to be avoided. Trust between the caregiving nurse and members of the community builds over time and is essential to the well-being of both.

Using knowledge of etic and emic care practices and information gained from the culturologic assessment, the nurse now uses the skills and competencies necessary to effect healthful outcomes for the clients in the community. Leininger has identified three modalities—preservation, accommodation, and repatterning—that "guide nursing judgments, decisions or actions so as to provide cultural congruent care that is beneficial, satisfying and meaningful to people nurses serve" (Leininger, 1994, p. 41). These modalities are defined in Table 3–3.

▶ **Box 3–2.** Pfifferling's Cultural Assessment Questions ◀

1. How would you describe the problem that brought you here today? Is there anyone else you can talk to about this problem? How would you describe the problem to them?
2. How long have you had this problem? Does anyone else know you have this problem? Describe them and their problem. Who does not have this problem?
3. What do you think is wrong, out of balance, causing your problem, etc?
4. Why do you think this happened to you, and why now? Why did you get sick and no one else did? Why has this happened to this part of your body?
5. What do you think will help clear this up?
6. Apart from the health care practitioner, who else can help you get better? Are there things that help you feel better, give you relief, that doctors do not know about?

Swiggum, P. (1995). Cultural diversity in care: The cultural assessment. *Creative nursing,* *1*(5), 9.

TABLE 3–3 • Leininger's Guidelines for Providing Culturally Congruent Care	
Modality	**Definition**
Cultural care preservation and/or maintenance	Refers to those assistive, supporting, facilitative, or enabling professional actions and decisions that help people of a particular culture to retain and/or preserve relevant care values so that they can maintain their well-being, recover from illness, or face handicaps and/or death
Cultural care accommodation or negotiation	Refers to those assistive, supporting, facilitative, or enabling creative professional actions and decisions that help people of a designated culture (or subculture) to adapt to or to negotiate with others for a beneficial or satisfying health outcome with professional care providers
Cultural care repatterning or restructuring	Refers to those assistive, supporting, faciltative, or enabling professional actions and decisions that help a client reorder, change, or greatly modify lifeways for new, different, and beneficial health care patterns while respecting the client's cultural values and beliefs and still providing beneficial or healthier lifeways than before the changes were coestablished with the client(s)

Cultural Care Preservation

The first of these modalities is cultural care preservation and/or maintenance. After careful assessment and observation, the nurse identifies those cultural care practices that are helpful to the client. The nurse then assists, supports, facilitates, or enables the client and family to preserve those actions or behaviors. For example, in the Amish community, the extended family, neighborhood, and church expect to assist and care for members within the community. The nurse working in this community encourages and supports enlisting the help of the extended community and facilitates ways to let the care needs be known (Wenger, 1988).

Cultural Care Accommodation

The second mode, cultural care accommodation or negotiation, refers to nursing actions and decisions that assist or enable the client/family to continue with practices that are meaningful to them but may be altered because of circumstances. For example, the nurse in the community may be setting up a referral for a client to be seen in a clinic for follow-up care. The client is Muslim and observes the practice of praying five times a day. The nurse will negotiate with the client as to times of day that would provide enough time between prayers for an appointment or help the client find a place within or near the clinic where these prayers may be said. In addition to assisting the client to carry out religious practices, the respect and care shown by the nurse toward the client enhance trust and feelings of caring support.

Cultural Care Repatterning

The third way in which nurses make decisions or intervene is cultural care repatterning or restructuring. When the nurse assesses the client/family/community and finds practices that may be detrimental to health and well-being, he or she will work with the client to change behaviors that are harmful. For example, in working within the Navajo community, the nurse may observe the practice of eating bread fried in fat as a staple in the diet. Knowing that this much fat soaked into the bread is detrimental to a community at risk for heart disease, the nurse may work with the Navajo women to explore ways to decrease the amount of fat in servings of fry bread. Together they may decide that placing the fry bread vertically or on paper towels before serving may decrease the amount of fat because it drips off before eating. Because the nurse works with the client to diminish risks to health, the changes are more likely to take effect.

Research Box 3–1 presents research that led to nursing actions providing culturally competent care using these three modes of action in an ambulatory care setting. Note how knowing the culture and learning the emic care can lead to simple but very important nursing actions and decisions that will be perceived by the clients as cultural care.

Whether the nurse is validating and supporting helpful existing cultural practices, helping clients to negotiate ways to maintain their practices, or working to identify and change harmful behaviors, it is essential to work with the community as a partner. When nurses show respect and are open, much can be learned from the wisdom of centuries of cultural health care practices predating modern medicine. Because optimum health care for all clients is the goal of nursing, these three modes of nursing actions and decisions, in close cooperation with the clients, can be enormously beneficial and satisfying to both the community and the nurse.

TRANSCULTURAL NURSING RESOURCES

These transcultural nursing books, listed in the bibliography, are excellent resources:

Andrews & Boyle, *Transcultural concepts in nursing care*

Giger & Davidhizer, *Transcultural nursing, assessment and intervention*

Purnell & Paulanka, *Transcultural health care: A culturally competent approach*

Another text, by the 2000 president of the Transcultural Nursing Society, is also recommended:

Spector, R. E. (2000). *Cultural diversity in health and illness.* Upper Saddle River, NJ: Prentice-Hall.

For a comprehensive look at transcultural nursing theory as developed by its founder, Dr. Madeleine Leininger:

Leininger, *Culture care diversity and universality: A theory of nursing*

Journals also address transcultural nursing care:

Journal of Transcultural Nursing, Sage Publications

Journal of Cultural Diversity, American Association of Critical Care Nurses (an on-line journal)

The Internet contains a wealth of information related to transcultural nursing and to various cultures. See What's on the Web for addresses and descriptions of some of these sites.

RESEARCH RELATED TO COMMUNITY-BASED NURSING CARE

Research Box 3–1 ▶ Research Informs Practice

The purpose of this study was to examine the cultural beliefs and practices of Puerto Rican families that influence feeding practices and affect the nutritional status of infants and young children. The goal of the study was to outline strategies that would enable nurses to provide culturally congruent care for this population. Resulting cultural care modalities are listed below.

Cultural Care Modalities for the Puerto Rican Client in an Ambulatory Care Setting

CULTURAL CARE PRESERVATION MODALITIES
Reinforce family caring values of nurturance and succorance.
Respect and understand use of religious symbols and protective care
 symbols.
Touch the infant or child and say "God bless you" if complimenting the
 child.
Treat the family with respect, use professional demeanor, maintain eye
 contact.
Promote continuity of care.

CULTURAL CARE ACCOMMODATION MODALITIES
Use the Spanish language to include the grandmother; reinforce intergenerational
 care giving.
Promote *respeto* (respect) and *confianza* (confidence, trust) by accommodation (or
 deference) to family and community values.
Encourage introduction of traditional, healthy foods—rice, beans, and eggs–at the
 appropriate time, linking their use with green vegetables and meat.
Encourage the generic folk practice of *Ponche* as needed, with additional health
 considerations.
Develop a comprehensive bilingual feeding assessment guide to improve
 anticipatory guidance.

CULTURAL CARE REPATTERNING MODALITIES
Include grandmother and kin in a collaborative participatory approach to
 feeding.
Emphasize the cultural ideology and beliefs. Explain how a new approach will
 contribute to a big, healthy baby.
Anticipatory guidance about overfeeding formula should begin at 2–4 weeks.
Anticipatory guidance about not adding solids to the bottle should be given at 4–8
 weeks before the practice is initiated. Stress the ease of feeding solids by
 mouth at 4–6 months of age.
Develop Spanish language pamphlets linking emic and etic feeding practices.
Provide nutrition and cooking demonstration classes with a cultural theme,
 linking emic and etic foods for mothers, fathers, and grandmothers.
Advertisements for classes on Spanish-speaking radio and TV stations.
Develop a nutritional outreach program including bilingual Puerto Rican mothers
 who are interested in nutrition and health.

Higgins, B. (2000). Puerto Rican cultural beliefs: Influence on infant feeding practices in western New York. *Journal of Transcultural Nursing,* 11(1), 19–30.

✳ CONCLUSIONS

All nurses, regardless of their own cultural background, are obligated to learn what is important to their clients. "Health and illness states are strongly influenced and often primarily determined by the cultural background of the individual" (Leininger, 1970, p. 22). Cultural awareness of one's own background, beliefs, values, and practices opens the nurse's mind to value and support the diversity of others. Cultural knowledge learned from books, formal coursework, and discussions with community members gives the nurse a background or framework in which to understand the cultural health care beliefs of a group. This information can then be validated or altered based on individual interactions. Cultural skill is the ability to conduct a culturologic assessment that will guide nursing actions and decisions. In the cultural encounter, the nurse reinforces, negotiates, or assists clients to repattern care practices for optimum health care.

An attitude of sensitivity, acceptance, and sincere desire to work with culturally diverse clients results in continuity and collaborative care and promotes a trusting relationship with the client. Nurses in the community setting must establish a bond based on trust with the home health care client to provide excellent care and do so cost effectively (Heineken & McCoy, 2000). Using knowledge of the generic or emic care practices of the cultural community and integrating these with professional or etic knowledge, the nurse assists in self-care by encouraging existing healthy behaviors and establishing preventive measures that are culturally congruent and acceptable in creating a healthy future for each community served.

What's on the Web

Center for Cross-Cultural Health

Internet address: http://www.crosshealth.com

This Minneapolis-based organization offers excellent information and resources for culturally competent medical and nursing care.

Diversity Calendar

Internet address: http://www3.kumc.edu/diversity

This Web site provides a calendar of ethnic, religious, and national celebrations for various cultural groups.

Ethnomed

Internet address: http://healthlinks.washington.edu/clinical/ethnomed

This Web site, through the University of Washington, offers information on selected African and Southeast Asian cultures.

Transcultural Nursing Society

Internet address: http://www.tcns.org

This is an excellent Web site with links to other resources, information about membership in the Transcultural Nursing Society, and transcultural nursing workshops, courses, and certifications. The site also provides an on-line index for all articles published in the Journal of Transcultural Nursing since 1989.

References and Bibliography

Andrews, M., & Boyle, J. (1999). *Transcultural concepts in nursing care*. Philadelphia: Lippincott Williams & Wilkins.

Campinha-Bacote, J. (1992). Voodoo illness. *Perspectives in Psychiatric Care, 28*(1), 11–17.

Campinha-Bacote, J. (1994). Transcultural psychiatric nursing issues. *Journal of Psychosocial Nursing, 32*(8), 41–46.

Campinha-Bacote, J. (1995). The quest for cultural competence in nursing care. *Nursing Forum, 30*(4), 19–25.

Campinha-Bacote, J. (1997). Understanding the influence of culture. In J. Haber, B. Krainovich, A. McMahon, P. Price-Hoskins (Eds.), *Comprehensive psychiatric nursing*. St. Louis: Mosby.

Fadiman, A. (1997). *The spirit catches you and you fall down*. New York: Noonday Press.

Fahie, V. P. (1998). Utilization of folk/family remedies by community-residing African American elders. *Journal of Cultural Diversity, 5*(1), 19–22.

Giger, J. N., & Davidhizer, R. E. (1995). *Transcultural nursing, assessment and intervention*. St. Louis: Mosby.

Grossman, D. (1996). Cultural dimensions in home health nursing. *American Journal of Nursing, 96*(7), 33–36.

Heineken, J., & McCoy, N. (2000). Establishing a bond with clients of different cultures. *Home Healthcare Nurse, 18*(1), 45–51.

Higgins, B. (2000). Puerto Rican cultural beliefs: Influence on infant feeding practices in western New York. *Journal of Transcultural Nursing, 11*(1), 19–30.

Horn, B. M. (1990). Cultural concepts and postpartal care. *Journal of Transcultural Nursing, 2*(1), 48–51.

Huff, R. K. (1999). *Promoting health in multicultural populations: A handbook for practitioners*. Thousand Oaks, CA: Sage.

Kozier, E., Erb, G., Blais, K., & Wilkinson, J. (1995). *Fundamentals of nursing, concepts, processes and practice*. Redwood City, CA: Addison Wesley.

Kudzma, E. G. (1992). Drug response: All bodies are not created equal. *American Journal of Nursing, 92*(12), 48–50.

Leininger, M. M. (1970). *Nursing and anthropology: Two worlds to blend*. Columbus, OH: Greyden Press.

Leininger, M. M. (1991). *Culture care diversity and universality: A theory of nursing*. New York: National League for Nursing Press; Publication No. 15–2402.

Leininger, M. M. (1994). *Transcultural nursing: Theories, concepts and practices*. Columbus, OH: Greyden Press.

Lipson, J. G., & Steiger, N. J. (1996). *Culture and nursing care: A pocket guide*. San Francisco: UCSF Nursing Press.

Lockhart, J. S., & Resnick, L. K. (1997). Teaching cultural competence: The value of experiential learning and community resources. *Nurse Educator, 22*(3), 27–30.

Napier, B. (1998). Culture and aging. *Home Care Provider, 3*(1), 38–40.

Narayan, M. C. (1997). Cultural assessment in home health care. *Home Healthcare Nurse, 15*(10), 663–670.

Pfifferling, J. H. (1981). A cultural prescription for mediocentrism. In L. Eisenburg, & A. Kleinman (Eds.), *The relevance of social science for medicine*. Boston: D. Rudd Publishers.

Poss, J. E. (1999). Providing cultural competent care: Is there a role for health promoters? *Nursing Outlook, 47*(1), 30–36.

Purnell, L. D., & Paulanka, B. J. (1998). *Transcultural health care: A culturally competent approach*. Philadelphia: Davis.

Raff, B., & Fiore, E. (Eds.). (1992). *Culturally sensitive caregiving and childbearing families, module 1*. New York: March of Dimes Birth Defects Foundation.

Stewart, E. M. (1991). *American cultural patterns* (Rev. ed.). Yarmouth, ME: Intercultural Press.

Swiggum, P. (1995). Cultural diversity in care: The cultural assessment. *Creative Nursing, 1*(5), 8–9.

Tripp-Reimer, T., Brink, P., & Saunders, J. (1984). Cultural assessment: Content and process. *Nursing Outlook, 32*(2), 78–82.

U.S. Department of Health and Human Services. (2000). *Healthy people 2010: National health promotion and disease prevention objectives, full report with commentary.* Washington, DC: U.S. Government Printing Office.

Wenger, A. F. (1988). *The phenomena of care in a high context culture: The old order Amish.* Doctoral dissertation. Wayne State University. Dissertation Abstracts International, 50/02B.

Wing, D. (1998). A comparison of traditional folk healing concepts with contemporary healing concepts. *Journal of Community Health Nursing, 15*(3), 143–154.

LEARNING ACTIVITIES

LEARNING ACTIVITY 3-1

▶ The Cultural Tree

Using the cultural tree in Figure 3–1, write down the ways in which your family of origin or your cultural background influences each area depicted on a branch. Discuss your findings with another student.

1. In what areas was culture a strong influence?
2. In what areas has acculturation or assimilation influenced your beliefs and preferences compared with what your grandparents may have answered?
3. What similarities and differences did you note in comparing your tree with another student's responses?
4. By participating in this activity, what awareness did you gain that may be helpful to you in caring for clients from other cultures?

LEARNING ACTIVITY 3-2

▶ Stereotyping

Make a list of various ethnic and minority or cultural groups (eg, Native Americans, Asians, the elderly, Latinos, WASPs, Jews, etc) and write down a stereotype you have or have heard about each group.

1. How does knowing these stereotypes exist make you more sensitive to clients about the barriers that may exist in daily living and access to health care?
2. In what way can nurses break through stereotypes to deliver the best possible care?

LEARNING ACTIVITY 3-3

▶ Clinical Thinking Exercise: American Cultural Values

Read the following list of American cultural values and reflect on how they may vary significantly from the values of other cultural groups. In your clinical journal:

1. Describe several of the values that are part of your everyday way of living.
2. How do those values influence how you see other cultural ways that differ?
3. Knowing that significant value orientation differences may exist between you and your clients in the community, describe accommodations you might make to provide culturally sensitive care within that setting.

AMERICAN CULTURAL VALUES

Doing—value of activity (ie, keeping busy)

Problem-solvers—conceive of more than one course of action

Achievement—personal, visible, measurable, materialistic

Choices—effects are preferably measurable, visible, materialistic

Practical—adjust to immediate situations without much thought for long-term effects

Exploration of values—"oughtness," "should"

Self-centered

Equality and fairness

Majority rule

Decision-makers—responsible for subsequent action, rational order to the world; cause and effect; world and nature are controllable

Separation of work from play

Hard work ethic

Time is money

Temporal orientation—toward the future, can improve on the present with effort and optimism; action and hard work = goal achievement (positive)

Training and education very important

Source of motivation lies in individual, not society

Need feedback—sensitive to praise and blame; need to be liked

Competitive—individual and ascriptive (team, country, etc)

Failure is the result of lack of will and effort of the individual

Individualism versus individuality

Limits role of authority—to providing services, protecting rights of individuals, inducing cooperation and adjudicating differences

Equality of opportunity

Social equality

Don't like obligations socially

Competition within cooperation

Cooperation to get things done more important than social relationship of doers

Physical comfort and health

Private property and free enterprise (Excerpted from Stewart, 1991)

LEARNING ACTIVITY 3-4

▶ **A Culturologic Assessment**

Using a cultural assessment guide referenced in the chapter, conduct a cultural assessment on a client from a cultural group that differs from your own. What specific information did you learn that would guide your nursing actions related to (1) cultural preservation, (2) cultural accommodation, and (3) cultural repatterning?

CHAPTER 4

Family Care

ROBERTA HUNT

- Recognize the relationships among family structure, family roles, family function, and culture.

- Differentiate between the concept of the family as the client and the care of the client in the context of the family.

- Identify family developmental tasks throughout the life span.

- Describe characteristics of healthy family functioning.

- Discuss the health–illness continuum and family needs during illness.

- Describe the role of the nurse in family assessment.

- Identify the steps of planning, implementing, and evaluating in family focused community-based nursing.

- Identify community agencies for family interventions at each level of prevention.

►KEY TERMS◄

affective interventions
behavioral interventions
cognitive interventions
developmental assessment
family developmental tasks
family functions
family health
family roles

family structure
family systems theory
functional assessment
genogram
healthy family functioning
role conflict
structural family
   assessment

Significance of Family Care

Nursing Competencies and Skills in Family Care

Conclusions

Not only is the family the basic social unit in American society, but it is also the most influential and dynamic unit. It has been the primary focus of nursing care in the community since the establishment of public health nursing in the late 19th century. The family performs a variety of key functions and has a central role in promoting and maintaining the health of its members.

Understanding family structure, roles, and functions is paramount in providing comprehensive nursing care. Knowledge of **healthy family functioning** allows the nurse to identify unhealthy functioning and take appropriate actions. In the current health care climate, the nurse must be cognizant of the needs, feelings, problems, and views of the family when providing care to the individual client.

Numerous models depict the relationship between nursing care and the family. These models reflect three ways to consider the family as it relates to nursing care.

Care of the individual in the context of the family. This point of view considers the family as it relates to the recovery of the individual client. Consequently, the client is the focus and the context is the family.

The family's impact on the recovery of the client. In this model, the influences that family structure, function, development stage, and interpersonal interactions have on the recovery of the client are considered.

Improvement of the family's collective health. This method focuses on the family as the unit of service. In this model, the nurse assesses the family, determines the family's health problems or diagnoses, and develops goals with the family that are intended to improve its collective health.

This chapter discusses all three models by which nursing care is provided to families. However, **family health** will be considered primarily in the context of the impact of the family on the health of the individual who has been identified as the client. Nursing process skills will focus on the health of the family as it relates to the health recovery of the individual client.

SIGNIFICANCE OF FAMILY CARE

Regardless of which method is used, it is evident the family and individual are closely interrelated. The individual's health affects the family, and the family's health affects the client.

Concepts

Definitions of family have evolved over the past several decades. Definitions usually include family structure, roles, and function. The definition currently accepted by most health care professions is that of a social group whose members share common values and interact with each other over time. Usually, but not always, they live together. In this text we will use this definition but also consider those whom the client has identified as family or significant others.

Family Structure

Traditionally, the family has been defined as the nuclear family, or a family with a mother, father, and two or more children. The characteristics of the "typical" family in the United States have changed markedly over the past 20 years. During that time, the typical family has evolved to the point where the traditional nuclear family—mother, father, and 2.2 children—no longer represents the majority of the population. Many different family structures exist. Table 4–1 lists the various **family structures** and their components; Figure 4–1 depicts different family structures.

In 1970, 85% of all children under age 18 were living with two parents; in 1993, only 71% were, and in 1998, 68% of all children were living with two parents. The proportion of children living with only one parent doubled between 1970 and 1993, rising from 12% to 24%. For white children, 77% were living with two parents in 1998; however, only 36% of African American children and 65% of Hispanic children lived with both parents (Federal Interagency Forum on Child and Family Statistics, 1999).

Marked differences in income are apparent among the different family structures. Children in married-couple families are much less likely to be living in poverty than children living only with their mothers. In 1997, 10% of children in married-couple families were living in poverty, compared with 49% in female-householder families. The contrast by family structure is especially pronounced among certain racial and ethnic groups. For example, in 1997, 13% of African American children in married-couple families lived in poverty, compared with 55% of African American children in female-householder families. Twenty-six percent of Hispanic children in married-couple families lived in poverty, compared with 63% in female-householder families. Most children in poverty are white, non-Hispanic. However, the proportion of African American or Hispanic children in poverty is much higher than the proportion of white, non-Hispanic children. Children under 18 continue to represent a very large segment of the poor populations (40%) even though they make up only about 25% of the total population. To complicate matters, in 1994, 15% of all Americans had no health insurance (Federal Interagency Forum on Child and Family Statistics, 1999). These statistics are important because the level of health and the quality of health care are affected by poverty. Those living in poverty, and consequently receiving poor health care, represent a large number of families in the United States.

TABLE 4–1 • Family Structures

Structure	Participants
Nuclear family	Married couple with children
	Unmarried couple, heterosexual or same sex with children
Nuclear dyad	Couple, married or unmarried; heterosexual or same sex
Single-parent family	One adult with children (separated, divorced, widowed, or never married)
Single adult	One adult
Multigenerational family	Any combination of the first four family structures
Kin network	Two or more reciprocal households (related by birth or marriage)

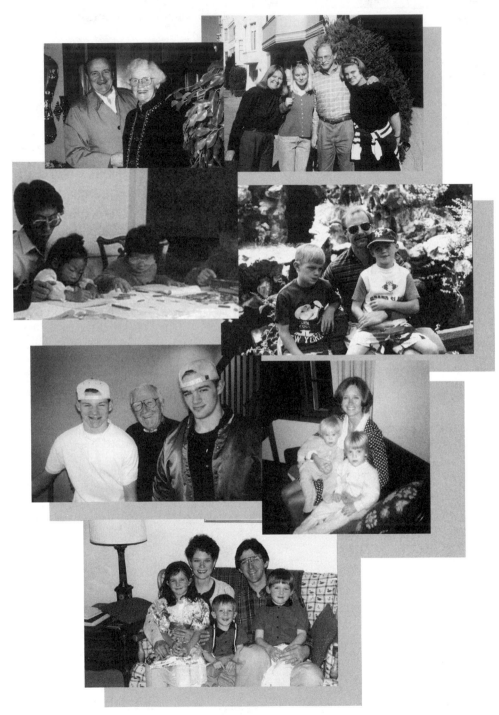

Figure 4–1. ▶ Various family structures.

Family Roles

A **family role** is an expected set of behaviors associated with a particular family position. Roles can be formal or informal. Formal roles are recognized by expectations associated with the roles, such as wife, husband, mother, father, or child. Examples of formal roles include breadwinner, housekeeper, child caretaker, financial manager, or cook. Informal roles are those that are casually acquired within a family. An example of an informal role would be the family member who plans the social schedule or who takes out the garbage, or the person in the family who pays the bills.

Role conflict may occur when the demands of one role conflict with or contradict another. This may also occur when one family member's expectations conflict with another's expectations. Role overload occurs when an individual is confronted with too many role responsibilities at one time. For instance, when a woman with children returns to school, she may have difficulty managing the roles of cook, driver, housekeeper, wife, and child care provider while keeping up with her schoolwork. The new role of student competes with the prior roles, and role overload occurs.

Illness or hospitalization of a family member causes role conflict or overload for all family members. Flexibility with family roles becomes particularly important during crises. Hospitalization and illness often require shifts in family roles and responsibilities. If one family member is ill, other family members may have to assume certain roles temporarily or permanently. In some situations this may mean a child's assuming a parental role if one of the parents becomes ill or is hospitalized. During illness, various family members' ability to take on different roles facilitates the family's adaptation or return to homeostasis. Role flexibility also allows the family to provide support to the family member who is recovering from an illness or injury. Similarly, role flexibility in a family may allow the ill family member to be more comfortable with giving up roles, thus facilitating recovery.

Family Functions

Family functions are defined as outcomes, or consequences, of family structure. They are the reason families exist. Functions are divided into several categories: affective, socialization, reproduction, economic, and health care, as shown in Figure 4–2.

The affective function of the family is defined as the family's ability to meet the psychological needs of family members. These needs include affection and understanding. This is considered by some as the most vital function of families.

Socialization and social placement is the second function. Socialization is the process of learning to adapt to life in a family and a community. This involves assisting children to adapt to the norms of the community and to become productive members of society. This socialization process is built into all cultures. Specific functions include a variety of day-to-day families and social experiences that prepare children to assume adult roles. These may include learning the norms of dress and hygiene and preparing and eating food.

The third function, reproductive, is procreation. It may be thought of as the family's providing recruits for society to ensure the continuity of the intergenerational family and society.

Economic functions encompass the allocation of adequate resources for family members. This entails the provision of sufficient income to provide for basic necessities. It also includes the allocation of these resources to all family members, especially those unable to provide for them.

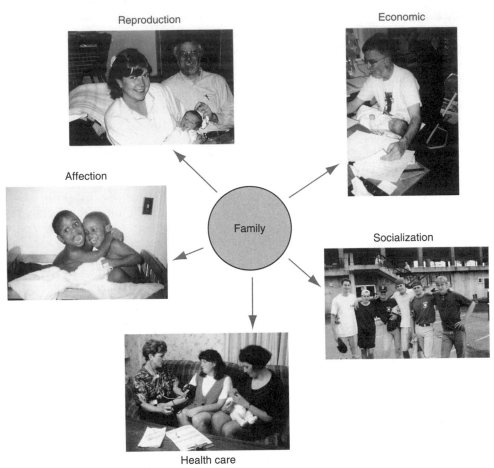

Reproduction

Economic

Affection

Family

Socialization

Health care

Figure 4–2. ▶ Basic family functions

Providing for health care and the physical necessities is the final family function. Physical care is the provision of material necessities such as food, clothing, and shelter. Family health care includes health and lifestyle practices such as nutrition, chemical use and abuse, recreation, and exercise and sleep practices.

Family functions can also be viewed in relationship to Maslow's Hierarchy of Needs. Maslow's theory is directionally based and presents the concept that the needs at the bottom of the model must be met before the next level can be addressed (Fig. 4–3). According to Maslow, the family must first meet physiologic needs (oxygen, food, fluids, shelter, sleep, and procreation) before members can consider any other opportunities in life.

Safety needs include both physiologic and psychological safety of family members. The infant experiences safety when held securely in the arms of the parent. The young child experiences safety in the family when the environment is sufficiently structured to protect the child from harm. Adolescents feel safe in an environment that allows freedom and provides responsibility and structure.

Physiologic and psychological safety remain important to adults. Physical safety includes living in a safe community. Increasingly, urban neighborhoods are more and more violent, resulting in residents' feeling unsafe. Psychological

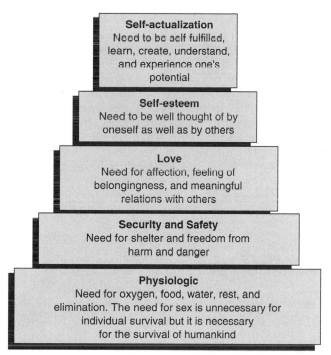

Self-actualization
Need to be self fulfilled,
learn, create, understand,
and experience one's
potential

Self-esteem
Need to be well thought of by
oneself as well as by others

Love
Need for affection, feeling of
belongingness, and meaningful
relations with others

Security and Safety
Need for shelter and freedom from
harm and danger

Physiologic
Need for oxygen, food, water, rest, and
elimination. The need for sex is unnecessary for
individual survival but it is necessary
for the survival of humankind

Figure 4–3. ▶ Maslow's hierarchy of needs. According to Maslow, basic physiologic needs must be met before the person can move on to higher-level needs. Adapted from Maslow, A. H. (1954). *Motivation and personality.* New York: Harper & Row.

safety evolves from living a relatively structured life with some definite social expectations of one's self and those around us.

Another family function is meeting love-and-belonging needs. We all need meaningful relationships with other people. In classic research by Spitz (1945), two groups of infants and children were studied. Both groups received excellent physical care, but the second group received little demonstrative affection. Members of the first group were talked to, held, and caressed. There was a higher mortality rate as well as impaired development among the infants and children of the second group who received no physical affection. This demonstrates the vital importance of meeting the love-and-belonging need.

Fulfillment of esteem needs is also a family function. Self-esteem comes from feeling that we are valued by those around us. The family introduces the child to self-esteem. Family members may assist one another to feel good about themselves through acceptance and approval.

Self-actualization is being "true to oneself," to fulfill one's potential. Self-actualization is not what one chooses to do in life, but how one feels about that choice. To joyfully do in life what one wants and is suited to do is self-actualization.

Family Systems Theory

The identification of the family as the unit of care is an emerging trend in family systems theory. **Family systems theory** defines family as a collection of people who are integrated, interacting, and interdependent. The actions of one member influence the actions of other members. The family system has a boundary; people recognize the family members. This boundary is selectively permeable according to the family's wishes, so items such as material goods, people, and information are allowed in or out according to the perceived needs of the system. Families with closed boundaries in one area may, for instance, be reluctant to use community resources.

After a crisis or during a transition from one developmental stage to another, the family system may experience disequilibrium. This imbalance causes a large amount of energy to be expended by individual family members in an attempt to cope with the discomfort. The family will attempt to return to the previous state of equilibrium. A nurse who is knowledgeable about family systems theory can facilitate healthy functioning.

The nurse considers the actions of family members as they apply to the health of the individual client. Family boundaries can be assessed to determine the likelihood that the family will use needed services. Similarly, disequilibrium of the family system as it pertains to the client can also be assessed.

Family Health

The Health–Illness Continuum and Family

The family's structure, roles, ability to fulfill family functions, culture, and developmental tasks all affect the way the family functions. When a family member is ill, adaptation depends on each of these areas. An individual's place on the wellness–illness continuum always affects family functioning. When an individual is ill, this illness has an effect on all members of the family and all interactions within the family.

Family structure also affects the health recovery of an individual. In a family with two adult members, recovery may be different from that in a family headed by one adult. Certainly, when an individual lives alone, there is a greater need to tap extended family and friends for support and assistance than when the family has other adult members.

Family roles have an impact on the health recovery of the individual, and the health of the individual affects family roles. It is difficult to fulfill the usual functions of the family during times of stress or illness. When a family member is hospitalized, it may be difficult to fulfill the family's basic physical necessities and care. Examples include the inability to provide meals, maintain a regular bedtime, or wash laundry.

Family Needs During Illness

Health care professionals are placing increased emphasis on the needs and roles of the family during a loved one's critical illness. Gravelle's (1997) research identified major recurring family needs that appear during illness, including the need to:

▶ Face and manage adversity
▶ Gain knowledge
▶ Plan and prepare
▶ Negotiate caregiving
▶ Use resources

Families require similar assistance from nursing staff during the course of a lifelong chronic condition. Taanila (1998) found from a 10-year study that families report they need quality information and advice at the time of diagnosis as well as ongoing communication concerning both emotional and factual issues. This research showed a relationship between the quality of information given to families and their feelings of insecurity and helplessness.

In addition to these needs, families experience stages or landmarks when a family member is ill (Marino & Kooser, 1986). As with any stage theory, these landmarks are not rigid pathways but, rather, a fluid progression. These stages could apply to chronic, acute, or terminal illness. Family needs during illness vary according to these stages. Table 4–2 outlines these needs.

In the first stage, the prediagnostic period, signs and symptoms of the disease appear. This tends to be a threat for the client and family. There may be concern about the future, along with misconceptions and misinformation, which compound existing fears. The nurse's role is that of counselor and educator.

In the second stage, a diagnosis is made. The client and family may experience a variety of responses—from denial and anger to guilt—as they attempt to cope with the diagnosis. During this stage, the family benefits from information about tests and treatment and emotional support.

The third stage, the treatment period, may be characterized by optimism, despair, anger, dependency, feelings of powerlessness, and fear of recurrence or long-term impairment. This is the stage of the "long, hard pull," which may last for months, but more often for years. Frequently, the nurse's role during the treatment period involves providing physical comfort measures, assisting with contacting and referring to resources, and giving positive feedback and encouragement.

The last stage is the end of life. Both terminal and chronic illnesses apply in this final stage. The client may have feelings of hopelessness and fear of abandonment; the family feels guilt, relief, or a profound sense of loss. The nurse provides support during this grieving process.

 ## NURSING COMPETENCIES AND SKILLS IN FAMILY CARE

Nurses are in the unique position among health care professionals in their close proximity to clients. As nursing has moved away from a task orientation, it has adopted a more holistic view of clients as individuals with a life beyond their illness.

TABLE 4–2 • Family Needs During Stages of Illness

Stage	Priority Family Needs	Role of the Nurse
Prediagnosis	Information	Counselor
	Relief from anxiety	Educator
	To be with and helpful to the client	
	Support and personal needs	
Diagnosis	Relief from anxiety	Support system
	Information	Educator
	To be with and helpful to the client	Assessor of family systems
	Support and personal needs	
Treatment	Relief from anxiety	Supporter for comfort measures
	Support and personal needs	Resource person
	Information	Supporter for emotions
End of life	Information	Supporter for comfort
	Relief from anxiety	Supporter for emotions
	To be with and helpful to the client	
	Support	

Adapted from Marino, L., & Kooser, J. (1986). The psychosocial care of clients and their families. Periods of high risk. In L. Marino (Ed.), *Current nursing* (pp. 53–56). St. Louis: Mosby.

The next step is to address the needs of families whose lives have been irrevocably changed by the illness of one member (Whyte & Robb, 1999). Providing nursing care to families is a logical development of the holistic approach to care of the client. It could become a cornerstone of nursing practice (Whyte & Donaldson, 1999).

The essential considerations when caring for individuals in the context of their families are as follows:

▶ One part of the family cannot be understood in isolation from the rest of the system.
▶ A family's structure and organization cannot be understood in isolation from the rest of the system.
▶ Communication patterns between family members are essential in the functioning of the family (Whyte & Robb, 1999).

Nurses need to be competent in using the nursing process as they work with clients and family members.

Family Assessment

The intent of the assessment process as it applies to the client in community-based nursing is to determine the nursing needs and intervene for the client. Initially a nurse collects information about the family to treat the client. Family interviewing, rather than family therapy, is an appropriate technique for intervention.

The Family Interview

The principles used in an effective interview with a client apply to a family interview. Effective communication is essential in the first step of establishing a trusting relationship. The interview might start with an informal conversation so all participants are put at ease. It is helpful to have all the family members present during this interview. It is also beneficial to encourage them all to participate.

Numerous family assessment tools are available. A short family assessment form is shown in Box 4–1. Many agencies have a standard form that they use for all family interviews.

The assessment may determine if a family's response is adaptive or maladaptive. This permits the nurse to identify problem areas and the need for additional assessment and referral. For example, after a family interview the nurse may share with the family concerns expressed by one member about family communication. The nurse may then suggest that the family explore this with a social worker, a public health nurse, a physician, clergy, or a counselor. A finding in assessment by the community-based nurse is the family's need for further assessment by a professional such as a family therapist or social worker with special expertise in family assessment and therapy. The intervention is the nurse's action to initiate a referral to an appropriate individual or organization.

The type of family assessment used depends on the focus of the treatment and the knowledge level of the care provider, as illustrated in Figure 4–4. Family members are asked questions regarding the client and the condition. The client is assessed within the context of the family with questions such as the following:

Question to the client: What is your understanding of a diabetic diet?

Question to the mother: What is your understanding of your son Jon's diabetes?

Question to the father: What is your understanding of your son Jon's diabetes?

(text continues on page 78)

▶ Box 4–1. Family Assessment Guide ◀

Family members

Member	Birth Date	Sex	Marital Status	Education

Genogram

Stage of Illness

What stage of illness is this family in? (See Table 4–2)

_____

_____

What are this family's priority needs?

_____

_____

What is the role of the nurse in this stage?

_____

_____

_____

(continued)

► **Box 4–1.** Family Assessment Guide *(Continued)* ◄

Development Assessment

What is this family's developmental stage?

_____

Is the family meeting the tasks of their stage?

_____

_____

_____

Does, or will, the client's health problem interrupt the family's ability to meet the developmental tasks? If yes, how does it interrupt?

_____

_____

_____

_____

_____

State nursing interventions to assist the family in meeting their developmental tasks.

_____

_____

_____

_____

Functional Assessment

Does the family meet the individual's need for affection, love, and understanding?

_____

_____

_____

_____

Does the family meet the individual's need for physical necessities and care?

_____

_____

_____

_____

_____

_____

(continued)

▶ Box 4–1. Family Assessment Guide *(Continued)* ◀

Does the family have the economic resources necessary to provide for the basic needs of the family?

_____

_____

_____

_____

Is the family meeting the function of reproduction as defined by the family?

_____

Is the family meeting the family function of socialization? Is the family fulfilling the function to socialize children to become productive members of society?

_____

_____

_____

Does the family attempt to actively cope with problems?

_____

_____

_____

_____

Assessment of Presence of Characteristics of a Healthy Family

Is communication between members open, direct, honest, and feelings and needs shared?

_____

_____

_____

_____

Do family members express self-worth with integrity, responsibility, compassion, and love to and for one another?

_____

_____

_____

_____

(continued)

▶ **Box 4–1.** Family Assessment Guide (*Continued*) ◀

Are family rules known to all members? _____

_____

Are rules clear and flexible, and do they allow individual members freedom?

_____

_____

_____

Does the family have regular links to society that demonstrate trust and friendship?

_____

_____

_____

_____

Do family members belong to various groups and clubs?

_____

_____

_____

_____

When the family is the client, other realms need to be assessed. These include family functions such as financial role responsibilities, the family's emotional system, and the meaning of the health event and its outcome to the family. Consequently, when the family is viewed as the client, individual members of the family are asked questions:

Question to the client: What impact do you think your illness has had on your family?

Question to the parents: How do you feel your family has adjusted to your son's illness?

Question to the parents: How has your son's illness affected your family's finances?

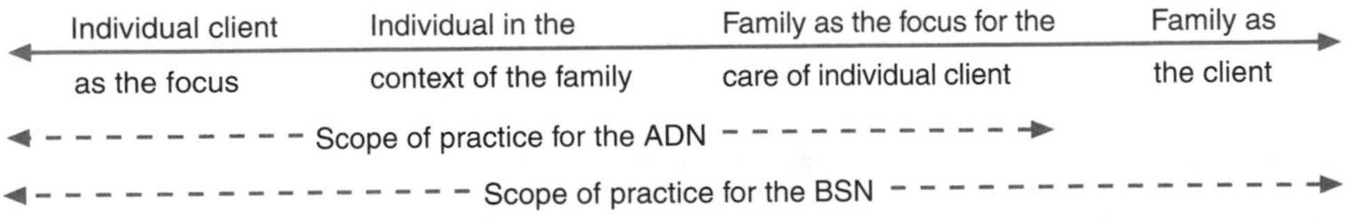

Individual client	Individual in the	Family as the focus for the	Family as
as the focus	context of the family	care of individual client	the client

◀ – – – – – – – – – – Scope of practice for the ADN – – – – – – – – – – ▶

◀ – – – – – – – – – – – – – Scope of practice for the BSN – – – – – – – – – – – – – – ▶

Figure 4–4. ▶ Focus of nursing care for individuals and families.

The first step in assessing the family as the client is to determine what the family's impact is on the recovery of the client. This is appropriate especially when the family's functioning is clearly impeding the recovery. Figure 4–5 illustrates the levels that are necessary in a comprehensive family assessment.

Overall, the intent of evaluating the family is to analyze the client's potential for recovery and self-care, given the familial conditions. To facilitate the client's return to the highest level of wellness, the circumstances in which the client lives must be considered.

Models of Family Assessment

DEVELOPMENTAL ASSESSMENT

The health of a family's functioning may be evaluated by a family **developmental assessment** considering normal **family developmental tasks.** As individuals have development stages that they must go through to move to the next stage of development, so do families. Duvall developed a commonly used theory of development stages of family life as it relates to nursing care. According to Duvall (1977), there are predictable stages within the life cycle of every family; each stage includes distinct family developmental tasks (Table 4–3). Stages of the family life cycle follow no rigid patterns. The family enters each stage with the birth of the first child or according to the age of the oldest child in the family. This model can be used as a guide to assessment by following these steps:

1. Determine the family's developmental stage. This can be done by determining the age of the oldest child in the family and correlating it with the level on Table 4–3.
2. Consider the family's health problems in the context of the tasks in their developmental stage. Is it likely that the health condition will interrupt the family's developmental tasks?
3. Determine if the family is meeting the tasks at their level of development.
4. Identify the nursing interventions that would assist the family in meeting their developmental tasks.

Because of the wide variety of family structures, not all families fit neatly into this family stage theory. For individuals who do not marry, remain childless,

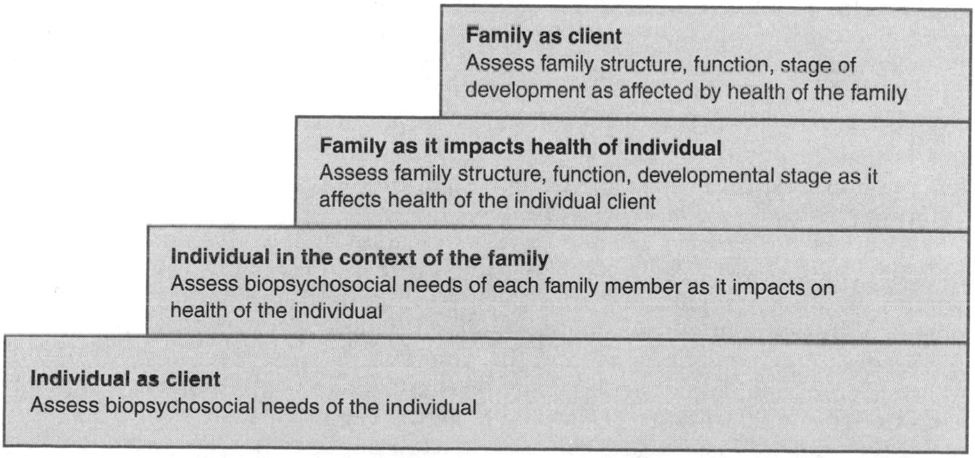

Family as client
Assess family structure, function, stage of development as affected by health of the family

Family as it impacts health of individual
Assess family structure, function, developmental stage as it affects health of the individual client

Individual in the context of the family
Assess biopsychosocial needs of each family member as it impacts on health of the individual

Individual as client
Assess biopsychosocial needs of the individual

Figure 4–5. ▶ Levels necessary to assess in a comprehensive family assessment.

TABLE 4–3 • Stages of the Family Life Cycle

Stage	Scope of the Stage	Family Developmental Tasks
Married couple	Couple makes commitment to one another	Establishing a mutually satisfying marriage Fitting into the kin network
Childbearing	Oldest child is infant through 30 mo	Adjusting to infants and encouraging their development Establishing a satisfying family life for both child and parent
Preschool	Oldest child is 2½–6 y	Adapting to the needs of preschool children in growth-producing ways Coping with lack of privacy and energy
Schoolage	Oldest child is 7–12 y	Fitting into age-appropriate community activities Encouraging the children's achievement
Teenage	Oldest child is 13–20 y	Balancing freedom with responsibility as teens mature and emancipate Establishing outside interests and career
Launching	First child leaves home to last child leaving home	Assisting young adults to work, attend school or military, with marriage, with appropriate rituals
Middle-aged parents	Empty nest to retirement	Rebuilding marital bond Cultivating kin ties with younger and older family
Aging family	Retirement to moving out of family home	Coping with loss and living alone Adapting to retirement and aging

Adapted from Spradley, B. W., & Allender, J. A. (1996). *Community health nursing: Concepts and practice* (4th ed.). Philadelphia: Lippincott-Raven.

or are in same-sex unions, or in divorced or blended families, the stages are viewed differently. In families where the stages of the family life cycle are disrupted, the emotional processes and issues relating to transition and development also differ from those set out in Duvall's stages.

Disruption of the family cycle because of a divorce causes additional steps to be taken to restabilize the family for further development. Family life cycle stages for divorced/disrupted families are compared with healthy families in Figure 4–6. In the postdivorce phase, the single custodial parent experiences a different emotional process and transition than the noncustodial parent. The developmental issues differ as well (Table 4–4).

Families with remarriage may experience emotional transitions or developmental issues as well (Table 4–5). Emotional transitions include attaining an adequate emotional separation from the previous marriage and accepting and dealing with fears about forming a new family. In addition, when beginning a blended family, members must find the time and patience necessary to permit another emotional adjustment. Resolving the feelings of attachment to a previous spouse and accepting the new family model require transitions by individuals. Developmental issues are also seen in each phase of the new marriage.

Family developmental tasks involve meeting the basic family functions dis-

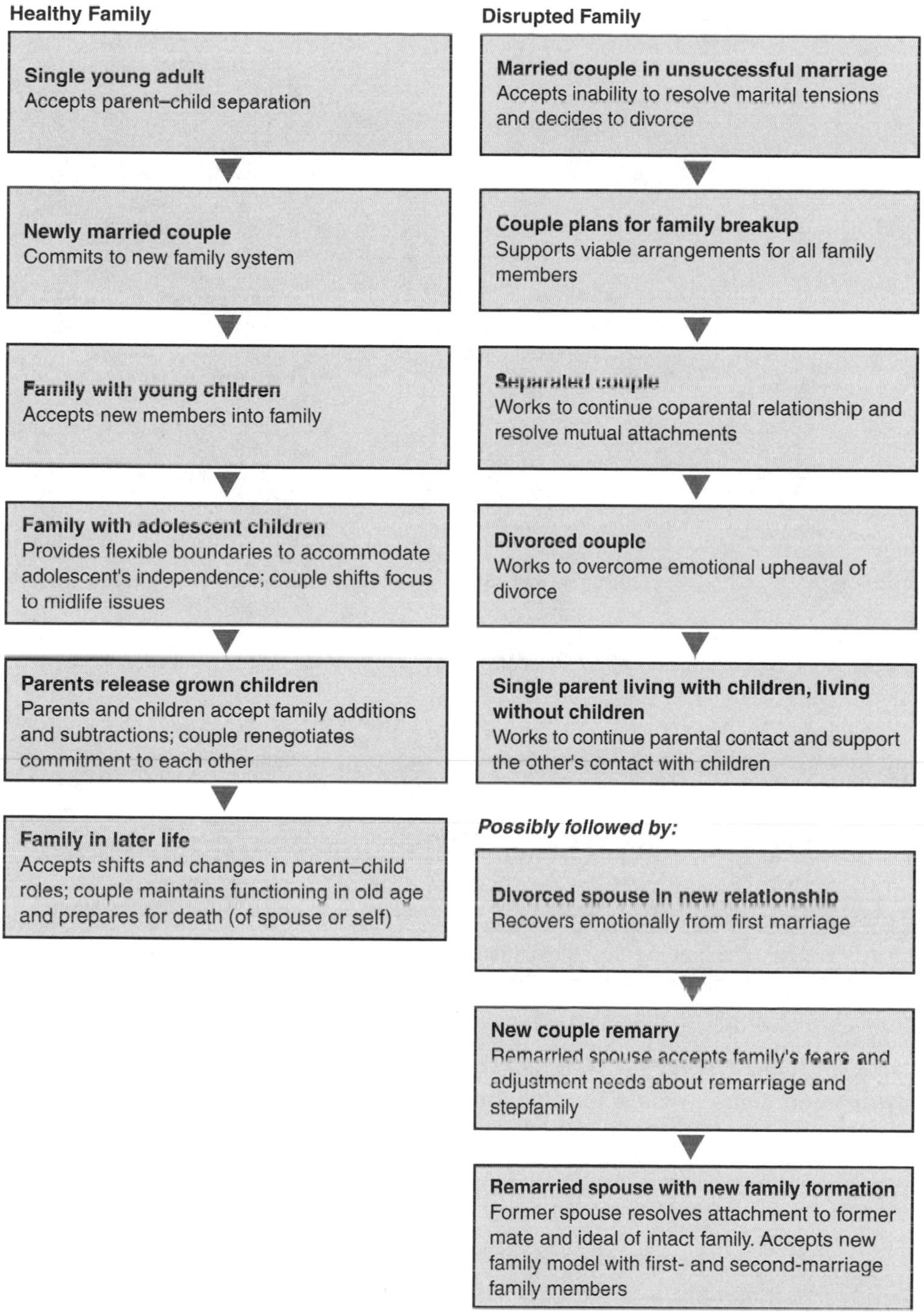

Healthy Family

Single young adult
Accepts parent–child separation

▼

Newly married couple
Commits to new family system

▼

Family with young children
Accepts new members into family

▼

Family with adolescent children
Provides flexible boundaries to accommodate
adolescent's independence; couple shifts focus
to midlife issues

▼

Parents release grown children
Parents and children accept family additions
and subtractions; couple renegotiates
commitment to each other

▼

Family in later life
Accepts shifts and changes in parent–child
roles; couple maintains functioning in old age
and prepares for death (of spouse or self)

Disrupted Family

Married couple in unsuccessful marriage
Accepts inability to resolve marital tensions
and decides to divorce

▼

Couple plans for family breakup
Supports viable arrangements for all family
members

▼

Separated couple
Works to continue coparental relationship and
resolve mutual attachments

▼

Divorced couple
Works to overcome emotional upheaval of
divorce

▼

**Single parent living with children, living
without children**
Works to continue parental contact and support
the other's contact with children

Possibly followed by:

Divorced spouse in new relationship
Recovers emotionally from first marriage

▼

New couple remarry
Remarried spouse accepts family's fears and
adjustment needs about remarriage and
stepfamily

▼

Remarried spouse with new family formation
Former spouse resolves attachment to former
mate and ideal of intact family. Accepts new
family model with first- and second-marriage
family members

Figure 4–6. ▶ Comparison of healthy family life cycle stages to disrupted family stages.
Liebermann, A. (1990). Community and home health nursing. Springhouse, PA:
Springhouse Corporation.

TABLE 4–4 • When Families Divorce

Phase	Emotional Responses	Transitional Issues
1. Stressors leading to marital differences	Reveal the fact that the marriage has major problems	Accept fact that marriage has major problems
2. Decision to divorce	Accept the inability to resolve marital differences	Accept one's own contribution to the failed marriage
3. Planning the dissolution of the family system	Negotiate viable arrangements for all members within the system	Cooperate on custody, visitation, and financial issues Inform and deal with extended family members and friends
4. Separation	Mourn loss of intact family Work on resolving attachment to spouse	Develop coparental arrangements/relationships Restructure living arrangements Adapt to living apart Realign relationship with extended family and friends Begin to rebuild own social network
5. Divorce	Continue working on emotional recovery by overcoming hurt, anger, or guilt	Give up fantasies of reunion Stay connected with extended families Rebuild and strengthen own social network
6. Postdivorce	Separate feelings about ex-spouse from parenting role Prepare self for possibility of changes in custody as children get older, be open to their needs Risk developing a new intimate relationship	Make flexible and generous visitation arrangements for children and noncustodial parent and extended family members Deal with possibilities of changing custody arrangements as children get older Deal with children's reaction to parents' establishing relationships with new partners

Spradley, B. W., & Allender, J. A. (1996). *Community health nursing: Concepts and practice* (4th ed., p. 360). Philadelphia: Lippincott-Raven.

cussed earlier in this chapter. The needs of the individual family members, family developmental tasks, and family functions must mesh.

Meeting these needs is not necessarily easy in families. The conflict that often occurs in families with adolescents illustrates this point. Typically, adolescents are attempting to break away from parents and spend more time with friends than family. Yet, parents may wish for the adolescent to participate as more of an adult in family activities. This conflict may be compounded, for instance, when family members need adequate rest to provide health care to a family member, but the adolescent's need is to stay out late and get support and approval from peers.

STRUCTURAL FAMILY ASSESSMENT

Structural family assessment considers the family's composition. A structural assessment defines the immediate family members, their names, ages, and the

TABLE 4–5 • Remarriage and Blending Families

Phases	Emotional Responses	Developmental Issues
1. Meeting new people	Allowing for the possibility of developing a new intimate relationship	Dealing with children's and ex-family members' reactions to a parent dating
2. Entering a new relationship	Completing an "emotional recovery" from past divorce Accepting one's fears about developing a new relationship Working on feeling good about what the future may bring	Recovery from loss of marriage is adequate Discovering what you want from a new relationship Working on openness in a new relationship
3. Planning a new marriage	Accepting one's fears about the ambiguity and complexity of entering a new relationship such as: New roles and responsibilities Boundaries: space, time, and authority Affective issues: guilt, loyalty, conflicts, unresolvable past hurts	Recommitment to marriage and forming a new family unit Dealing with stepchildren as custodial or noncustodial parent Planning for maintenance of coparental relationships with ex-spouses Planning to help children deal with fears, loyalty conflicts, and membership in two systems Realignment of relationships with exfamily to include new spouse and children Restructuring family boundaries to allow for new spouse or stepparent
4. Remarriage and blending of families	Final resolution of attachment to previous spouse Acceptance of new family unit with different boundaries	Realignment of relationships to allow intermingling of systems Expanding relationships to include all new family members Sharing family memories and histories to enrich members' lives

Spradley, B. W., & Allender, J. A. (1996). *Community health nursing: Concepts and practice* (4th ed., p. 360). Philadelphia: Lippincott-Raven.

relationship between those who live together. A **genogram** is constructed to clarify the relationship and information about each member of the family. Symbols often used for the genogram are shown in Figure 4–7.

Genograms can be helpful to nurses in many settings. An inpatient nurse can quickly sketch a genogram and identify family members; this helps to define which family members should be involved in the collaboration of planning care, including being present at care conferences with professional staff. Genograms may also be used in discharge planning by identifying the need for support and assistance when the client returns home. Genograms may help the home care nurse clarify the dynamics of the family in relation to the recovery of the client.

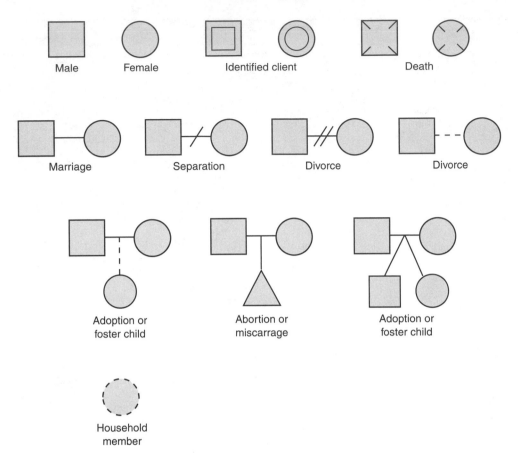

Figure 4–7. ▶ Symbols used in genograms.

FUNCTIONAL ASSESSMENT

Six family functions must be considered during **functional assessment:** affective, health care and physical necessities, economics, reproduction, socialization and placement, and family coping.

Through interviews, the nurse collects information about the family member's perceptions of how well the family is fulfilling basic functions. To assess family functions the nurse may ask questions from each of the above categories.

Is the family meeting the individual's need for affection, love, and understanding?

Is the family meeting the individual's need for physical care?

Does the family have the economic resources required to provide for basic needs of the family?

Is the family meeting the function of reproduction, as defined by the family?

Is the family meeting the family function of socialization? Is the family fulfilling the function of socialization of its children for them to become productive members of society?

Does the family attempt to actively cope with problems?

Using Characteristics of a Healthy Family for Assessment

The characteristics of a healthy family can be used as the baseline for family assessment. Family health depends on the ability of family members to share and to understand the feelings, needs, and behavior patterns of each individual (Satir, 1972). Healthy families demonstrate the following characteristics:

▶ There is a facilitative process of interaction among family members.
▶ The family enhances the development of its individual members.
▶ Role relationships are structured effectively.
▶ The family actively attempts to cope with problems.
▶ The family has a healthy home environment and lifestyle.
▶ The family establishes regular links with the broader community.

In addition, interactions in a healthy family are defined as having the following qualities:

▶ Communication among members is open, direct, and honest, with shared feelings.
▶ Family members express self-worth with integrity, responsibility, compassion, and love to, and for, one another.
▶ Family rules are known to all members. Rules are clear and flexible and allow individual members their freedom.
▶ The family has regular links with society, which demonstrate trust and friendship.
▶ Family members belong to various groups and clubs.

Nursing Diagnosis: Identifying Family Needs

After the family interview and assessment is completed and analyzed, the nurse can identify family strengths and needs. Again, the primary focus in community-based nursing is the care of the client. Assessment and identification of the needs of the family are focused on the family's effect on the care and recovery of the client.

The process of identifying the needs of the family follows the same steps as those used for the client. By comparing the collected data about the family with defining characteristics of the North American Nursing Diagnosis Association (NANDA) diagnosis, the nurse can arrive at the appropriate diagnosis for the client in the context of the family.

Maslow's model is valuable in individualizing and prioritizing care for individuals in the context of the family. Again, food and shelter, the most basic family needs, must be met first. When these needs are met, the priority of care can shift to safety and then on up the hierarchy of needs. The priorities of the family can change as the circumstances of the family change.

Planning: Expected Outcomes

The process of planning care for families is similar to planning for an individual's care. The primary goal is to define expected outcomes in relation to the recovery of the client. The family may benefit from these established expected outcomes; however, the primary intent is to enhance the recovery of the client.

Mutual goal setting in which the client and the family are included is the cornerstone of effective planning in relation to families. Examples of outcomes for family interventions are listed in Box 4–2. It is essential that family members be

▶ **Box 4–2.** Examples of Outcomes for
Commonly Used Nursing Diagnoses ◀

Decisional Conflict: The client or family will state advantages and disadvantages of choice by ————— (date).

Anticipatory Grieving: The client and/or family will express grief by ————— (date).

Dysfunctional Grieving: The client and/or family will share grief with significant others by ————— (date).

Parental Role Conflict: The parents will demonstrate control over decision-making regarding the child and collaborate with health professionals in making decisions about the health/illness care of the child by ————— (date).

Social Isolation: The client and/or family will state the reasons for his or her feelings of isolation by ————— (date).

Altered Parenting: The parent will demonstrate increased attachment behaviors such as holding infant close, smiling and talking to the infant, seeking eye contact with infant, and holding the infant by ————— (date).

Risk for Violence: The client or family member will experience control of behavior with assistance from others by ————— (date). The client and/or family will identify factors that contribute to violence ————— (date).

Ineffective Disabling Family Coping: The client and/or family will discuss the physical assault by ————— (date). The client and/or family will identify factors that contribute to violence by ————— (date).

Impaired Adjustment: The client and/or family member will identify the temporary and long-term demands of the situation by ————— (date).

Relocation Stress Syndrome: The client and/or family member will identify the most difficult aspect of relocation.

Adapted from Carpenito, L. (2000). *Nursing diagnosis: Application to clinical practice* (8th ed.). Philadelphia: Lippincott Williams & Wilkins.

a part of the planning process because ultimately it is the family members who are the primary caregivers and implement the plan of care. The process of goal setting has a positive effect on the health care provider's interactions with families. Mutual goal setting also has a positive effect on family interactions and compliance and accountability with the plan of care. Like individual clients, family members tend to resist being told what to do; they are much more likely to work toward goals they have chosen and support.

Nursing Interventions

Nursing interventions fall into three levels of family functioning: cognitive, affective, and behavioral. **Cognitive interventions** involve the act of knowing, perceiving, or understanding. An example is teaching a client or family member about the exchange system for a diabetic diet. **Affective interventions** have to do with feelings, attitudes, and values. Helping family members to understand their fears about a loved one's diagnosis of diabetes is an illustration of an affective intervention. **Behavioral interventions** are those that have to do with skills and behaviors. Teaching clients about giving themselves insulin injections and beginning a group exercise program for newly diagnosed diabetic clients are examples of behavioral interventions. Like other steps of the nursing process, interventions must be directed primarily toward the health recovery of the client.

TABLE 4–6 • Examples of Expected Outcomes and Nursing Interventions for Commonly Used Nursing Diagnoses for Family Intervention

Nursing Diagnosis	Expected Outcome	Nursing Intervention
Ineffective Management of Therapeutic Regimen	Client and family will describe disease process, causes, and factors contributing to symptoms and regimen for disease or symptom control by ———— (date).	Promote learning by providing information to client or family regarding strategies to enhance symptom control.
Health-Seeking Behavior	Client and family will state benefits of abstinence from tobacco use by ———— (date).	Promote learning by providing written information regarding the benefits of abstinence from tobacco.
Impaired Home Maintenance Management	Client and family members will identify factors that restrict self-care and home management by ———— (date).	Provide referral sources that the family agrees are appropriate to assist with household tasks.
Knowledge Deficit	Client and family members will demonstrate using aseptic technique when using a heparin lock by ———— (date).	Demonstrate and provide written information about aseptic technique when using a heparin lock by ———— (date).

Adapted from Carpenito, L. (2000). *Nursing diagnosis: Application to clinical practice* (8th ed.). Philadelphia: Lippincott Williams & Wilkins.

Nursing interventions provide specific directions and a consistent, individualized approach to the client's care. They are written as instructions for others to follow. Obviously, interventions in community-based care require the active involvement of the client and the family to determine the appropriate interventions. The client or family will often be responsible for implementing the interventions at home. As with goal setting, the client and family are more likely to comply with the plan of care if they are active participants in the planning of interventions. Examples of expected outcomes and nursing interventions appear in Table 4–6.

The Internet is an excellent resource for researching appropriate nursing interventions for families. For example, the Bright Futures for Families Web site (http://www.brightfutures.org), supported by the Maternal and Child Health Bureau, U.S. Department of Health and Human Services, offers tools to prepare families for health supervision to make them full participants in the process, to demonstrate the value of health supervision, and to inform families about what to expect from health professionals.

Nursing interventions for families may include strategies in primary, secondary, and tertiary prevention. Primary prevention encompasses nursing interventions that obviate the initial occurrence of a disease. When attempting to implement interventions for individual clients, it is often necessary to involve family members because they are affected as well. An example is family planning.

(text continues on page 91)

▶ **Box 4–3.** Family Assessment ◀

Family members

Member	Birth Date	Sex	Marital Status	Education
Becky	7/15/71	F	Married	college grad
Jack	11/10/69	M	Married	college grad
Joe	9/18/97	M		
Kevin	2/15/00	M		
Michael	2/22/02	M		

Genogram

Lives a block from Becky, has arthritis

John — Jan

Eugene — Ila — Stephen

In good health, live in another state

Jack — Becky

32-years-old, in good health

30-years-old, has cancer

Live in another state

Joe　Kevin　Michael

4 years　2 years　2 months

Stage of Illness

What stage of illness is this family in? (See Table 4–2)

　Diagnosis stage

What are this family's priority needs?

　relief from anxiety information, to be with and helpful to the client, and support for personal needs

What is the role of the nurse in this stage?

　emotional support, educator, assessor of family

(continued)

▶ Box 4–3. Family Assessment (*Continued*) ◀

Developmental Assessment

What is this family's developmental stage?

Preschool age stage

Is the family meeting the tasks of their stage?

No, the added energy depletion of Becky's illness has caused profound exhaustion for all members of the family

Does, or will, the client's health problem interrupt the family's ability to meet the developmental tasks? If yes, how does it interrupt?

Becky's illness has interrupted the family meeting the developmental tasks. Becky and Jack state they are
"unable to keep up the demands of the kids, the baby, and rigors of daily living."

State nursing interventions to assist the family in meeting their developmental tasks.

1. Identify specific parental roles that Becky and Jack want to retain.

2. Identify parental responsibilities that they are willing to give up to someone else.

3. Identify possible support persons who could assist more with child care.

4. Determine other household tasks which can be assumed by family members or community services.

Functional Assessment

Does the family meet the individual's need for affection, love, and understanding?

Both Becky and Jack continue to be very affectionate and loving to each other and their children. This is evident in
the way they interact with each other and with the children, hold the children, explain things to them, and comfort
them. The children are in turn affectionate to Becky. Becky states "My sister has provided me with alot of
emotional support."

Does the family meet the individual's need for physical necessities and care?

Jack is able to continue working, and still has opportunity to take some time off if necessary. Becky is unable to
fulfill her prior role responsibilities of homemaker, which included the responsibilities of cooking, cleaning,
marketing, and most of the child care. Becky states that she is "exhausted and able to only participate in a limited
manner in the care of the children and the work of running the household." Becky states "I want to be able to bathe
the kids, read them their bedtime story. I also want to continue to give Michael his bottles." Note disorderly
surroundings with the children's toys, dirty clothes, and dirty dishes scattered in all of the rooms. The children
are cranky and the baby cries most of the visit.

(continued)

> ▶ Box 4–3. Family Assessment (*Continued*) ◀

Does the family have the economic resources necessary to provide for the basic needs of the family?

Jack states "My job is very secure, I have been lucky that I have a job which allows me to provide so well for my family, I have a lot of vacation time saved up because we were going to take a big family vacation next summer,"

Is the family meeting the function of reproduction as defined by the family?

Yes

Is the family meeting the family function of socialization? Is the family fulfilling the function to socialize children to become productive members of society?

Becky states "It is very hard to provide guidance and discipline for Joe because I am so tired, He wears me down, Maybe he should be in day care a few days a week, There is a day care at our church, which is only a few blocks away,"

Does the family attempt to actively cope with problems?

Becky says "Jack does not want to talk about the future and what the doctor has said about my prognosis, He believes that I will be better by summer, He has been so angry since the diagnosis," Jack says "I believe that Becky will be better by summer, She has the best doctor in the Midwest, and people survive from cancer all the time,"

Assessment of Presence of Characteristics of a Healthy Family

Is communication between members open, direct, and honest, and are feelings and needs shared?

Becky says "It is hard for Jack to share his feelings with me, I think he talks to his dad but not to me, Sometimes his dad tells me what he has said, It's hard for me to tell him what I really think because it seems like then I am giving up," Jack says "I have a close relationship with my dad, It is so hard for me to talk to Becky about my fears because I want to be upbeat and hopeful, I don't want her to have to comfort me,"

Do family members express self-worth with integrity, responsibility, compassion, and love to and for one another?

Both Becky and Jack express love and concern for each other, They are so concerned about each other that Becky states "our concern for each other gets in the way of open communication,"

Are family rules, known to all members? *Becky and Jack describe the family in precisely the same way— "Becky is responsible for the care of the children and the home and Jack is the breadwinner,"*

(*continued*)

► **Box 4–3.** Family Assessment (*Continued*) ◄

Are rules clear, flexible, and do they allow individual members freedom?

Both state that before Joe was born, Becky worked full-time and the home maintenance was shared. Becky says that since she became ill, Jack has assumed many of the responsibilities at home. Becky states "He is working too hard and is exhausted. We need help!"

Does the family have regular links to society that demonstrate trust and friendship?

During the home visit, three neighbors came over with food and two people called. There were many plants, cards, and flower arrangements in the house. Becky stated "Our friends have been wonderful. They have offered to take the kids, brought food, and visited."

Do family members belong to various groups and clubs?

The family is active in a church and Jack is involved in an environmental group. Becky has many friends in the neighborhood.

EXAMPLE OF A CLIENT SITUATION

► **Intervention at the Primary Prevention Level**

Pam is a nurse working in a clinic whose clients are primarily from Southeast Asia. When she first began teaching female clients about family planning, Pam did not include the husband or significant other. Over time, she discovered that the use of birth control for many of her clients was decided by the male partner. By involving the male partner in planning (choosing a method of birth control and teaching the couple about its use), the couples were more likely to comply.

Secondary prevention is early detection and treatment of a condition. In some families, lack of information may be a barrier to seeking services related to secondary prevention.

EXAMPLE OF A CLIENT SITUATION

► **Intervention at the Secondary Prevention Level**

Tom is a nurse working in a day care center for older adults. One of the clients who comes to day care, Irene, is having problems with her eyesight and is from a family with a history of glaucoma. Tom has been encouraging her to have her eyes tested. Although Irene has severe arthritis, she is alert and cognitively intact. Irene tells Tom that she does not want to ask her son to take her to any more clinic visits. The son is unaware of his mother's vision problems. Tom learns that only by involving another family member (Irene's son) will the secondary prevention strategy (vision screening) occur.

Tertiary prevention is seeking treatment and rehabilitation for maximizing recovery. In some situations, the family is compliant with nursing care but is not aware of resources in the community that may provide support for the client's care.

EXAMPLE OF A CLIENT SITUATION

▶ Intervention at the Tertiary Prevention Level

Kristi is a staff nurse working on a medical-surgical unit in a hospital. Her situation illustrates tertiary prevention. Kristi is in charge of Barb's discharge planning. Barb has had a fusion of three cervical vertebrae and will be discharged from the hospital in 4 days. She lives alone; however, her daughter (the mother of five children) lives in town an hour from Barb's home. After discharge, Barb will need assistance with activities of daily living for at least 2 weeks at home, will not be permitted to drive for 6 weeks, and will receive physical therapy four times a week starting 2 weeks after discharge. Kristi, Barb, and Barb's daughter sit down together to plan for the care and assistance Barb will need at home. They also discuss what community services may be of assistance to transport Barb to physical therapy until she is permitted to drive.

Evaluation

Evaluation has a profound effect on the quality of care in community-based nursing. It is a joint effort among the nurse, family, and other caregivers. As is true in an acute care setting, this leads to more assessment or refinement of the goals set out in the care plan and results in the identification of additional diagnoses, expected outcomes, or interventions.

Questions for reflection that may be useful during evaluation of the family care plan include:

What additional data are required to evaluate progress?

Did the nursing diagnosis focus on the most important problem for this family as it relates to the potential for the client to do self-care?

What other nursing problems apply to this family and client?

Were the diagnosis, expected outcome, and intervention realistic and appropriate for this client and family?

Were the family strengths considered when the expected outcomes and interventions were defined? If not, how could these strengths be used to enhance the outcome?

Are the nurse, client, and family satisfied with the outcome? If not, what would provide satisfaction?

The nursing process continues in an ongoing, circular, and dynamic manner. Information gained from asking the above questions is used to define a new problem and identify new or additional expected outcomes and interventions as the ongoing process of providing care and evaluating its effect continues.

Documentation

Complete and accurate information is an essential element of nursing care of the client or family. Creating a clear account of what the nurse saw and did related to the family's care provides a record of that care. This includes documentation of the client's and family's strengths and needs. Charting is used to determine eligibility for care needed and for reimbursement for care provided.

EXAMPLE OF A CLIENT SITUATION

The Family and Nursing Process

Jane, a home health care nurse, is assigned to care for Becky, a 30 year old homemaker who is the mother of three preschool children (Joe, age 4, Kevin, age 2, and Michael, age 2 months). Becky has been diagnosed with liver cancer. Jack, Becky's husband, is a 32-year-old accountant with his own accounting firm. Jack's parents are in good health and live in another city. Ila, Becky's mother, lives in the same neighborhood as Jack and Becky. Becky's father died 10 years ago and Ila remarried Stephen last year. Ila has severe arthritis. Becky also has a sister and brother who both live out of state.

As Becky's home care nurse, Jane completes a family assessment during the first visit. She begins the family interview by getting acquainted with all of the family members. Joe shows her the new toy his grandmother sent for his birthday; Kevin is very shy and sits in Becky's lap during the home visit. Jack holds the baby. Jane hopes to be able to identify how much support the family will be able to provide to Becky from this family assessment. She is also interested in identifying any problem areas where intervention is needed. The completed family assessment is shown in Box 4–3.

Identification of the Nursing Diagnosis

Jane reviews her family assessment as well as Becky and Jack's responses. She identifies the family strengths as:

The family and a large number of supportive friends are willing to assist with care of the children and the home.
A strong marital bond between Becky and her husband is apparent; they show mutual support and love.
The family has a stable financial status.

She identifies the family needs as:

There is difficulty managing the home and child care of three preschool children. This was evident when Becky stated she needed help managing the family's daily needs. Jane also observed that the house was very disorganized.
There is the potential for ineffective family coping. This was evident when Becky and Jack were unable to be honest and open when discussing Becky's illness and prognosis.
Becky has difficulty in performing her role of child caretaker because of her disabling illness.

Setting Priorities

To identify the priority of family needs, Jane uses Maslow's Hierarchy of Needs. Recognizing that the family and client must have their basic needs addressed first, she concentrates on the family's difficulty in managing the home and the child care.

As a result, Jane believes that Becky's and Jack's priority problem is:

Impaired Home Maintenance Management related to Jack's complex care regimen as evidenced by a disorderly home environment and Becky's statement, "I can only care for the kids a few minutes at a time. We need help."

Planning

At the second home visit, Jane, Becky, and Jack discuss the family assessment. Jane shares her conclusion about their primary problem. She asks Becky and Jack what their impressions are and they agree with her that the major concern is the care of the home and the children. Becky adds, "I am concerned about being able to continue to provide care for the kids. I'm also worried about Jack and me having time together and being able to talk."

The three decide to address the problems about home management and save the discussion about communication for the third visit. Jane suggests that if some of the issues regarding care of the home and family are addressed, Becky may have more energy for the children.

Expected Outcomes

Jane, Becky, and her husband define the following outcomes that address impaired home maintenance. The goal is to accomplish them by the third visit.

1. Becky and Jack will identify home maintenance tasks that need to be done daily and weekly.
2. Becky and Jack will compile a list of family members and friends who are able and willing to assist with these tasks.
3. Becky and Jack will match the list of tasks with the list of people and contact them within the next 3 days.
4. Becky will call Jane with the list of tasks that their family and friends can do.
5. Jack will contact the list of community agencies that Jane gave him to see what assistance they can provide.

Nursing Implementation

Jane lists the specific nursing interventions she has identified for the plan of care:

1. Jane will assist the family in determining a realistic plan for both health care and home maintenance.
2. Jane will identify resources in the community that can assist with the tasks that the family and friends cannot do. She will contact Jack and give him the list of resources and telephone numbers.
3. Jane will schedule periodic home visits to evaluate the effectiveness of the plan and identify any changes that occur in Becky's condition that may need intervention.

Evaluation

At the third home visit, Jane, Becky, and Jack evaluate the plan to date. The first four outcomes were met; however, Jack did not contact the community agencies. He will contact them next week. Jane and the family agree on the plan and the method for evaluating the plan. Jane also reviews the list of community resources with Becky and Jack. They all agree on which one to contact. They agree to discuss Becky's concern about caring for her children at the next visit.

CONCLUSIONS

The family is the basic social unit of American society and has long been the primary focus of nursing care in the community. Understanding family structure, roles, and functions is essential in providing comprehensive nursing care both in the acute care and community-based setting. Knowledge of healthy family functioning permits the nurse to identify unhealthy functioning and take appropriate action, including referring to community resources. Often, families with an ill family member are in crisis and require nursing intervention or referral.

Today, more than ever, the nurse must be cognizant of the needs, feelings, problems, and views of the family when providing care for the individual client. Community-based nursing requires the nurse to provide care in the context of the client's family to enhance self-care. This is accomplished by assessing the client in the context of the family.

To provide continuous care with a preventive focus, the nurse must consider the family's ability and needs. The care of the client in the context of the family is enhanced by following the principles of community-based care.

References and Bibliography

Brumfield, R. (1997). A family system approach to case management in a rural community setting. *Home Care Provider, 2*(4), 180–185.

Carpenito, L. (2000). *Nursing diagnosis: Application to clinical practice* (8th ed.). Philadelphia: Lippincott Williams & Wilkins.

Carter, E. A., & McGoldrick, M. (Eds.). (1980). *The family life cycle.* New York: Gardner.

Dixon, E. (1999). Community health nursing practice and the Roy adaptation model. *Public Health Nursing, 16*(4), 290–300.

Duvall, E. M. (1977). *Marriage and family development* (5th ed.). Philadelphia: Lippincott.

Duvall, E. M., & Miller, B. (1985). *Marriage and family development* (6th ed.). New York: Harper & Row.

Federal Intragency Forum on Children and Family Statistics. (1999). *American's children: Key national indicators of well-being, 1999.* Federal Intragency Forum on Child and Family Statistics. Washington, DC: U.S. Government Printing Office.

Friedemann, M. (1989). The concept of family nursing. *Journal of Advanced Nursing, 14,* 211–216.

Gravelle, A. (1997). Caring for a child with a progressive illness during the complex phase: Parents experience facing adversity. *Journal of Advanced Nursing, 25*(4), 738–745.

Green, C. (1997). Teaching students how to "think family." *Journal of Family Nursing, 3*(3), 230–246.

Hartrick, G. (2000). Developing health-promoting practice with families: One pedagogical experience. *Journal of Advanced Nursing, 31*(1), 27–34.

Kulbok, P, Gates, M., Vicenzi, A., & Schultyz, P. (1999). Focus on community: Directions for nursing knowledge development. *Journal of Advanced Nursing, 29*(5), 1188–1196.

Liebermann, A. (1990). *Community and home health nursing.* Springhouse, PA: Springhouse Corporation.

Marino, L., & Kooser, J. (1986). The psychosocial care of cancer clients and their families: Periods of high risk. In L. Marino (Ed.), *Cancer nursing* (pp. 53–66). St. Louis: Mosby.

Pillitteri, A. (1999). *Maternal & child health nursing: Care of the childbearing & childrearing family* (3rd ed.). Philadelphia: Lippincott Williams & Wilkins.

Satir, V. (1972). *People making.* Palo Alto, CA: Science and Behavioral Books.

Shyu, Y. (2000). Patterns of caregiving when family caregivers face competing needs. *Journal of Advanced Nursing, 31*(1), 35–53.

Spitz, R. (1945). Hospitalization: Inquiry into genesis of psychiatric conditions in early childhood. *Psychoanalytic Study of the Child, 1.*

Taanila. A., Kokkonen, J., & Jarvelin, M. (1998). Parental guidance and counselling by doctors and nursing staff: Parents' views of initial information and advice for families with disabled children. *Journal of Clinical Nursing, 7*(6), 505–511.

Williams, S. (1999). Family nurses: Europes's future? *Nursing Standard, 13*(13), 29.

Whyte, D., & Donaldson, I. (1999). All in the family: Activating family support can dramatically improve care. *Nursing Times, 95*(32), 47–48.

Whyte, D., & Robb, Y. (1999). Families under stress: How nurses can help. *Nursing Times, 95*(30), 50–52.

Wright, L., & Leahey, M. (1999). Maximizing time, minimizing suffering: The 15-minute (or less) family interview. *Journal of Family Nursing, 5*(3), 259–274.

LEARNING ACTIVITIES

LEARNING ACTIVITY 4-1

▶ **Client Care Study:** Chemical Dependency Day Treatment

You are working in a chemical dependency day treatment unit for adolescents. Your primary patient is Chris, a 16-year-old boy, admitted yesterday. Chris was brought in by his father, Michael, and his stepmother, Joanna, after a family fight. Michael says that Chris's grades in school have been on a downhill slide since his sophomore year began 6 months ago. Both parents have noticed that Chris's behavior has changed. He is spending more time in his room; his appearance has become disheveled; and he is increasingly more listless, fatigued, hostile, and erratic. Michael describes his son as a cheerful, focused boy—until this year.

Chris has a 13-year-old brother, and both boys live a week with their mother, Lori, and a week with their father, Michael, and his second wife, Joanna. Lori and Michael have been divorced for 4 years. Michael and his new wife have a 1-year-old daughter. Lori visited Chris this morning. While at the treatment center, she mentions that she is suing Michael for money he owes her. After lunch, you are visiting with Michael and he relates to you that two of Lori's brothers are lawyers and the family is always suing someone for something. Last year, he says, Lori claimed that she had lupus and collected disability payments until the insurance company discovered it was a phony claim.

During the initial family conference, Lori blames Michael for Chris's problems, maintaining that Michael has suffered from depression over the past years. Michael talks about his feelings: that the ongoing battle between him and Lori is stressful for their children. He wants the conflict to end.

1. Construct a genogram for this family.
2. Identify which stage of crisis this family is in. List data that led you to this conclusion.
3. Describe additional information you will need to plan care.
4. Identify the developmental stage of each member of the family. Explain how you will use this information.
5. Identify the developmental stage of each family. Explain how you will use this information when planning care for Chris.
6. Detect which family functions are not being met.
7. Develop outcomes you hope to see with this family.
8. Propose referrals you could initiate.

LEARNING ACTIVITY 4-2

▶ **Critical Thinking Exercise:** Family Development

1. In your clinical journal, discuss a situation you have observed or in which you have been the caregiver in which the family enhanced or interrupted the client's self-care or return to maximum functioning. What was the family doing to influence the client's health? What else could they have done? Use theory from this chapter to support your ideas.
2. What did you do (or would you have done) as a nurse to facilitate family involvement in this situation? What did you learn from this experience? What would you do differently next time? Use theory from this chapter to support your ideas.

UNIT II

Skills for Community-Based Nursing Practice

 Now that you understand the concepts of community-based nursing, including the importance of a healthy community, understanding cultural surroundings, and care of the family, you are ready to explore how you can develop skills in applying your knowledge. Skills in assessment, teaching, case management, and continuity of care are all important to practice in community-based nursing. Although you probably have studied them previously, in this unit they are discussed in their specific relationship to community-based health care.

Chapter 5 opens with a discussion of the significance of assessment to community-based care. Assessment of the individual client, family, and community is addressed. A section on community assessment includes concepts, methods, and application. The chapter ends with a discussion of the nurse's role as an advocate in public policy making.

The importance of client teaching along with teaching theory and developmental considerations in Chapter 6 leads to a discussion of the relationship of the nursing process to the teaching process.

Chapter 7 discusses the role of the case manager in community care.

Continuity of care, addressed in Chapter 8, is a concept central to quality of care in the community. It can be easy for the client and family to get lost in the new health care system, but responsible professionals build bridges between settings and people. Entering and exiting the system are covered, along with the skills and competencies involved in continuity of care.

Assessment: Individual, Family, and Community

R O B E R T A   H U N T

▶ L E A R N I N G   O B J E C T I V E S ◀

- Identify components essential to assessment of the individual client in community-based settings.

- Discuss health needs commonly assessed in community-based settings.

- Outline the components of a holistic assessment.

- Identify the components of the 15-minute family interview.

- Discuss the value of community assessment.

- Review concepts of people, place, and social systems in a healthy community.

- Discuss methods for collecting community data.

- Apply concepts of assessment to a client situation, including the individual client, the family, and the community.

▶ K E Y   T E R M S ◀

activities of daily living (ADL)
assessment
community assessment
community health need
constructed survey
demographics
environmental assessment
epidemic
functional assessment
holistic assessment

informant interviews
instrumental activities of daily living
  (IADL)
participant observations
power system
secondary data
social system
spiritual assessment
windshield survey

Significance of Assessment

Assessment of the Individual Client in the Community

Assessment of the Family in the Community

Assessment of the Community

Advocacy in Public Policy-Making

Conclusions

 SIGNIFICANCE OF ASSESSMENT

Nursing has long understood the significance of the community in the health of the individual and family. Florence Nightingale set the scene early for involvement of health care professionals in assessing and intervening in establishing healthy communities. Her analysis of 1861 census data became the foundation of England's sanitary reform acts (Woodham-Smith, 1950). Much of Nightingale's work focused on assessment of the physical and social environment and its role in causing or contributing to illness. She identified how sanitation, nutrition, and rest contribute to successful recovery from injury and illness. She also determined the relationship among adequate housing, recreation, employment, and health.

Assessment is a dynamic, ongoing process that uses observations and interactions to collect information, recognize changes, analyze needs, and plan care. Physicians primarily use assessment to determine pathology. Hospital-based nurses use assessment as the first step in the nursing process, for ongoing monitoring of acute conditions, and as an essential component in ensuring continuity with discharge planning. In community-based settings, assessment provides baseline information to help evaluate physiologic and psychological normality and functional capacity and to identify environmental factors that may enhance or impair the individual's health status (Barry, 1998). Because the community-based nurse sees clients only periodically and the status of conditions varies over time, thorough assessment is the cornerstone of quality community care. Assessment of the individual client, family, and community is discussed in this chapter.

 ASSESSMENT OF THE INDIVIDUAL CLIENT IN THE COMMUNITY

To perform an accurate assessment, the nurse must communicate effectively, observe systematically, and interpret the collected data accurately (Carpenito, 2000). Typically, the health assessment consists of the interview and health history. The focus and parameters of the assessment depend on the scope of the service provided by the agency and the role of the nurse in that service. However, the first contact is always extremely important because it acts as the foundation for the nurse–client relationship. Establishing trust beginning with the first contact is imperative.

Community care differs from nursing care provided in tertiary care settings. Because the client and family are in charge of most aspects of care most of the time, the nurse is primarily a facilitator of self-care rather than solely a care provider. Thus, the assessment process is intended both to assess the client, whether it be the individual client, family, or community, and to identify needs and strengths and proceed accordingly. It is a continuous process that occurs in the context in which the response occurs. Thus, the response must be considered within the environment, whether it be family, culture, immediate physical environment, or community environment. A holistic assessment often requires collaboration of many professionals. This approach expands the usual definition of holistic assessment—body, mind, and spirit—to an even broader view.

This comprehensive view is used across the life span. The nurse in community-based settings is always diligent to complete a comprehensive assessment but is particularly attentive when caring for vulnerable populations. Thus, when assessing a newborn during a home visit, the nurse will bear in mind that a holistic assessment of the physical and psychological condition of the newborn, the immediate environment, and the skill of the primary caregivers is essential to the normal growth and development and protection of the infant from harm. The newborn is unable to speak on his or her own behalf, so a thorough assessment is the primary way the nurse initiates advocacy for the infant. Thus, comprehensive assessment is essential to injury and disease prevention as well as health promotion and maintenance.

Assessment of the Individual Across the Life Span

Infants and Children

When assessing the infant and toddler, the nurse should begin by interviewing the primary caregiver. Typically the areas covered include nutrition, growth and development, and vision and hearing. Monitoring growth and development is

COMMUNITY-BASED NURSING CARE GUIDELINES

Personalizing Nursing Care to Promote Attachment

The following are interventions, which are directed to parents to assist them to develop attachment with their newborn.

- Explore with the mother and father their feelings of moving from pregnancy to postpartum
- Ask the parents what they see now in the newborn which were behaviors they recognized from baby being in utero.
- Remind the parents that the newborn knows their voice from hearing it when the baby was in utero.
- Tell the parents that newborns like being flexed and close to them as they were positioned before they were born
- Emphasize to the partner/dad their role in nurturing the mother to nurture the newborn
- Encourage the partner/dad to get support for themselves as needed
- Compliment the mother on her ability to read her newborns cues, ie, need for comfort, nourishment, diaper change. Bring to the mother's attention the infants response to her care.
- Make positive comments regarding the newborn's progress
- Ask about the mother's well being

O'Leary, J. (1998). *After loss: Parenting in the next pregnancy*. Minneapolis: Allina Publishing.

easily done by weighing the infant and measuring length and head circumference, and plotting the results on a growth grid. Psychological status should also be assessed. Development of the infant, toddler, and preschooler is assessed by the Denver Developmental Screening Tool.

Infants and toddlers are not routinely screened for vision and hearing until 3 years of age. However, a parent's observations may indicate possible presence of vision and hearing problems. For assessment of vision with an infant over 6 weeks of age, ask the parent the following questions:

Does the infant return your smile?

Do the infant's eyes follow you as you walk past or move around the room?

Do you have any concerns that the infant is unable to see?

To assess for evidence of the need to screen the vision of toddlers, ask the parents the following questions:

Does the child cover one eye when looking at objects?

Does the child tilt his or her head to look at things?

Does the child hold toys, books, or other objects very close or very far away to look at them?

Does the child rub his or her eyes, squint, frown, or blink frequently?

Infants at high risk for hearing impairment should be screened at birth. These include infants with the following:

▶ Family history of childhood hearing impairment
▶ Perinatal infection (eg, cytomegalovirus, rubella, herpes, toxoplasmosis)
▶ Anatomic malformations of the head or neck

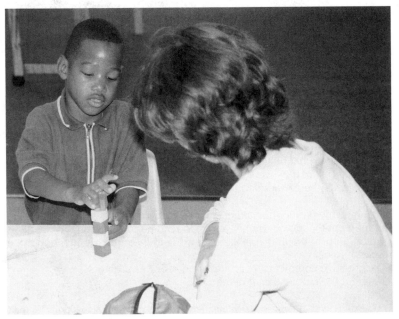

Figure 5–1. ▶ The Denver Developmental Screening Tool uses a series of tasks to screen children for developmental delays.

▶ Low birth weight (less than 1,500 g)
▶ Hyperbilirubinemia exceeding indications for exchange transfusion
▶ Bacterial meningitis
▶ Birth asphyxia, infants with Apgar score of 0 to 3, failure to breathe
   spontaneously in 10 minutes, or hypotonia of 2 hours past birth

To determine if a toddler should be screened for hearing impairment, ask if the child has had frequent ear infections or has the same risk factors listed previously for infant screening. Also assess the child's speech. Hearing impairments often become apparent when the child begins to talk and are evidenced by the child's difficulty with pronunciation, resulting in speech that is hard to comprehend.

Periodic assessment of preschool- and school-aged children includes a health history and physical and developmental evaluation. As with the infant and toddler, height, weight and head circumference are important indicators of growth. Not only does this measure determine if the child is following a normal growth curve, but it also reflects whether the child's weight is proportional to height. Obesity is on the increase, with more than 11% of children between the ages of 6 and 19 years overweight. Because obesity substantially increases the risk of illness from high blood pressure, high cholesterol, type 2 diabetes, heart disease and stroke, arthritis, sleep disturbances, and cancer (breast, prostate, and colon), it is important to identify overweight children early to allow for early intervention. Nutrition assessment is also an important portion of a health assessment.

Adults and Elderly Adults

Assessment of the adult client requires application of the same principles discussed in the preceding paragraphs. Increasingly, the caseload of nurses working in community-based settings will reflect the graying of the population. By 2030, 20% of the population will be older than 65 years, and the number of people older than 85 will triple (AARP, 1997). Because contact with the nurse is intermittent in community-based settings, it is essential that the assessment be comprehensive. A **holistic assessment** includes environmental, cultural, spiritual, and nutritional factors, as well as functional and physical aspects of the client.

The functional assessment requires the nurse to determine whether there are environmental, cognitive, or neurologic or behavioral barriers to independent function and self-care. Societal and cultural factors may also create barriers. The primary consideration of the functional assessment is whether the client needs the assistance of another person for daily function. The client's ability to conceptualize an activity is just as important as the client's physical ability to perform the activity.

The **environmental assessment,** or evaluation of the client's home and neighborhood environment, is the first component of the functional assessment. The client may be physically, cognitively, or emotionally disabled, yet able to function independently except for the limitations created by barriers in the home. The next areas assessed are neurologic status, cognitive and emotional status, integumentary status, and respiratory status. Last, the individual's abilities to complete **activities of daily living** (ADL) and **instrumental activities of daily living** (IADL) should be assessed. ADL are a standard method for evaluating ability to perform the activities that are essential for independent living. They include grooming, dressing, bathing, toileting, transferring, walking, and feeding or eating. IADL involve planning and preparing light meals, traveling, doing laundry, housekeeping, shopping, and using the telephone. Box 5–1 presents a complete functional assessment.

► **Box 5–1.** Functional Assessment ◄

Environmental Assessment

Structural Barriers

Do stairs in the home limit the client's independent mobility to reach the
  bathroom, kitchen, and bedroom?
Check for presence of:
  Handrails on stairs and in the bathroom and tub
  Narrow doorways
  Unsafe flooring or floor covering
  Inadequate lighting
  Safe gas and electrical appliances
  Improperly stored hazardous materials

Neurologic Status

Perceptual Function

Is the client able to perceive his or her immediate environment?

Sensory Function

Does the client have impaired vision/?
Does the client have impaired hearing and ability to understand spoken
  language?
Is the client able to participate in an appropriate conversation 10 to 15 minutes
  long?
Is the client experiencing chronic pain?

Cognitive and Emotional Status

Does the client make eye contact with the visitor, greet the visitor, and appear to
  be well groomed or have made an attempt to be?
Assess if the client is oriented to person, place, and time. Work these questions
  into the conversation.
Ask the client to perform a simple task as getting the nurse a glass of water (but
  without putting the client on the spot or acting as if this is a test).

Integumentary Status

If the client is unable to perform ADL or IADL because of a wound, dressing, or
  pain, then the wound impairs the client's functional ability.

Respiratory Status

Respiratory status is impaired if the client's respiratory status, typically
  shortness of breath or dyspnea, prevents functioning. Specifically:
  If the client stops or slows down the activity before it is completed
  If the client sits down midway through or after the activity
  If the client complains of chest tightness, pain or breathes in quick shallow
    breaths

Adapted from Neal, L. (1998). Functional assessment of the home health client. *Home
Healthcare Nurse, 16*(10), 670–677. In R. Hunt (Ed.). (2000). *Readings in community based
nursing* (pp. 168–177). Philadelphia: Lippincott Williams & Wilkins

Screening Across the Life Span

Nutrition screening is an important part of providing care for clients across the life span in community-based settings. A screening tool that may be used in home settings is found in Box 5–2. This tool screens all types of home care clients for nutritional risk. After assessing the client's nutritional risk, the nurse, client, and family will devise a plan together to address the identified needs. If the client requires a level II assessment, a nurse specially trained in nutrition assesses the client.

Assessing medication knowledge and practice is an important aspect of comprehensive assessment. Polypharmacy, the use of multiple medications, is common among older people because of the multiple chronic illnesses they experience. However, correct use of medication is a concern across the life span. The tool in Box 5–3 can be used in a community-based setting to assess a client's medication use. After assessing the client's knowledge base, the nurse and client then devise a plan to address identified learning needs.

Culture and the impact culture has on health and health beliefs are discussed in Chapter 3. A cultural assessment is always a part of the health history. It is important to start with the client's understanding of health-related issues. One way to begin is to ask the following questions:

How is this kind of illness treated in your culture (or home country)?

How would you describe this problem you have?

What does this sickness do to you?

How long have you had this problem?

Why do you think the problem began when it did?

What has been done so far?

What do you think will help your problem clear up?

What does the family think should be done?

What else do you think can be done to help you get better?

How serious do you think this situation/problem is? (Heineken & McCoy, 2000)

Further, a psychosocial assessment in tandem with the cultural assessment will help the nurse understand the client in the context of family as defined by the client's culture. This may involve exploring the topics of family decision-maker, sick role behavior, language barriers, and community resources as they relate to the client's culture. This assessment may simply address the following issues:

Who is the decision maker in the family?

What are the characteristics of the sick role in the client's culture?

Do any language barriers exist?

What resources are available in the community that are sensitive to the client's culture?

A simple cultural assessment guide is seen in Box 5–4. After the assessment if complete, the nurse, client and family devise a plan of care, which is built around the identified cultural considerations.

An **environmental assessment** is an essential aspect of any assessment across the life span and across settings. Figure 5–2 and Box 5–5 are useful when completing an environmental assessment.

(text continues on page 108)

▶ **Box 5–2.** Level I Nutrition Screen ◀

Signature HOME CARE	LEVEL I NUTRITION SCREEN	PATIENT		
		PAYOR	TEAM	MR#
		DATE		TIME

BODY WEIGHT AND HEIGHT (*Measure height to the nearest inch and weight to the nearest pound*):
PRIMARY DIAGNOSIS: _____   Weight (lbs):_____ Height (in): _____
OTHER DIAGNOSIS: _____   Special diet. Type:_____ Calorie limitations: _____

Check any boxes that are TRUE for the individual:
● ☐ Has lost or gained 10 pounds (or more) in the past six (6) months without wanting to.

EATING HABITS

■	☐ Has appetite changed?	●	☐	Has difficulty chewing or swallowing.
■	☐ Consumes dairy or dairy products once or not at all daily (and does not take calcium supplement).	◆	☐	Has pain in mouth, teeth or gums.
			☐	Anorexia.
■	☐ Consumes fruit or drinks fruit juice once or not at all daily.		☐	Has more than one alcoholic drink per day (woman); more than two drinks per day (man).
■	☐ Does not have adequate fluid intake (less than 4 glasses [8 oz] per day).		☐	Usually eats alone.
◆	☐ Eats vegetables two or fewer times daily.	●	☐	Does not have enough food to eat each day.
◆	☐ Eats breads, cereals, pasta, rice, or other grains five or fewer times daily.	◆	☐	Does not eat anything on one or more days each month.

LIVING ENVIRONMENT

◆	☐ Lives alone.		☐	Does not have a stove and/or refrigerator.
■	☐ Are there more than 6 people living in household?		☐	Lives in a home with inadequate heating or cooling.
■	☐ Is housebound.	●	☐	Is unable or prefers not to spend money on food (< $25–30 per person spent on food each week).
■	☐ Does not have significant caregiver.			

FUNCTIONAL STATUS

Usually or always needs assistance with: (*check each that apply*)

◆	☐ Walking or moving about.	Other Problems:		
■	☐ Eating.	● ☐ Nausea. ☐ Vomiting.		
■	☐ Preparing food.	●	☐	Diarrhea (> 3–5 per/day for > 2 days).
	☐ Shopping for food or other necessities.	●	☐	Constipation (> 2 weeks).
		◆	☐	Over 80 years of age.

INSTRUCTIONS: To be completed within 5 days from Start of Care date. Repeat Level I screen at least every 120 days (every other recertification).
HIGH RISK:
● Proceed to Level II Nutritional Screen.
◆ 5 or more "◆", proceed to Level II Nutritional Screen.
■ 8 more "■" go to Level II Nutritional Screen.

TOTALS:
● _____
◆ _____
■ _____

Categories left blank should be addressed by the Signature Nutrition Screener or go to Level II.

Signature of Screener: _____ | Date:

▶ Box 5–3. Medication Assessment ◀

Note to administrator: The sequence of the interview, along with the instructional statements, are merely suggestions, and should be considered guidelines when using the interview. It is acceptable to reword statements or change the format to better meet the needs of the individual, yet all topics must be included in the assessment.

Start Time: _____ Who is the respondent? ☐ Patient ☐ Spouse
☐ Other (list) _____

Please Check The Appropriate Response.

Administrator: "*I need to see all of your medications. Please show me those you take every day, and those you take occasionally. Don't forget to show me eyedrops, insulin, laxatives, vitamins, antacids, ointments or any over-the-counter drugs you sometimes use. Are there any other medications that you regularly take that are not here today?*" (Attach copies of medication profiles to document drugs.)

I. Medication Administration and Storage

☐ Yes ☐ No Can patient open a pill bottle? (Have patient demonstrate.)
☐ Yes ☐ No Can patient break a pill in half? (Have patient demonstrate. Omit if not applicable.)
☐ Yes ☐ No Does someone help you take your medicine?
☐ Yes ☐ No Do you use any type of system to help you take your pills, such as a pill box, or a calendar?
List: _____
☐ Yes ☐ No Do you have problems swallowing your pills?
Where do you store your medicines? _____

II. Medication Purchasing Habits

What drug store do you use? _____
☐ Yes ☐ No Does the drug store you use deliver the medications to your home?
If no, then how do you get your medications? _____
_____
☐ Yes ☐ No Do you always use the same drug store? If no, explain: _____
☐ Yes ☐ No Do financial difficulties ever prevent you from buying your medications?

III. Attitudes

☐ Excellent How would you describe your health? _____
☐ Good What do you see as your health needs? _____
☐ Fair _____
☐ Poor _____
☐ Yes ☐ No Does taking your medications upset your daily routine? If yes, explain: _____
☐ Yes ☐ No Do side effects from your medications upset your daily routine?
☐ Yes ☐ No Do your medications help you?
☐ Don't Know
☐ Yes ☐ No Do you ever share your medications with anyone else?

(continued)

▶ **Box 5-3.** Medication Assessment (*Continued*) ◀

IV. Lifestyle Habits

TIMES PER WEEK

_____ How often do you drink coffee, tea, colas, or eat chocolate?
_____ How often do you use cigarettes, snuff, or tobacco products?
_____ How often do you consume beer, wine, or liquor?
_____ How often do you use recreational drugs such as marijuana?

V. Home/Environment

Who else stays at your residence? (List relationship and age) _____
_____

If someone else lives in home, does that person participate in your
health care?_____

VI. Medication Profile

Record each medication separately on the form below: (Attach additional sheets
as necessary.)_____

(MEDICINE NAME, DOSAGE, ROUTE, EXPIRATION DATE EXACTLY AS PRINTED ON LABEL)

☐ Yes   ☐ No   Can you read the name, dosage, and expiration date of this
                medicine? Why do you take the medication?_____
                _____

                How long have you taken this dosage? _____
                _____

                When do you take the medicine and how many do you take?____
                _____

                Do you know what the side effects are? List: _____
                _____

☐ Yes   ☐ No   Does the medicine cause you any problems or side effects? ____

                What do you do if you experience side effects? (Stop the pills,
                call the doctor, etc.)_____
                _____

_____

Adapted with permission from DeBrew, J., & Tesh, A. (1998). Assessing medication
knowledge and practice in older adults. *Home Healthcare Nurse, 16*(10), 686–692.

The primary consideration of any environmental assessment is to identify
safety concerns. Again, vulnerable populations, the very young and very old, and
those with serious chronic conditions are most at risk for safety issues. Many
communities have home safety check kits available through the Red Cross or local fire department to assess for unsafe conditions in the home.

Numerous studies show that religious practice is correlated with greater health
and longer life. Assessing spiritual health and intervening according to the client's
values may be one of the most important areas to address in community-based care.
A **spiritual assessment** allows the nurse to determine the presence of spiritual distress or identify other spiritual needs. A spiritual needs protocol is shown in Box
5–6. The results of this assessment can be used mutually by the nurse, client, and
family to identify spiritual issues and incorporate them in the plan of care.

(*text continues on page 113*)

► Box 5–4. Cultural Assessment Guide ◄

Patient _____ Patient Number _____ Team _____
Cultural/Ethnic Identity _____ Religion _____
Etiquette and Social Customs _____
_____

Nonverbal Communication Patterns _____
_____

Client's Explanation of Health Problem _____
_____
_____
_____

Traditional Treatments/Healers _____
_____

Expectations of Nurse/Care Providers _____
_____

Pain Assessment

Cultural Patterns/Patient's Perception of Pain Response _____
_____

Nutrition Assessment

Meal patterns _____
_____

Sick foods _____
_____

Food Intolerances/Taboos _____
_____

Medication Assessment

Patient's Perceptions of Medications _____
_____

Possible Pharmacogenetic Variations _____
_____

Psychosocial Assessment

Family Structure and Decision-making Patterns _____
_____

Sick Role Behavior _____
_____

Language Barriers and Resources _____
_____

Cultural/Ethnic/Religious Resources/Supportive Systems _____
_____

Adapted with permission from Curry, M. (1996). Cultural assessment in home healthcare.
Home Healthcare Nurse, 15(10), 664–671.

Environmental Assessment Checklist

Patient _____ Patient Number _____ Team/Person Completing Form _____			
Date and initial as each assessment area is addressed. Describe unsafe/unmet needs. Suggest modifications.			
Assessment Areas	**Safe/Meets Client's Needs**	**Unsafe/Needs Adaptation**	**Recommended Modifications and Possible Referral**
Physiologic and Survival Needs Food/Fluids/Eating			
Elimination/Toileting			
Hygiene/Bathing/Grooming			
Clothing/Dressing			
Rest/Sleeping			
Medication			
Shelter			
Safety and Security Mobility and Fall Prevention			
Fire/Burn Prevention			
Crime/Injury Prevention			
Love and Belonging Caregiver			
Communication			
Family/Friends/Pets			
Self-Esteem, Self-Actualization Enjoyable/Meaningful Activities			

Figure 5–2. ► Environmental assessment checklist (see Box 5–5 for questions for each category). Adapted with permission from Narayan, M., & Tennant. J. (1997). Environmental assessment. *Home Healthcare Nurse, 15*(11), 799–805.

▶ Box 5–5. Questions To Complete:
Environmental Assessment Checklist ◀

Physiologic and Survival Needs
Food and Fluids/Eating

What does the patient plan to eat? Drink? Who will prepare the food?
Is there food in the home? Who will do the grocery shopping?
Is the food properly stored? Does the refrigerator work?
Is there drinkable water?
Does the kitchen have barriers to the patients actually preparing the food?
Are the pathways clear? Can the items be reached? Are there clean dishes?

Elimination/Toileting

Can the patient get to the bathroom? Is the pathway clear? Is a bedside commode
  indicated?
Do assistive devices (wheelchairs, walkers) fit through the doorways and can the
  patient turn?
Will the patient have a hard time getting up and down from the commode? Would
  a raised toilet seat help? Grab bars? (Towel racks, if used for steadying, can
  pull away from the wall.)
Will the patient be able to wash hands? Able to turn water off and on?

Hygiene/Bathing/Grooming

What is the plan for bathing? Bathtub? Shower? Shower chair? At the sink?
  Requires help?
Is there hot and cold running water? Is the water temperature 120° or less?
Are there grab bars next to the tub and shower?
Are there nonskid tiles/strips/appliques/rubber mats on tub bottom and shower
  floor?
Are the bathroom and fixtures clean?
What provisions are there for mouth care? Hair care?

Clothing/Dressing

Does the patient have shoes or slippers which are easy to put on, fit properly
  with nonskid soles?
Will the patient be able to change clothes?
Are the clothes so baggy that they could trip the patient?
Are there clean clothes? How will the laundry be washed?

Rest/Sleeping

Where will the patient sleep? Would the patient benefit from a hospital bed? A
  trapeze?
How far is the bed from the floor? Can the patient get in and out of the bed?
How much time will the patient spend in bed? Does the patient need a special
  mattress?
How far is the bed from the bathroom? From other family members?

Medications

Does the patient have a plan for taking the right medications at the right time?
Is there a secure place to store the medications? Are they safe from children and
  the cognitively impaired?
Can the patient reach the medications needed? Open the container? Read the label?
Is there adequate lighting where the patient will be preparing medications?
Is there a safe way to dispose of syringes? Medical supplies?

(continued)

▶ **Box 5–5.** Questions To Complete:
Environmental Assessment Checklist (*Continued*) ◀

Shelter

Is the house clean and comfortable for the patient? Who will do the housework?
Are the plumbing and sewage systems working?
Is there a safe heat source? Are space heaters safe? Are the electrical cords in
  good condition?
Is there adequate ventilation?
Is the house infested with roaches, other insects, or rodents?

Safety and Security

Mobility/Fall Prevention

Is the patient able to get around the home? Does the patient have good balance?
  Steady gait?
Is the caregiver thinking of using restraints? What sort of restraints? Are they
  necessary?
Does the patient use assistive devices (walkers, canes) correctly? Are they the
  right height?
Do the devices fit through the pathways without catching on furnishings?
Are the pathways, hallways and stairways clear? Are there throw rugs?
Are there sturdy handrails on the stairs? Are the first and last steps clearly marked?
Is there adequate lighting in hallways and stairways? Is the path to the bathroom
  well-lighted at night?
Are the floors slippery? (Floors should not have a high gloss or be highly waxed.)
Are there uneven floor surfaces?
Are the carpets in good repair without buckles or tears that could cause
  tripping?
Can the patient walk steadily on the carpets? (Thick pile carpets can cause
  tripping if the patient has a shuffling gait.)
Are the chairs the patient uses sturdy? Are they stable if the patient uses them to
  prevent a fall?
Does the patient use furniture or counters for balance when walking? Are these
  sturdy enough to withstand the pressure?
Are there cords or wires that could cause the patient to trip?

Fire/Burn Prevention

Is there a smoke detector on each level of the home? Is there a fire extinguisher?
Is there an escape plan for the patient to get out of the house in case of fire?
Is the patient using heating pads and space heaters safely?
Are wires and plugs in good repair?
If the patient smokes, are there plans to make sure the patient smokes safely?
Are there signs of cigarette burns? Burns in the kitchen?
Are oxygen tanks stored away from flames and heat sources?

Crime/Injury Prevention

Are there locks on the doors and the windows?
Can the patient make an emergency call? Is the telephone handy? Are emergency
  numbers clearly marked?
Are firearms securely stored in a locked box? Is the ammunition stored and
  locked away separately?
Is there evidence of criminal activity?

(continued)

▶ **Box 5–5.** Questions To Complete:
Environmental Assessment Checklist *(Continued)* ◀

Love and Belonging

Caregiver

Is there a caregiver? Is the caregiver competent? Willing? Supportive?
Does the caregiver need support?
Can the caregiver hear the patient? Should there be an intercom? "Baby
  Monitor?" Handbell?

Communication

Is the telephone within easy reach of the patient?
Should the telephone have an illuminated dial? Oversized numbers? Memory
  feature? Audio enhancer?
Are needed numbers clearly marked? Police? Fire? Ambulance? Nurse? Doctor?
  Relatives? Neighbors?
Is there a daily safety check system? Should there be an alert system like
  Lifeline?
How will the patient obtain mail?

Family/Friends/Pets

Are the neighbors supportive?
Does the patient have family, friends, church/synagogue members to help and
  visit?
Is the patient able to take proper care of any pets? Are pets well-behaved?

Self-Esteem and Self-Actualization

Are there meaningful activities the patient can do? Listening to music/book
  tapes? Interactive activities?
What kind of activities does the patient enjoy? Are there creative ways that these
  activities can be brought to the patient?

Adapted with permission from Narayan, M., & Tennant, J. (1997). Environmental
assessment. *Home Healthcare Nurse, 15*(11), 799–805.

ASSESSMENT OF THE FAMILY IN THE COMMUNITY

Changes in health care delivery, budget constraints, and staff cutbacks have all
contributed to enormous pressure on nurses to do more in less time. A simple
family assessment, completed in 15 minutes or less, may actually save the nurse
time, allowing the nurse to identify issues early and prevent problems later. The
key ingredients to a simple family interview are using good manners, using therapeutic communication, constructing a family genogram, asking therapeutic
questions, and commending the family and individual on their strengths (Wright
& Leahey, 1999).

In many ways, modern culture has experienced a decline in civility and good
manners. Nursing has not been immune to this phenomenon. The professional
relationship requires that the nurse introduce himself or herself to the client and
family and set a contract with the client and family. Following basic elements of
establishing a therapeutic relationship, such as calling the client and family by

▶ Box 5–6. Spiritual Needs Protocol ◀

Illness often triggers spiritual wrestling in addition to emotional, mental, and physical pain. Spiritual care is an integral part of holistic care. The health care team must be comfortable with and receptive to these needs for them to emerge and be addressed. The concept of presence implies self-giving by the health care provider to the patient. It means being available and listening in a meaningful way. It also means having an awareness that it is a privilege to be invited into a person's life in this way, as well as an ethical responsibility.

Assessment

Assess spiritual/religious preference and request to see chaplain using database on admission.
Listen for verbal cues regarding spiritual/religious orientation:

- patient refers to God or Higher Power
- patient talks about prayer, church, synagogue, spiritual/religious leader

Look for visual cues on patient's person and in room regarding spiritual/religious orientation:

- Bible, Torah, Koran, or other spiritual books
- symbols such as the cross or Star of David
- articles such as prayer beads, medals, or pins

Listen for significant comments, eg, "It's all in God's hands now" or "Why is this happening to me?"
Assess for signs of spiritual concerns:

- discouragement
- mild anxiety
- expressions of anticipatory grief
- inability to participate in usual spiritual practice
- expressions of concern about relationship with God or Higher Power

- inability to obtain foods required by beliefs

Assess for signs of spiritual distress:

- crying
- expressions of guilt
- disturbances in sleep patterns
- disrupted spiritual trust
- feeling remote from God or Higher Power
- moderate to severe anxiety
- anger toward staff, family, God, or Higher Power
- challenged belief or value system
- loss of meaning and purpose in life

Assess for signs of spiritual despair:

- loss of hope
- refusal to communicate with loved ones
- loss of spiritual belief
- death wish
- severe depression
- flat affect
- refusal to participate in treatment regimen

Assess for special religious concerns such as diet, refusal of blood.

Interventions

Convey a caring and accepting attitude.
Provide support, encouragement, and respect.

Provide presence.
Listen actively.
Use therapeutic communication techniques such as restatement, clarification, or silence.
Join in prayer or reading scripture if comfortable.
Use therapeutic touch with the patient's permission.
Include family/significant other in spiritual care.
Consult physician for medications as needed for anxiety or depression.

Reportable Conditions

Notify physician of severe anxiety, or depression that may require pharmacologic or psychiatric intervention.
Notify chaplain, priest, rabbi, pastor or spiritual leader of spiritual concerns, distress or despair with patient's permission.

Documentation

Document assessment on database and flow sheet.
Document significant comments, behaviors of patient/family/significant other, interventions, physician notification, and referrals to chaplain or other religious leader on nurse's notes.
Document initiation of protocol on plan of care.

Adapted with permission from Sumner, C. (1998). Recognizing and responding. *American Journal of Nursing, 48*(1), 26–50.

name and involving the client and family in the care, are essential to establish-ing a trusting relationship with the client (Wright & Leahey, 1999).

Therapeutic communication is the second element of a simple family as-sessment. From the start of a brief family assessment, conversation is purpose-ful and time limited. Often, listening, showing compassion, and emphasizing strengths are the most powerful therapeutic interventions that a nurse can use. Some of the most basic suggestions include the following:

▶ Invite families to accompany the client to the unit/clinic/hospital.
▶ Involve families in the admission procedure or interview.
▶ Encourage families to ask question during the client orientation or first visit.
▶ Acknowledge the client and family's expertise in self-care or assisting in self-care.
▶ Ask about routines at home and incorporate in plan of care.
▶ Encourage the clients to practice interactions that may come up in the future related to health regimens (eg, have a parent practice telling a diabetic child that she may not eat ice cream at a birthday party).
▶ Consult with clients and family about their ideas for treatment and discharge. (Adapted from Wright & Leahey, 1999, p. 264.)

A genogram is an essential element of the quick family interview. See Chap-ter 4 for detailed information on completing genograms.

Asking therapeutic questions is the next element of the brief family inter-view. Numerous examples are found in Chapter 4. Additional questions are listed below (Wright & Leahey, 1999):

Who of your family or friends would you like us to share information with, and who not?

How can we be most helpful to you and your family or friends as we provide care for you?

What has been most/least helpful to you in past hospitalization, home visits, or clinic visits?

The last aspect of the simple family interview is to focus on strengths rather than on needs and problems. Strength-based nursing validates the client's and family's assets. In every encounter with a family, the acknowledgment of the re-sources, competencies, and efforts observed allows the family and client to real-ize their strengths and develop new perspectives of themselves and their abilities.

In summary, this framework recommends the following steps:

1. Use good manners to engage or re-engage; introduce yourself by offering your name and role and orienting family members to the purpose of a brief family interview.
2. Assess key areas of internal and external structure and function; obtain genogram information and key external support data.
3. Ask three key questions to family members.
4. Commend the family on two strengths.
5. Evaluate usefulness of the interview and conclude (Wright & Leahey, 1999, p. 272).

 ## ASSESSMENT OF THE COMMUNITY

All nurses have a role in community assessment, ranging from identifying ap-propriate resources for referral to determining the need for a new hospital. Be-cause community assessment varies in levels of complexity, the role of the nurse depends on the nurse's educational preparation and expertise. The associate degree nurse uses community assessment primarily as it relates to the care of the individual client in the context of the community. For example, a nurse working in the acute care setting may want to find placement for a client with mental illness, but the agencies generally used by the referring facility are not appropriate. Thus, the nurse may conduct a simple community assessment to determine available, accessible, and appropriate community resources for referral.

Public health nurses typically use community assessment to determine needs for particular services or programs in a given geographic area or neighborhood. An example is the community health nurse who uses community assessment to determine the need for flu shot clinics in a neighborhood.

A more complex example is the use of community assessment in influencing public policy. The nurse with a graduate degree, or a nurse statistician or epidemiologist, may be contracted by a state or local government to do a community assessment to determine the number and percentage of citizens in a particular geographic area who are not insured or are underinsured.

Concepts in Community Assessment

Through **community assessment,** the nurse determines how a community influences the health of its residents. Community assessment is a technique that may be used to determine the health status, resources, or needs of a group of individuals. Similar to basic nursing process, the nurse collects information about the physiologic, psychological, sociocultural, and spiritual health of the community. Community assessment allows the nurse to explore the relationship between a variety of community variables and the health of its occupants. Professionals from a number of disciplines participate in community assessment activities. These professionals include nurses, social workers, therapists, community health workers, public health nurses, physicians, epidemiologists, statisticians, and public policy makers.

Chapter 1 describes the community as made up of people, place, and social systems and discusses the characteristics of a healthy community. Just as the characteristics of healthy families can be used in assessment, the characteristics of a healthy community can be used as a simple tool to assess a community's level of health.

Community assessment reflects a problem-solving process similar to the nursing process that uses steps similar to those used to assess the individual client or family. All three dimensions of the community are assessed: the people, the place, and the social systems, as shown in Box 5–7.

▶ **Box 5–7.** Basic Components of Community Assessment ◀

People	Social Systems	
Vital statistics	Social systems	Legal
Population characteristics	Health	Communication
Mortality characteristics	Economic	Community dynamics
Morbidity characteristics	Education	What are the community values?
	Religious	How do things get done in
Place	Welfare	the community?
Physical	Political	Who has the power
Environmental	Recreation	in the community?

People

A community can be assessed by analyzing the characteristics of the people in that community. These characteristics are defined through the **demographics** of the community, which include the number, composition by age, rate of growth and decline, social class, and mobility of the people in the community. Other vital statistics include the birth rate, overall death rate, death rate by cause and by age, and infant mortality rate. Of these, the infant mortality rate is considered to be the most important statistical indicator regarding the level of maternal–infant health in a community. These vital statistics are the "vital signs" of the community.

Place

Place or location is where the community is located and its boundaries. It may include the type of community, such as rural or urban; location of health services; or climate, flora, fauna, and topography. Assessment of location is important because it determines what services are accessible and available to the people living within that area.

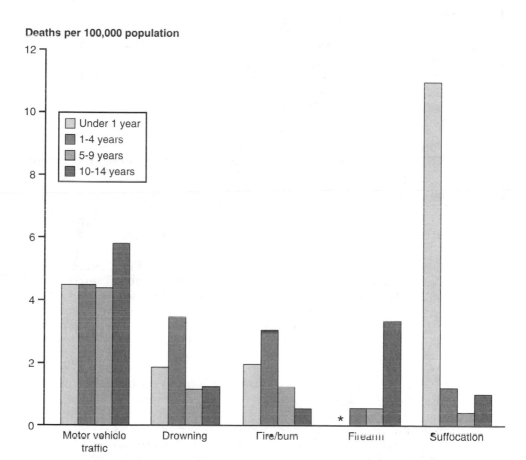

Deaths per 100,000 population

* Rate is based on fewer than 20 deaths.

SOURCE: Centers for Disease Control and Prevention, National Center for Health Statistics, National Vital Statistics System.

Death rates for leading causes of injury among children under 15 years of age by age: United States, 1995

Social Systems

Social systems are assessed as economic, educational, religious, political, and legal systems. Further, human services, opportunities for recreation, and communication systems are components of a community's social systems. **Power systems** within a community must also be assessed as part of the overall social system—how power is distributed throughout a particular social system. Determining how decisions are made and how change occurs are essential in planning.

Methods in Community Assessment

Many methods can be used to collect data in a community. Five methods are discussed here: windshield survey, informant interviews, participant observations, secondary analysis of existing data, and constructed surveys. These assessments are typically in the domain of the public health nurse; however, it is helpful for community-based nurses to understand these methods, because they may be asked to participate in community assessment.

Windshield Survey

A common method of community assessment is a **windshield survey.** The windshield survey is the motorized equivalent of a simple head-to-toe assessment. The observer drives through a chosen neighborhood and uses the five senses and powers of observation to conduct a general assessment of that neighborhood. Conclusions from a windshield survey reveal common characteristics about the way people live, where they live, and the type of housing that exists in a given neighborhood. An example of a windshield survey is seen in Box 5–8.

Informant Interviews

Informant interviews involve community residents who are either key informants or members of the general public. Key informants are individuals in positions of power or influence in the community, such as leaders in local government, schools, and the religious or business community. General public interviews may include random telephone or person-on-the-street interviews. Interviews are typically unstructured and are conducted to collect general information.

Nurses working in acute care settings use the equivalent of informant interviews to elicit information from the client, family members, social workers, and spiritual leaders. Nurses may also use this technique as they talk to other nurses about potential community resources that may be appropriate for referral purposes. If hospital or agency follow-up telephone calls are used after discharge, informant information about referral sources is elicited.

Participant Observations

The third method of data collection is **participant observations.** The nurse observes formal and informal community activities to determine significant events and occurrences leading to conclusions about what is happening in selected settings. Formal gatherings would include government, city council, county board, and school board meetings; informal gatherings occur at the local coffee shop or cafe, barber shop, or school. This type of assessment can be effective in determining the values, norms, and concerns of a community. It may also offer an opportunity to identify the power systems within the community. Recognizing how power is distributed throughout the community social system, and how de-

► Box 5–8. Windshield Survey ◄

This assessment has been designed to assist the nurse traveling around the neighborhood to identify objective data related to people, places, and social systems that help define the community. This information may help identify trends, stability, and changes that may affect the health of the individual living in the community.

People

Who is on the street (eg, women, children, men)?
How are they dressed?
What are they doing?
Are the people African American, white, Asian?
How are the different racial groups residentially located?
How would you categorize the residents: upper, upper middle, middle, lower class? How did you come to this conclusion?
Is there any evidence of communicable diseases, alcoholism, drug abuse, mental illness? How did you come to this conclusion?
Are there animals on the street? What kind?

Place

Boundaries

Where is the community located?
What are its boundaries?
Natural boundaries?
Humanmade boundaries?

Location of Health Services

Where are the major health institutions located?
What health institutions may be necessary for a community of this size but are not located in the community (eg, a large community with few or no acute care or ambulatory care facilities)?
Are there geographic features that may pose a threat?
What plants or animals could pose a threat to health?

Human-Made Environment

Do you see major industrial areas with heavy industrial plants?
Do the roads allow easy access to health institutions? Are those roads marked by easily seen and understandable signs?

Housing

What is the quality of the housing?
How old are the houses?
Are there single or multifamily dwellings?
Are there signs of disrepair and decay? If so, explain.
Are there vacant dwellings? If so, explain.

Social Systems

Are there schools in the area? Are they in good repair?
Are there parks and outdoor recreation opportunities?

(continued)

▶ **Box 5–8.** Windshield Survey *(Continued)* ◀

Social Systems

What churches are located in the community?
What schools, community centers, clinics, or other services for the community
  are provided by the churches?
Does the community have public transportation that provides accessible
  service?
What supermarkets and stores are available in the neighborhoods?
Is there evidence of police and fire protection in the area?
Are there social agencies, clinics, hospitals, dentists, or other health care
  providers?

cisions are made, provides important insight into how change occurs in a community.

Nurses in inpatient settings use this technique when they observe a client in physical therapy, occupational therapy, or any activity off the unit. These observations may tell the staff nurse something about the client's values and behavior. Home visits conducted with clients after discharge from the acute care setting to assess their ongoing needs, or before admission to an acute care setting, are examples of participant observation. During the home visit the nurse collects information about the client in the context of the family and the community.

Secondary Data

Sources of **secondary data** for analysis include records, documents, and other previously collected information. Depending on the community, an abundance of demographic data may be available to describe the health status of its members. These may include databases from schools, departments of health at the city and state levels, county data, private foundations, and state universities. Health data kept by the state may be thought of as the health record of the citizens of that state. Secondary data provides the statistics that are the vital signs of the community.

An example of secondary data may be seen in a clinic setting. Last week you noticed that many of the adults seen in the clinic where you work were admitted with the diagnosis of bronchitis. You calculate that last week 30 of 100 clients who came to the clinic had bronchitis. You wonder if this is an epidemic (the occurrence of a disease that exceeds normal or expected frequency in a community or region). To determine if it is, you look at the clinic statistics for the year before and find that during the same week last year, 20 of 60 adults were admitted for bronchitis. Are you seeing an epidemic this year? Nurses in acute care and clinics use secondary data when they consult old charts and past notes, vital signs, orders, and other indicators of client progress documented in the client's chart.

Constructed Surveys

Constructed surveys may be used to collect information about communities. This model is typically time-consuming and expensive. A random sample of a targeted population asks a list of specific questions. Data collected are analyzed for patterns and trends.

TABLE 5–1 • Examples of Community Assessment in Community-Based Care

People	Place	Social Systems
	Self-Care	
Assess the client related to people in immediate environment and surrounding community to determine ability to enhance or detract from the client's ability to maintain self-care.	Determine where the client lives and how the home, neighborhood, and community may contribute to the client's ability to maintain self-care.	Assess available, appropriate, and accessible community resources to support self-care.
	Context of Client, Family, and Community	
Assess the values, attitudes, and norms of people in the client's immediate environment and surrounding community.	Determine where the client lives; both the immediate environment and surrounding community.	Identify if social systems provide support or detract from the individual's potential for recovery.
	Prevention	
Consider the people in the immediate environment and surrounding community to determine support or disregard for a preventive focus.	Assess the location and whether it supports or disregards a preventive focus.	Assess the social systems for evidence of a preventive focus.
	Continuity	
Determine if the people in the immediate and surrounding community support continuity.	Identify if the location enhances or detracts from continuity.	Describe the available, accessible, and appropriate community resources that support continuity.

Application

Community assessment may be accomplished by using any one, or a combination, of the methods discussed. These methods are applied to the three dimensions of community: people, place, and social systems. One simple method of assessment is to use the characteristics of a healthy community. Another way to assess a community is to use an assessment guide with specific assessment questions. Once information is collected, the nurse reviews it for repeating patterns that may appear in all three areas of assessment. At this point, a community health need may be identified. A third way to assess people, place, and social systems is to use the components of community-based care, as outlined in Table 5–1.

EXAMPLE OF A CLIENT SITUATION

Addressing Community Needs in the School

Maria is the school nurse for Harmony High School, which has an enrollment of 2,300 students. To determine the health needs of the students attending Harmony, she is conducting an assessment of the school community. She has collected the following information about the school district and the students at Harmony High.

Windshield Survey

First, Maria spent time traveling around the school district completing a windshield survey. This is what she discovered.

Most of the people on the street during the day are women and small children. Based on the way they are dressed and the cars they are driving, they appear to be middle class. Most of the people are Mexican American or white. There is no evidence of drug abuse or problems with communicable diseases.

Harmony is a community of 20,000 people located at the outer suburban ring of Metropolitan City, which has a population of 3,000,000; it is a predominantly suburban community with 10% of the citizens in rural areas. There is little pollution of any type in the area. There are no hospitals or clinics in the community. The houses are primarily well-kept, single-family dwellings between 5 and 20 years old.

In evaluating the social systems, Maria found that there are primary, secondary, and tertiary health care services nearby. However, because there is no public transportation, it is difficult for students to gain access to these services. In addition, none of the health services is targeted at adolescents. For instance, 100% of the prenatal classes are attended by suburban, middle-class couples. The closest facility in which pregnant adolescents can receive confidential pregnancy testing, prenatal care, or prenatal classes is 45 minutes away by car.

Informant Interviews

Maria then interviews some of the key informants in the community. She asks them what they think are the primary health issues among high school students in their community. The county public health nurses, counselor, and principal of the high school and parish nurse all agree that many pregnant adolescents do not receive prenatal care. The fire chief and mayor believe there is a need for more emergency medical services.

Participant Observations

Based on the students who come to her office for care, Maria has identified two categories of students who frequently need health care. One group consists of students with somatic complaints related to personal or family stress. The second group consists of students who have questions about sexuality or who are pregnant and need referral. The girls who are pregnant have a great deal of difficulty getting early prenatal care.

Maria attends the school board meetings where issues of health are occasionally discussed. All of the school board members are concerned about cost containment, and two members are particularly sensitive about including sexuality in the school's curriculum. The superintendent is committed to curricula sensitive to community values.

Secondary Data

Maria collects secondary data on the community from the state health department. She discovers demographic facts about Harmony and compares them with data on all the high school students in the state. Harmony has a lower rate of prenatal care among adolescents and a higher percentage of infant mortality and low-birth-weight newborns.

Community Health Need or Problem Statement

Maria decides that the community health care need in Harmony High School is early identification of pregnancy and provision of prenatal care for pregnant adolescent girls.

Outcome and Interventions

Maria defines the outcomes she hopes to establish and the interventions as follows:

Outcome after 6 months
Establish a task force made up of a teacher, a counselor, a public health nurse, and a member of the school board to determine how the school and community can address this need.

Interventions after 6 months

1. Establish and convene a task force every 2 weeks.

2. Present a summary of the results of the community assessment to the school board, public health nurses, teachers, and counselors.
3. Keep the key players apprised of the progress of the task force.

Outcome after 1 year

1. Develop a method for referring all pregnant adolescents seen by school and community personnel to the school's prenatal program.
2. Develop a prenatal course to be offered in the school.
3. Develop a list of community referral sources for prenatal adolescents.
4. Develop a mechanism for follow-up after birth.

Interventions during year 1

1. Present the results of the task force to the school board, public health nurses, teachers, and counselors.
2. Ask for input and involvement of all key players.

Interventions after year 2

1. Streamline a method for referral.
2. Evaluate the prenatal program including the number and percentage of pregnant students attending the classes, satisfaction with the program, and total percent now receiving prenatal care, infant mortality rate, and rate of low-birth-weight infants.
3. Increase community awareness about the prenatal program.

Actual Outcome After 2 Years

	Harmony		
	Expected	Actual	**State**
Number live births per 1,000 per year	15	15	15
Percent pregnant teens with prenatal care	80%	70%	90%
Percent pregnant teens with prenatal care first trimester	15%	15%	30%
Percent of births with low-birth-weight infants	12%	13%	9%
Percent of births to teens under 16	45%	45%	45%
Percent of births requiring NICU	10%	11%	7%
Infant mortality rate per 1,000 live births	11	12	10

Evaluation

Are the outcomes met?

1. Yes: Continue with the interventions.
2. No: Revise the interventions:
   Reconvene the task force.
   Reassess the community.

Reassessment

To reassess the community, Maria answers the following questions:

1. What additional data do we need to collect to evaluate the program?
2. Did the problem statement focus on the most important problems for the individuals living in the community?
3. What other problems are important to this community?
4. Were the problem statement, expected outcome, and interventions realistic and appropriate for this community?
5. Are the individual members of the community satisfied with the outcome?

Statement of a Concern or Problem and Expected Outcomes

Formatting statements of the community's health concerns or problems, as well as its strengths, concludes the assessment phase. It is important to document the data that support the problem and the overall processes used for the identification of the problem.

From the problem statement, the nurse defines expected outcomes. These outcome statements are specific and based on measurable criteria. Examples with possible outcomes are given here.

Example 1: When the Individual is the Client

Nursing diagnosis: *Ineffective Airway Clearance* related to asthma as manifested by respiratory rate of 28/min and wheezes in all lung fields.

Expected outcome: The client will demonstrate a respiratory rate of 16/min and cessation of wheezes in all lung fields.

Example 2: When the Community of the School District is the Client

Problem statement: The number of children between the ages of 5 and 18 years with asthma in the school district of Rosie Mountain increased from 3/1,000 in March 1995 to 6/1,000 in March 2005.

Expected outcome: Reduce the number of children between the ages of 5 and 18 years in Rosie Mountain with the diagnosis of asthma from 6/1,000 in 2000 to 3/1,000 by the year 2005.

Example 3: When the Community of the County is the Client

Community problem: The infant mortality rate for Normaldale County was 11/1,000 births in 2000, compared with the state infant mortality rate of 7/1,000 and the national rate of 8/1,000.

Expected outcome: Reduce the infant mortality rate for Normaldale County to 9/1,000 births by 2005.

Example 4: When the Community of the Hospital is the Client

Community problem: In March 2001, at Normaldale County Hospital, 65% of the nursing staff washed their hands between clients. The recommended percentage is 90%.

Expected outcome: By March 2003, 85% of the nursing staff will wash their hands between clients.

Intervention

Interventions at the community level are directed primarily toward health protection, health promotion, and disease prevention. These interventions fall under the categories of education, enforcement, or engineering (Salmon-White, 1983). Educational interventions are programs aimed at achieving the expected outcome, including programs that give information or seek to change attitudes about health issues. Enforcement interventions include legislated mandates such as seatbelt laws or restricted smoking in public places. Engineering interventions protect by design. Toys are engineered to be safe for specific age categories. Air bags are designed for the safety of the automobile driver; the intervention has been engineered into the product.

Evaluation

Community interventions are evaluated, just as nursing interventions for individual clients and families are evaluated. The expected outcome is compared with the outcome achieved at the end of the established time frame. Similar to the nursing process, community assessment is cyclical and continuous. Evaluation is not an end point. It usually begins the assessment step of the next phase of community assessment.

ADVOCACY IN PUBLIC POLICY-MAKING

Public policy may appear, at first glance, to evolve primarily from the government. However, policy-makers consider many sources when developing public policy. Nurses are valued professionals whose opinions and input are often sought by those who participate in the policy-making process. The nurse may participate in policy making in a variety of ways. These activities may range from calling or sending a letter to a city, state, or federal lawmaker, to testifying at a public hearing, to informing a client about proposed changes in the law related to health care. Often, through public education, the nurse may influence public opinion and in turn public policy. It is a professional responsibility of the graduate nurse to stay current on health care issues and to share that expertise with other members of the community.

Evidence of public opinion affecting public policy is seen in maternal care (Fig. 5–3). Until the late 1970s, third-party payers allowed a postpartum woman to stay in the hospital from 3 to 5 days. Gradually, reimbursement reduced the length of stay to 2 to 4 days, and eventually to 24 hours to 3 days. As the negative consequences of early discharge on the mother and newborn became common knowledge through the medical and nursing community's disapproval and advocacy for longer stay, this policy was changed. By the late 1990s, many states extended the 24-hour stay to 48 hours.

Numerous issues offer nurses the opportunity to act as advocates for individuals, families, and communities. Through advocacy and education, the nurse may influence public opinion and health care public policy.

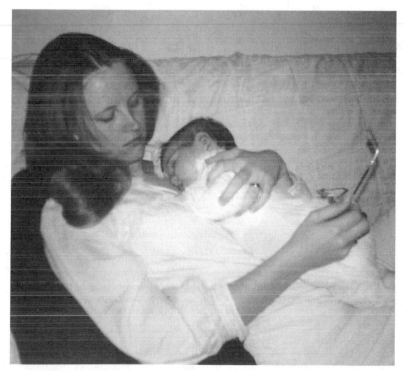

Figure 5–3. ▶ Public opinion and advocacy led to increased postpartal care.

CONCLUSIONS

Assessment in community settings has long been a part of nursing practice. Assessment is directed toward individual clients across the life span, families, and communities. Holistic assessment considers not only physical and psychosocial factors, but also cultural, functional, nutritional, environmental, and spiritual aspects of the client. Family assessment maybe abbreviated but is always essential to quality community care. Community assessment helps the nurse become aware of problems in the community that directly or indirectly affect the lives of clients and their families. Although the community-based nurse is infrequently asked to do a formal community assessment, the nurse may, along with other health care professionals, participate in some aspect of community assessment. Communities are assessed by using the nursing process to determine how people, place, and social systems influence health. As health care and nursing shift from the acute care setting to the community setting, the role of the nurse in community assessment will continue to expand.

References and Bibliography

AARP (1997). *A profile of older Americans–1996.* (p. 2) (Brochure). Washington, DC: Author.

Allen, D. (1999). People, not statistics. *Nursing Standard, 13*(34), 22–23.

Barry, C. (1998). Assessing the older adult in the home. *Home Healthcare Nurse, 16*(8), 519–529.

Carpenito, L. (2000). *Nursing diagnosis: Application to clinical practice* (8th ed.). Philadelphia: Lippincott Williams & Wilkins.

Dahl, R. (1995). The development of a community-based nursing practice: Shifting the focus to health promotion. *Advanced Practice Nursing Quarterly, 1*(3), 1–6.

Debrew, J., Barba, B., & Tesh, A. (1998). Assessing medication knowledge and practices of older adults. *Home Healthcare Nurse, 16*(10), 686–692.

Dossey, B., & Dossey, L. (1998). Attending to holistic care. *American Journal of Nursing, 98*(8), 35–38.

Heineken, J., & McCoy, N. (2000). Establishing a bond with clients of different cultures. *Home Healthcare Nurse, 18*(1), 45–51.

Lindell, D. (1997). Community assessment for the home healthcare nurse. *Home Healthcare Nurse, 15*(9), 618–627.

Lyman, B., & Marquardt, P. (1997). Nutrition screening tool for home care patients: Development and utilization. *Home Healthcare Nurse, 15*(12), 835–831.

Murray, R., & Wentner, J. (1997). *Health assessment and promotion strategies through the life span* (6th ed.). Stamford, CT: Appleton & Lange.

Narayan, M. (1996). Cultural assessment in home healthcare. *Home Healthcare Nurse, 15*(10), 664–671.

Narayan, M., & Tennant, J. (1997). Environmental assessment. *Home Healthcare Nurse, 15*(11), 799–805.

Neal, L. (1998). Functional assessment of the home health client. *Home Healthcare Nurse, 16*(10), 670–677.

O'Leary, J. (1998). *After loss: Parenting in the next pregnancy.* Minneopolis: Allina Publishing.

Pillitteri, A. (1999). *Maternal and child health nursing: Care of the childbearing and childrearing family* (3rd ed.). Philadelphia: Lippincott Williams & Wilkins.

Rijswij, L. (1998). Assessing the risk of foot ulcers. *Home Healthcare Nurse, 16*(1), 25–32.

Salmon-White, M. S. (1982). Construct for public health nursing. *Nursing Outlook, 30*, 527–530.

Sumner, C. (1998). Recognizing and responding. *American Journal of Nursing, 98*(1), 26–30.

Vogelzang, J. (1999). Elusive hunger. *Home Healthcare Nurse, 17*(4), 261–262.

Woodham-Smith, C. (1950). *Florence Nightingale.* London: Constable.

Wright, L., & Leahey, M. (1999). Maximizing time, minimizing suffering; the 15 minute (or less) family interview. *Journal of Family Nursing, 5*(3), 259–274.

LEARNING ACTIVITIES

LEARNING ACTIVITY 5-1

▶ **Client Care Study:** Assessment of the Individual Client

Nhu is a home care nurse who is making a home visit to Marion, an 85-year-old women who has just been discharged from a transitional hospital after a hip replacement. After completing the agency admission intake interview, Nhu takes a few minutes to assess Marion's functional capacity.

What areas will Nhu assess?

Nhu learns that Marion is able to perform all ADL, her home environment is basically safe, her sensory and perceptual function is intact, and her cognitive, emotional, integumentary, and respiratory status are all within normal limits and sufficient to allow her to live independently. However, as Nhu is assessing function, Marion tells her, "I was doing fine until the physician changed my medication for high blood pressure. Now I am dizzy all the time."

What does Nhu assess next?

LEARNING ACTIVITY 5-2

▶ **Clinical Thinking Exercise:** Self-Evaluation

A. INDIVIDUAL CLIENT ASSESSMENT

In your clinical journal, describe a situation in which you used an assessment guide from this chapter to assess a client in a community-based setting.

What did you learn from this activity?

What benefit do you think you created for your client?

What did you do that didn't work?

What will you do differently next time?

B. FAMILY ASSESSMENT

In your clinical journal, describe a situation in which you used an assessment guide from this chapter to assess a family in a community-based setting.

What did you learn from this activity?

What benefit do you think you created for the family?

What did you do that didn't work?

What will you do differently next time?

C. COMMUNITY ASSESSMENT

In your clinical journal, describe a situation in which you used an assessment guide from this chapter to assess a community.

What did you learn from this activity?

What benefit do you think you created for the community or could create for the community?

What did you do that didn't work?

What will you do differently next time?

Client Teaching

ROBERTA HUNT

▶ L E A R N I N G   O B J E C T I V E S ◀

- Define the teaching role.
- Discuss teaching and learning theory, learning domains, and successful teaching techniques as related to community-based nursing.
- Discuss assessment, planning, and teaching methods that are required in determining learning needs.
- Summarize Medicare reimbursement guidelines for teaching.
- Identify barriers to successful teaching.
- Explore the characteristics of successful teaching.
- State methods used in teaching the client who is not adhering to the treatment plan.
- Discuss specific teaching techniques for each level of prevention.

▶ K E Y   T E R M S ◀

affective learning
cognitive learning
learning domains
learning needs
learning objective

need to learn
psychomotor learning
readiness to learn
reimbursement requirements

Significance of Teaching

Teaching and Learning Theory

Learning Domains

Developmental Considerations

Nursing Competencies and Skills in the Teaching Process

Conclusions

At no other time in nursing history has client teaching been so important. Owing to the decreased length of stay in all acute care settings and increased amount of care provided in community settings, teaching is a central role for nurses in all settings. One example is seen in teaching prior to discharge from acute care settings. As many as 20% of clients discharged from hospitals do not even fill their prescriptions after discharge. Of those who do, between 40% and 60% do not follow the prescribed regimen, either increasing or decreasing the dose, not taking the correct dose or at the prescribed time, or not taking the entire dose. These errors may both result in serious health complications as well as cost $100 billion every year in unnecessary hospitalization, treatment, and lost work time (Dunbar-Jordan, 1999). As care is more community based, our clients provide most of their own health care, with up to 80% of all illnesses managed by clients or family members (London, 1999). It is the nurse's responsibility to promote quality self-care through teaching. Quality teaching is essential in community-based nursing care.

With this in mind, this chapter addresses quality teaching. The benefits of teaching are presented in light of the current health care system. Teaching and learning theory are discussed along with learning domains. A large section of the chapter is devoted to helping the nursing student develop skills and competencies in teaching, discussing teaching as it follows the nursing process, and sharing useful teaching techniques. The chapter ends with activities to be used in further developing understanding and skills in teaching. Because of its importance, teaching is also addressed in other chapters.

 SIGNIFICANCE OF TEACHING

In the 21st century, more care will be provided outside the acute care setting. Clients are discharged from the hospital "quicker and sicker," or they are not being admitted to an acute care facility at all. The days of progressive teaching in the acute care setting are past. Teaching now begins at whatever point the client enters the system. In fact, many clients and families receive their initial teaching from the home care nurse. Table 6–1 gives examples of important teaching opportunities. Benefits of quality teaching include better outcomes, improved satisfaction, continuity of care between settings, and cost containment while maintaining quality care.

The first and most important goal of teaching in community-based care is to assist the client and family in achieving independence. Quality teaching enhances the ability of the client and family to be successful in providing for their own needs. When client learning needs are considered within the context of the client, family, and community, better outcomes will result. These outcomes include improved care, facilitated recovery, reduction of postoperative complications, and resumption of activities of daily living.

Good teaching improves client and family satisfaction. Clients and families are more likely to feel confident about discharge and follow-up care if they believe they have some knowledge about their condition and their questions have been answered satisfactorily. Teaching often increases a client's sense of con-

TABLE 6–1 • Important Teaching Opportunities in Community-Based Nursing Care

Opportunity	Possible Learning Need
Admission	Facility policies, how to work call light and bed, specific treatments that have been ordered and why
New medication	Action of drug, possible side effects, frequency, and any special considerations
Diagnostic procedure	Preparation that is necessary before procedure, what will be experienced during procedure, any restrictions or special considerations after procedure
Surgery	Preoperative preparation, postoperative protocols (eg, deep breathing, leg exercises), pain control, how to get out of bed and turn easily
Discharge	Limitations on activity or diet, procedures such as wound care, when to call the physician

trol through mutual participation in care planning. Staff satisfaction improves when teaching results are positive. It is professionally satisfying to prepare a client for discharge and receive feedback later that the discharge was satisfactory. Likewise, it is professionally satisfying for the home care nurse to prepare a client to successfully manage self-care at home. On the other hand, it is stressful when a nurse sees a client with inadequate preparation trying to manage home care unsuccessfully.

Quality health education provides continuity between settings of care. When health care professionals give clear instructions, one setting can confidently discharge a client into another setting.

A final benefit to quality instruction is more efficient use of resources. One national report indicates that 2% of all hospital readmissions are a result of a need to re-educate caregivers (Leske & Pelczynski, 1999). Rehospitalization of clients is costly to the client, family, and third-party payers. It is frustrating to the client, family, and care providers when teaching has to be repeated several times because it was not done well the first time. Furthermore, concern for cost containment while maintaining quality care requires that all teaching incorporate prevention strategies, which further allow resources to be used efficiently.

TEACHING AND LEARNING THEORY

To be a successful teacher in any setting, the nurse must understand and apply basic teaching and learning principles. Learning depends on both the **readiness to learn** and the **need to learn** and is influenced by the individual's life experiences (Knox, 1985).

Need to Learn

Learning is facilitated when the client perceives information as needed or relevant for immediate application. For example, a postoperative client is scheduled to go home in 2 hours with a client-controlled analgesia pump. The client learns quickly how to use the pump and administer medication to control postoperative pain. This learning is facilitated by the need for pain relief and the immediate application of learning.

Readiness to Learn

Learning depends on readiness. Readiness involves such factors as emotional state, abilities, and potential. Examples of these are listed in Box 6–1.

An example of lack of learning readiness follows. You are doing preadmission teaching with a 30-year-old woman, an attorney with a busy law practice who has outpatient surgery scheduled for the next day. She is thinking about the important trial she has beginning that afternoon after surgery. She may not hear you when you tell her she should not drive or make important decisions for a full day after surgery with general anesthesia. Because of her distracted mental state she is not ready to learn.

Motivation is a strong determinant of learning readiness. Motivation starts with the client's need to know and then provides the drive or incentive to learn. Because so many things can affect motivation, motivation can change from day to day. For instance a young woman who drinks alcohol becomes pregnant, and her health care provider tells her alcohol is harmful for the fetus. Because she is concerned for the fetus' welfare, she discontinues drinking. The motivation is strong enough to make her stop. However, at a party her friends insist that she join them in a drink. "One drink won't hurt you," they say. Now the woman is motivated to drink. Her decision depends on which motivation is stronger.

Life Experiences

Both differences and similarities between past and present life experiences influence learning. For example, you are doing discharge planning from a maternity center for a multipara who delivered her second child yesterday evening. Her delivery was complicated by a 1,000-mL blood loss and a fourth degree laceration. She has an 18-month-old toddler at home. Her husband is an accountant. It is tax season and he presently works 12 or 13 hours a day. Neither set of grandparents nor any other family or friends live nearby. Your client is going home this afternoon and insists that she does not need help at home because she did not need help after her first child. The client does not understand the difference between her first delivery and the circumstances complicating the second one.

▶ **Box 6–1.** Factors That Affect Readiness to Learn ◀

- Physiologic factors: Age, gender, disease process currently being treated intactness of senses (hearing, vision, touch, taste), preexisting condition
- Psychosocial factors: Sociocultural circumstances, occupation, economic stability, past experiences with learning, attitude toward learning, spirituality, emotional health, self-concept and body image, sense of responsibility for self
- Cognitive factors: Developmental level, level of education, communication skills, primary language, motivation, reading ability, learning style, problem-solving ability
- Environmental factors: Home environment, safety features, family relationships/problems, caregiver (availability, motivation, abilities), other support systems

LEARNING DOMAINS

Teaching and learning occur in three **learning domains:** cognitive, affective, and psychomotor. Teaching strategies are listed in Box 6–2. All three domains must be considered in all aspects of the teaching and learning process. Thus, the nurse must assess the client's need, readiness, and past experience in the cognitive, affective, and psychomotor domains.

Cognitive learning involves mental storage and recall of new knowledge and information for problem solving. Sometimes this domain is referred to as the critical thinking or knowledge domain. An example is the client who has recently been diagnosed with insulin-dependent diabetes. Not only will this person need information about diet, insulin, and exercise, but this client also needs to use that information to formulate menus and an exercise plan. In addition, as blood sugar levels fluctuate, a client with diabetes must alter food intake and exercise. All this requires cognitive learning.

Affective learning involves feelings, attitudes, values, and emotions that influence learning. This is also referred to as the attitude domain. For example, the client who has just been identified as being diabetic may have to talk about feelings related to fears or concerns about having diabetes before he or she is ready to learn about insulin.

Psychomotor learning consists of acquired physical skills that can be demonstrated. This may be referred to as the skill domain. For example, the newly diagnosed insulin-dependent diabetic client must learn to give self-injections. Self-injection will require learning the skill of using syringes.

DEVELOPMENTAL CONSIDERATIONS

It is helpful for the nurse to understand various theories of development. Appendix 6–1 outlines intellectual development as well as other developmental stages and nursing implications related to them. Just as the need to learn will be different at various age levels, the cognitive domain will differ and life experiences will differ. For example, teaching a 6-year-old girl about insulin administration will be different from teaching a 24-year-old woman, which would in turn

---

▶ Box 6–2. Suggested Teaching Strategies
for the Three Learning Domains ◀

Cognitive Domain	Affective Domain	Psychomotor Domain
Lecture or discussion	Role modeling	Demonstration
Panel discussion	Discussion	Discovery
Discovery	Panel discussion	Audiovisual materials
Audiovisual materials	Audiovisual materials	Printed materials
Printed materials	Role playing	
Programmed instruction	Printed materials	
Computer-assisted instruction programs		

Taylor, C., Lillis, C., & LeMone, P. (1997). Fundamentals of nursing: The art and science of nursing care (p. 395). Philadelphia: Lippincott-Raven.

be different from teaching a 69-year-old woman. The nurse must consider these factors.

Affective learning and psychomotor learning will also differ. The 6-year-old girl will approach insulin administration differently emotionally than the 24-year-old woman. The 6-year-old girl may not have fine motor skills needed to administer insulin. On the other hand, the older woman may have arthritis and not have the dexterity needed to fill the syringe or insert the needle in the site. Signs and symptoms associated with age-related changes and diseases that can interfere with the client teaching–learning process are shown in Figure 6–1. Chronologic age does not always indicate maturity. A young child may respond more maturely to health teaching than a 28-year-old client. Much depends on the client's responses to changes and stress in life experiences.

Nurses may need to show adults why they need to learn before the actual teaching can begin. Many adults have not been involved in educational programs for many years. Often they show a hesitancy to learn something new, perhaps be-

Signs and Symptoms	Age-Related Changes	Cataracts	Macular Degeneration	Diabetic Retinopathy	Glaucoma
Diminished visual acuity	●	●	●	●	●
Distorted central vision			●		
Blurred or clouded vision	●	●		●	
Loss of visual field	●				●
Loss of central vision			●		● (LATER STAGE)
Loss of peripheral vision					●
Reduced accommodation	●				
Glare	●	●	●	●	●
Decline in depth perception	●				
Decreased color perception	●		●	●	
Decreased contrast sensitivity		●		●	●
Decreased light/dark adaptation	●			●	●
Scotomas			●		
Reduced night vision	●	●			
Slower processing of visual input	●				

Figure 6–1. ▶ Signs and symptoms associated with age-related changes and disease that can interfere with the client teaching–learning process. Used with permission from Barry, C. (2000). Teaching the older client in the home: Assessment and adaptation. *Home Healthcare Nurse, 18*(6), 379. Adapted from Jarvis, 1996, pp. 306, 332; Miller, 1999, pp. 208–212; Stanley & Beare, 1999, pp. 93–94, Stone, Wyman, & Salisbury, 1999, pp. 516–519, 524–525.

COMMUNITY-BASED NURSING CARE GUIDELINES

Teaching the Older Learner

General Teaching Tips
- Meet in a quiet room where there is no background noise.
- Make sure the room is brightly lit and glare free.
- Face the learner with light on your face rather than light behind you.
- Speak in a low, slow voice.
- Include family members if agreeable to the client or when necessary.
- Limit sessions to no more than 20 to 30 minutes.
- Use analogies.
- Use visual aids with large letters and bright colors.
- Relate new information to past experiences if possible.
- Repeat information frequently; use frequent summaries.
- Watch for feedback and its implications for positive or negative learning.
- Watch for cues indicating inadequate hearing, lack of attention, tiredness.
- Provide written materials as reinforcement when possible.
- Compliment the client for adaptability to learning session.

Teaching Related To Medication
- Be sure client understands what each medication is for.
- Be sure client knows how many pills to take and when.
- Be sure client knows what to do if a dose is missed.
- Be sure client has written medication instructions in appropriate language.

Adapted from Rice, R. (1996). Patient education in the home. In R. Rice (Ed.), *Home health nursing practice: Concepts and applications* (2nd ed.). St. Louis: Mosby–Year Book.

cause they are afraid of failing. Added to this is the older client's concern about memory loss. The nurse needs to develop rapport and be an honest and open communicator to encourage, or give the client self-confidence, to learn something new.

The nurse should never assume that all clients can read and write. Illiteracy is found in every walk of life, among all races and cultures, and at all socioeconomic levels. Educational level is not a true determinant of a person's ability to read or write. Literacy or illiteracy must be assessed as part of the client's readiness to learn.

NURSING COMPETENCIES AND SKILLS IN THE TEACHING PROCESS

Teaching and learning follow several prescribed steps, similar to the steps of the nursing process, as shown in Table 6–2. It is essential to assess the learner to determine need to learn, readiness, and past life experiences. A comprehensive assessment helps the teacher identify learning needs. Learning outcomes, which both direct the learning plan and provide outcome criteria, arise from the learning needs. Once the learning objectives or outcomes are defined, then the teacher will determine teaching strategies or tools and methods appropriate for the learner. After implementation of the plan, evaluations are made to determine the success of teaching. The process is outlined in Figure 6–2.

TABLE 6–2 • Relationship Between Nursing Process and Teaching and Learning

Steps	Nursing Process	Teaching and Learning
Assessment	Assessment of client/family/caregiver determines need for nursing care.	Assessment of client/family/ caregiver determines need for nursing care.
Diagnosis	Statement of nursing problem	Statement of learning need
Expected outcome	Expected outcome for client or family	Learning objectives/goals for the learner
Planning	Nurse and client work together to develop plan of nursing care.	Nurse and client work together to develop learning plan.
Interventions	A variety of actions can be used to implement the plan.	A variety of actions in cognitive, affective and psychomotor learning are used to augment plan.
Evaluation	Nurse and client evaluate success of outcomes; nurse determines why plan was not successful (if so); nurse and client revise and set new objectives and plan.	Nurse and client evaluate success of outcomes; nurse and client determine weakness of plan; new objectives and plan are written.

Assessment

The first assessment begins with assessment of the learning needs, readiness, and life experiences of the client, family, and caregiver. Numerous factors must be considered when assessing these areas. Assessment must incorporate the three learning domains: cognitive, affective, and psychomotor. It is essential also to consider the nursing implications for various developmental stages, listed in Appendix 6–1.

Successful teaching is positively associated with a nonjudgmental attitude. This is especially true of clients from minority groups or from cultures different from the nurse's culture. A nonjudgmental attitude is enhanced when the nurse does the following:

▶ Recognizes and accepts differences between the nurse and client
▶ Tries to understand the cultural or value basis for client behavior
▶ Listens and learns before advising or teaching
▶ Empathizes with the client regardless of differences in attitudes and values

A cultural assessment tool will help the nurse determine how learning need is influenced by culture. Various types of cultural assessment tools are discussed in Chapter 3.

A learning assessment guide can be used to assess the learning need of the client. Such a guide is printed in Box 6–3. Documentation is integral to the teach-

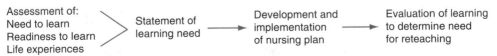

Assessment of:
Need to learn
Readiness to learn
Life experiences
→ Statement of learning need → Development and implementation of nursing plan → Evaluation of learning to determine need for reteaching

Figure 6–2. ▶ Diagram of the teaching process. The nursing process and the teaching process have some similarities.

▶ Box 6–3. Learning Assessment Guide ◀

Client name _____

Health condition requiring health education_____

Primary caregiver _____

Learner_____ Relationship to client_____

Age_____Gender _____Occupation _____

Developmental Stages and Implications for Learner_____

   Psychosocial stage_____

_____

_____

   Cognitive stage_____

   Language _____

How does the caregiver or client feel about the responsibilities of self-care _____

_____

_____

Describe any disabilities or limitations of the learner (including sensory disabilities) _____

_____

_____

Describe any preexisting health conditions of the learner_____

_____

_____

List sociocultural factors that may impede learning_____

_____

_____

State learner behaviors that indicate motivation to learn_____

_____

_____

Can the learner read and comprehend at the reading level required by the task?

_____

_____

Does the learner show an ability to problem solve at a level that provides safe care in the home? _____

_____

Is the home environment conducive to the learning required by the care?_____

_____

If not, what modifications are necessary?_____

_____

(continued)

▶ **Box 6–3.** Learning Assessment Guide *(Continued)* ◀

If the learner is not able to carry out the care, are other caregivers available for backup support? _____

_____

If so, please name. _____
Phone number _____
Address _____
What other support is available for the client and caregiver? _____

_____

_____

---

ing process. All assessment is documented. After the client, family, and caregiver needs, readiness to learn, and past life experiences have been assessed and documented, the learning need can be determined.

Identification of the Learning Need

The nurse, based on the assessment, draws some inferences and conclusions. Table 6–3 illustrates this process. A list of **learning needs** and problems emerges, which leads to identification of priority needs. When lack of knowledge, attitude, or skill hinders a client's self-care, a nursing diagnosis can be used to name the problem or strength. The list of the North American Nursing Diagnosis Association (NANDA) can help identify the learning needs of the individual, family member, or caregiver. According to Carpenito (2000), knowledge deficit does not represent a human response, alteration, or pattern of dysfunction, but rather a related factor. All nursing diagnoses incorporate teaching as a part of the diagnosis, as follows:

- ▶ Risk for Ineffective Management of Therapeutic Regimens related to lack of knowledge of management, signs, and symptoms of complications of diabetes mellitus
- ▶ Decisional Conflict related to lack of knowledge about advantages and disadvantages of infant circumcision
- ▶ Risk for Impaired Home Maintenance Management related to lack of knowledge of home care and community resources
- ▶ Risk for Injury related to lack of knowledge of bicycle safety

It is also useful to consider learning domains. Learning needs can be determined in one, two, or all of the learning domains. Consider the learning domains in the following example.

EXAMPLE OF A CLIENT SITUATION

▶ **Newborn Circumcision**

Pat, a primipara, delivered a boy yesterday afternoon. The newborn is to be circumcised this afternoon before Pat and her newborn are discharged. Despite the fact that you have gone over the teaching outline about circumcision twice with Pat, she states, "How will the penis look in 3 days?" She is also unable to demonstrate the application of the dressing to the site and states, "Maybe we shouldn't have the baby circumcised if it will hurt the baby."

For this scenario an example of a learning need in the affective domain is:

Anxiety related to lack of knowledge as manifested by the mother's statement, "Maybe we shouldn't have the baby circumcised if it will hurt the baby."

An example of a learning need in the psychomotor domain is:

Risk for Impaired Home Maintenance Management related to lack of knowledge and ability to demonstrate dressing change.

An example of a nursing diagnosis in the cognitive domain is:

Altered Parenting related to lack of knowledge and inexperience as manifested by the mother's statement, "How should the circumcision site look in 3 days?"

After the learning need is identified, the nurse determines if the teaching needed by the client is reimbursable. Referral may depend on reimbursement. In most situations, nurses providing teaching to clients in the home are restricted by **reimbursement requirements.** Medicare/Medicaid and most other third-party payers reimburse skilled nursing care. The specific requirements are defined in the Medicare Guidelines, Revision 222, Section 205.13. A summary is given in Box 6–4.

It is imperative that the nurse be familiar with the reimbursement requirements of the various third-party payers for teaching at the agency where he or she works. Agencies will not receive payment for teaching if the nurse does not follow the requirements as specified by the particular payer.

Planning

Planning for learning involves developing a teaching plan. Teaching plans are similar to nursing care plans—both follow the steps of the nursing process. In some agencies standardized teaching plans are used and may include a computerized teaching plan. If standardized teaching plans are used, the plan must be individualized to the client and his or her needs. Teaching plans are also incorporated into critical pathway documentation.

Planning skills are essential in the development of individualized teaching plans. The teaching plan identifies learning objectives that reflect the specifics of the ongoing care at home. Often, the goal of teaching is to ensure the client's safety and total reliance on self-care. The planning of the care is a mutual process among the nurse, client, and family caregivers. Planning is based on the three learning domains.

▶ *Cognitive objectives:* Relate to learning activities that strengthen comprehension regarding the illness and its treatment
▶ *Affective objectives:* Relate to learning activities that enhance the acceptance of the illness and subsequent treatment
▶ *Psychomotor objectives:* Relate to learning activities that demonstrate management of the treatment procedures

A **learning objective** is the same as a client goal or expected outcome used in the nursing process. Each includes a subject, action verb, performance criteria, target time, and special conditions.

The following learning objective contains these components:

Client will state three signs and symptoms of infection by (date)_____, and know which complications require contacting the nurse on call.

TABLE 6–3 • Examples of Inferences Made from Assessment Data

Factors to Consider When Assessing Readiness to Learn	Data	Inference
Physiologic Factors		
Age	85	Elderly client may have special needs
Gender	Male	Men and women each have special needs
Disease process currently under treatment	Newly diagnosed diabetic	New diabetics have many teaching needs
Intactness of senses— hearing, vision, touch, taste	Hearing and vision are impaired	Teaching must be modified considering sensory deficit
Preexisting conditions	Cataract surgery 2 y ago	Vision may still be partially impaired or may be corrected
Psychosocial Factors		
Sociocultural	Hmong refugee	Teaching must consider diet common to this culture
Occupation	Retired	
Cognitive Factors		
Motivation	Learner states "I am interested in learning about _____."	Learner is motivated
Reading ability	Observed reading the newspaper	Shows ability to read
Learning style	Observer, doer, or by listening	Tailor teaching to style
Problem-solving ability	Learner can come up with concepts and alternatives	Learner can problem solve
Environmental Factors		
Home environment	Home cluttered with no place to sit or set up for teaching	Environment must be modified before teaching
Caregiver Availability	Client a widow or spouse works full-time	No caregiver available
Motivation	Caregiver states "I can't handle hearing about that device."	Caregiver not motivated
Abilities	Caregiver is unable to follow simple instructions or directions	Caregiver has limited ability to provide care
Other support	Client is active in his or her church	Church may be another source of care and support

Subject: client

Action verb: state

Performance criteria: signs and symptoms of infection

Target time: (date)

Special conditions: when to contact the nurse on call

▶ Box 6–4. Medicare Guidelines ◀

". . . activities which require skilled nursing personnel to teach a beneficiary, the beneficiary's family or care givers how to manage his treatment regimen constitutes skilled nursing services. Where the teaching or training is reasonable and necessary to the treatment of the illness or injury, skilled nursing visits for teaching would be covered. The test of whether a nursing service is skilled relates to the skill required to teach and not to the nature of what is being taught. . . . Skilled nursing visits for teaching and training activities are reasonable and necessary where the teaching or training is appropriate to the beneficiary's functional loss, or his illness or injury." From Medicare Guidelines Coverage of Services Revision 222 Section 205.13.

Summary of Medicare Reimbursement Requirements for Teaching

Teaching is reimbursed when it is:

* Teaching how to manage treatment.
* Reasonable and necessary to the treatment of the illness or injury.
    Reasonable and necessary = teaching to the client's functional loss or his illness or injury
    To determine the number of necessary and reasonable visits
        Initial teaching = number of visits depends on the *complexity* of the tasks and the *ability* of the learner
        Reinforcement teaching = number of visits depends on *retained knowledge* and *anticipated learning progress*

Teaching is not generally reimbursed if:

* It becomes apparent after a reasonable period of time the client, family, or caregiver is NOT able to learn.
* The reason that learning did not occur is NOT documented.

Adapted from Medicare Guidelines Coverage of Services Revision 222 Section 205.13.

Examples of learning objectives in the three learning domains are:

▶ *Cognitive objectives:* Family or caregiver will state three signs and symptoms of infection by (date)_____.
▶ *Affective objectives:* Family or caregiver will express feelings about having to be in charge of client's port-a-cath care by (date)_____.
▶ *Psychomotor objectives:* Family or caregiver will demonstrate aseptic technique when cleaning and flushing sites on port-a-cath by (date)_____.

Action verbs that can be used when writing learning objectives are listed in Box 6–5.

In most situations, the nurse and the client plan a series of small, incremental learning objectives through a series of lessons based on the specific needs of the client. The overall goal of planning is to assist the client to have enough understanding to be safe with self-care. For many clients, the ultimate goal is independence through total reliance on care from family or other caregivers for others. The goal of teaching is to maximize individual potential or quality of life.

▶ Box 6–5. Active Verbs for Learner Objectives ◀

Cognitive Domain	Affective Domain	Psychomotor Domain
categorize	answer	adapt
compare	choose	arrange
compose	defend	assemble
define	discuss	begin
describe	display	change
design	form	construct
differentiate	give	create
explain	help	manipulate
give example	initiate	move
identify	join	organize
label	justify	rearrange
list	relate	show
name	revise	start
prepare	select	work
plan	share	
solve	use	
state		
summarize		
write		

Intervention

The nurse carries out the teaching plan according to the client or family caregiver learning needs. This is accomplished in one or more teaching sessions. Interventions may vary according to learner readiness, perceived need, and past life experience, all of which fluctuate throughout an individual's life span. Specific interventions for children are shown in Box 6–6, and nursing implications are given in Appendix 6–1. It is essential to incorporate nursing interventions that are designed to deal with existing barriers to successful teaching. Some of these barriers are discussed in the next section.

The basic principles of teaching and learning discussed so far apply in both community-based and acute care settings. However, there are some differences between the two settings. These differences are discussed in relation to discharge planning and teaching. Barriers to successful teaching are presented first and followed by characteristics of successful teaching.

Discharge Teaching in the Acute Care Setting

BARRIERS TO SUCCESSFUL TEACHING

Because clients are discharged from the hospital "quicker and sicker," or have complicated procedures done on an outpatient basis and are sent home, the need for comprehensive discharge teaching is accentuated. Discharge teaching, however, does not always result in learning. In a questionnaire designed to evaluate the quality of discharge teaching, only one of five family caregivers reported feeling adequately prepared to care for the client at home (Leske & Pelczynski, 1999). Their retention of information may diminish owing to the anxiety experienced with the client's homecoming. Barriers to successful discharge teaching are shown in Table 6–4.

> ▶ Box 6–6. Cognitive Stages and Approaches
> to Patient Education With Children ◀

Cognitive Stage	Approach to Teaching
Ages Birth to 2 y—Sensorimotor Development	
Begins as completely undifferentiated from environment	Orient all teaching to parents.
Eventually learns to repeat actions that have effect on objects	Make infants feel as secure as possible with familiar objects in home environment.
Has rudimentary ability to make associations	Give older infants an opportunity to manipulate objects in their environments, especially if long hospitalization is expected.
Ages 2–7 y—Preoperational Development	
Has cognitive processes that are literal and concrete	Be aware of explanations that the child may interpret literally (eg, "The doctor is going to make your heart like new" may be interpreted as "He is going to give me a new heart"); allow child to manipulate safe equipment, such as stethoscopes, tongue blades, reflex hammers; use simple drawings of the external anatomy because children have limited knowledge of organs' functions.
Lacks ability to generalize	Comparisons to other children are not helpful, nor is it meaningful to compare one diagnostic test or procedure to another.
Has egocentrism predominating	Belief that he causes events to happen may result in guilty thoughts that he caused his own pain, hospitalization, and so forth; reassure child that no one is to blame for his pain or other problems.
Has animistic thinking (thinks that all objects possess life or human characteristics of their own)	Anthropomorphize and name equipment that is especially frightening.
Ages 7–12 y—Concrete Operational Thought Development	
Has concrete, but more realistic and objective, cognitive processes	Use drawings and models; children at this age have vague understandings of internal body processes; use needle play, dolls to explain surgical techniques and facilitate learning.
Is able to compare objects and experiences because of increased ability to classify along many different dimensions	Relate his care to other children's experiences so he can learn from them; compare procedures to one another to diminish anxiety.

(continued)

▶ **Box 6–6.** Cognitive Stages and Approaches
to Patient Education With Children *(Continued)* ◀

Ages 7–12 y—Concrete Operational Thought Development

Views world more objectively and is able to understand another's position

Has knowledge of cause and effect that has progressed to deductive logical reasoning

Use films and group activities to add to repertoire of useful behaviors and establish role models.

Use child's interest in science to explain logically what has happened and what will happen; explain medications simply and straightfowardly (eg, "This medicine [insulin] unlocks the door to your body's cells just as a key unlocks the door to your house. By unlocking the door to the cell, the insulin can deliver the food and energy in your blood to the cell.").

London, F. (1999). *No time to teach: A nurse's guide to patient and family education.* Philadelphia: Lippincott Williams & Wilkins. Adapted from Petrillo, M., & Sanger, S. (1998). *Emotional care of hospitalized children.* Philadelphia: Lippincott-Raven (pp. 38–50) and Kolb, L. C. (1977). *Modern clinical psychiatry* (9th ed., pp. 90–91). Philadelphia: Saunders.

TABLE 6–4 • Combating Barriers to Successful Discharge Teaching

Barriers	Sample Nursing Interventions
Timing (client's physical or psychological conditions do not allow learning to occur)	Document client's lack of mastery of the material. Update physician or nurse practitioner on an ongoing basis to plan discharge. Refer for follow-up if learning is not adequate for safe self-care.
Past experiences impede perceived learning readiness or need.	Identify past experiences. Determine and clarify misconceptions. Determine if past experience will interrupt or enhance new learning.
Retention of information impeded by anxiety of going home or leaving security of health care environment.	See interventions for timing. Break learning into small, easily mastered segments. Use positive reinforcement and praise.
Cultural differences between nurse and client or family impede learning or understanding.	Work to build a trusting relationship with client and family. Show respect for the client's culture and incorporate it in discharge planning. Use resources to overcome a language barrier.
Lack of adherence	Establish trust. Identify reasons for lack of adherence. Clarify misinformation. Use formal and informal contracting.

The average length of stay for all clients in acute care settings has decreased significantly in the past 10 years. Postpartum client stay has decreased from 5 days to 24 hours. Many procedures that used to be performed in the acute care setting are now performed on an outpatient basis. Consequently, time for teaching is now grossly limited in the acute care setting.

Women in the immediate postpartum period are not receptive to learning (Rubin, 1984). The typical postpartum client who has just delivered is not ready to learn because of normal physical and psychological conditions of the postpartum status. Seventy-two hours after delivery, mothers are in a stage where they need reinforcement from professionals. Now, because of early discharge, 72 hours falls after they have left the hospital and are at home. As a result of the unreadiness to learn and the shortened stay, almost no learning or teaching occurs. In addition, the recent trend to limit postpartum stay to 24 hours has resulted in an increased incidence of serious complications for newborns. These complications include an increase in hyperbilirubinemia and dehydration, which frequently require hospitalization or clinic follow-up. Inadequate breastfeeding and weight loss have also resulted from early postpartum discharge.

Clients may speak a language different from the nurse's or have sight, comprehension, or retention problems. Suggestions for communicating with these clients are given in the Community-Based Nursing Care Guidelines boxes.

A major area of discharge teaching that has been identified as problematic is compliance with medications after discharge. Numerous studies have shown a high rate of nonadherence with the medication regimen after discharge from an inpatient setting. This may result in rehospitalization, clinic follow-up, or admission to home care. Comprehensive discharge teaching regarding medication management at home prevents or reduces this problem. Strategies to help clients get full benefit from drug therapy are shown in Box 6–7. As the primary client educator, the nurse is in a vital position to promote adherence to prescribed treatment regimens.

Discharge teaching does not always result in good learning. Timing is an issue, because readiness to learn may be impeded by physical or psychological conditions. Retention of information is often a problem. Compliance with the nursing regimen is another. Cultural differences between the nurse and the client may also interfere with effective discharge teaching. These barriers to successful discharge planning and possible nursing interventions are summarized in Table 6–4.

SUCCESSFUL TEACHING

The first and most essential component of successful teaching is building a trusting relationship with the client and family. As trust is built, barriers to accurate communication between the nurse and the client and family are removed. This results in increased client adherence to the prescribed regimen and enhanced learning (Riley & Theilan, 1999). It is important that the nurse and client jointly determine the learning plan. Joint planning leads to better adherence to treatment regimens. This process requires forming a partnership, building an alliance, and working together toward a shared goal. It takes time to build trust and know the client, but this is the only way to individualize care (London, 1999). Strategies for better adherence to treatment regimens are shown in Box 6–8. A discharge teaching program that is successful in overcoming many of the barriers to successful teaching is shown in Research Box 6–1.

Meticulous documentation is an essential component of a successful discharge teaching program. Methods of documentation vary, but the trend is toward

COMMUNITY-BASED NURSING CARE GUIDELINES

Providing Health Information to a Client or Family Member with English as a Second Language

- Listen carefully to what the client and family is telling you. Present one idea at a time, use simple, uncomplicated sentences, and use concrete examples to enhance learning.
- Assess the client's and family members' understanding of the illness being treated.
- Include the client and family in the plan of care.
- Assess the client's and family members' understanding of the agreed-on treatment plan.
- Use materials printed in the client's or family members' first language, when possible.
- Validate the correct use of folk medicines and home remedies. Be aware of and discuss the contraindications for concurrent use of medications with the client and family.

Adapted from Wilson, A., & Robledo, L. (1999). Listening to Hispanic mothers: Guidelines for teaching. *Journal of Society of Pediatric Nurses, 4*(3), 125–127.

COMMUNITY-BASED NURSING CARE GUIDELINES

Working With Interpreters

- Determine the language the client speaks at home.
- Use qualified, professional interpreters.
- Avoid using interpreters from rival tribes, states, regions, or nations.
- Use an interpreter of the same gender as the client, if possible. In general, an older interpreter is preferred to a younger interpreter.
- Allow enough time for the interpreted session.
- Look directly at the client, addressing your questions to him or her.
- Speak in a normal tone of voice, clearly and slowly, using words and not just gestures.
- Keep your sentences simple and short; pause often to permit interpretation.
- Ask only one question at a time.
- Give the interpreter freedom to interrupt for clarification.
- Ask the interpreter to take notes if needed when the interview gets too complex.
- Be prepared to repeat yourself, use different words, rephrase as necessary for understanding. Be patient.
- Use the simplest vocabulary; avoid slang, jargon, and unfamiliar medical terminology.
- Check to see if the information has been understood. Have the interpreter tell you what the client has said he or she understands. Be direct and expect directness.

Adapted from Andrews, M., & Boyle, J. (1999). *Transcultural concepts in nursing care* (p. 40). Philadelphia: Lippincott Williams & Wilkins.

COMMUNITY-BASED NURSING CARE GUIDELINES

Communicating With Clients With Special Needs

Strategies for Visually Impaired Clients
- Speak to the client when approaching.
- Avoid speaking from behind the client.
- Identify yourself by saying your name or gently touching the client to alert him or her to your presence.
- Ask other people in the room to introduce themselves—this allows the client to hear each person's voice.
- Describe the room and the position of furniture to familiarize the client with the surroundings.
- Explain procedures precisely.
- Inform the client when you are leaving the room; let the client know what you are doing and where you are located at all times.
- Use adaptive devices for the partially impaired client such as large-print materials (telephone dials, thermostat dials) and a magnifying glass.

Strategies for Hearing Impaired Clients
- Provide a well-lit environment.
- Face the client; speak slowly and deliberately.
- When entering a room, place yourself in front of the client so he or she can see you, or lightly touch the client.
- Always ask if the client uses a hearing aid and if it is working properly; ask if the client needs assistance with inserting the hearing aid and if he or she wears the aid.
- Ask the client if he or she desires an auditory amplifier in the telephone, a TDD telecommunications device for the hearing impaired, or a light on the telephone to alert client of a caller.
- Write down points you make and give the list to the client.

Strategies for Clients With Speech and Language Deficits (Aphasia)
- Provide services for communication such as a letter board so the client can spell words, word boards (nurse or client points to word), picture charts (nurse or client points to object), or a computer.
- Be patient; supply needed support when the client falters in communication attempts.
- Provide regular mental stimulation.
- Praise all efforts and encourage practicing what is learned in treatment.

Adapted from Anderson, C. (1990). *Patient teaching and communication in an information age.* Albany, NY: Delmar; Arnold, . & Boggs, . (1995). *Interpersonal relationships. Professional communication skills for nurses* (2nd ed.). Philadelphia: Saunders.

the use of clinical pathways that outline teaching needs by diagnosis or procedure and include learning outcomes, content, methods, and strategies for teaching. Successful discharge teaching also involves care of the client in the context of the community. Careful assessment of the family, their culture, and the community environment can result in a comprehensive teaching plan. Discharge teaching objectives must focus on all levels of prevention. Continuity of teaching strengthens discharge teaching and improves outcomes.

▶ **Box 6–7.** Effective Medication Counseling: 26 Steps ◀

1. Explain the purpose of the counseling session.
2. Obtain pertinent initial drug-related information (eg, allergies, other medications, age).
3. Warn client about taking other medications, including over-the-counter medications, herbals/botanicals, and alcohol, that could inhibit or interact with the prescribed medication.
4. Assess the client's understanding of the reason(s) for therapy.
5. Assess any actual and/or potential concerns or problems of importance to the client.
6. Discuss the name (generic and trade) and indication of the medication.
7. Explain the dosage regimen, including scheduling and duration of therapy, when appropriate.
8. Assist the client in developing a plan to incorporate the medication regimen into his or her daily routine.
9. Explain how long it will take for the drug to show an effect.
10. Discuss storage recommendations and ancillary instructions (shake well, refrigerate, etc).
11. Inform client when/if the medication is to be refilled.
12. Emphasize the benefits of completing the medication as prescribed.
13. Discuss potential (significant) side effects.
14. Discuss how to prevent or manage the side effects of the drug should they occur.
15. Discuss precautions (activities to avoid, etc).
16. Discuss significant drug–drug, drug–food and drug–disease interactions.
17. Explain in precise terms what the client should do if a dose is missed.
18. Explore with the client potential problems in taking the medication as prescribed.
19. Use language that the client is likely to understand.
20. Use appropriate aids to enhance teaching.
21. Respond with understanding/empathy.
22. Use open-ended questions.
23. Display effective nonverbal behaviors.
24. Verify that the client understands via feedback.
25. Summarize by acknowledging and/or emphasizing key points of information.
26. Provide an opportunity for final concerns or questions.

———. (2000). Effective medication counseling: 26 Steps. *Home Healthcare Nurse, 18*(3), 157–160.

Teaching in the Community-Based Setting

BARRIERS TO SUCCESSFUL TEACHING

A number of barriers to successful teaching in community-based care exist (Table 6–5). These barriers interrupt the coordination of and consistency in teaching and communication with the caregiving team.

The primary difference between teaching in the acute care setting and the community-based setting is the need for independent decision making in the unstructured community-based setting. The nurse's role changes from client care manager to health care facilitator. Because of this difference, nurses may feel as if they have lost control of outcomes. The nurse has to focus on enhancing self-care for the client rather than giving care to the client, which is the norm within the structured context of the acute care setting.

Client resistance to following the treatment regimen is a barrier to successful teaching in the home. Nursing students often express dismay over their di-

> **► Box 6–8.** Steps to Improve Treatment Adherence ◄

Assess for potential problems

- Past adherence issues
- Presence of psychological stress
- Present knowledge base

Start teaching during hospitalization

- Review medications during each administration
- Begin discharge planning at admission
- Introduce self to family members at admission

Discuss typical schedule at home and requirements of treatment

- Determine how regimen can fit into typical schedule

Promote self-monitoring

- Include family in teaching
- Use techniques to enhance compliance (eg, calendar, pamphlets, teaching sheets, phone numbers)

Follow-up after discharge

- Follow-up phone call
- Referral to home care follow-up

Adapted from Dunbar-Jacob, J. (1999). Five steps to better treatment adherence. *Nursing 99, 29*(11), 32hm14.

minished control of client behavior when providing care in settings other than the acute care setting. For instance, teaching in the home often requires adaptation to the particular home environment with the client in control.

The need to bring all necessary supplies to the home interferes with to successful teaching. Unlike the acute care or inpatient setting where all teaching supplies are on the unit, teaching in the home requires the nurse to carry a supply of teaching materials.

Another barrier relates to difficulty in coordinating client teaching among multiple providers. Often, many care providers are involved with the client's care. Other professionals may include other nurses, physical therapists, social workers, home health aides, nurse practitioners, and physicians. It is difficult to maintain ongoing communication among multiple caregivers in several diverse settings.

Wide age variations among clients and family members create differences in cognitive and developmental levels. This makes teaching difficult in community-based nursing. Further, most home care clients are older; consequently their particular learning needs are different. Cultural barriers also impede successful teaching in the community-based setting.

Lack of time is also a barrier to home care teaching. The time factor in acute care settings may prohibit teaching, and many home care referrals come from clinics or physicians' offices. As a result, the first teaching, in many cases, may be done in the home. Home care nurses are also pressed for time. It may be difficult for the home care nurse to feel teaching is ever complete or even adequate.

SUCCESSFUL TEACHING

As in the acute care setting, the first and most essential component of successful teaching is building a trusting relationship with the client and family. Successful

RESEARCH RELATED TO COMMUNITY-BASED NURSING CARE

Research Box 6–1 ▶ Teaching Video Effect on Renal Transplant Patient Outcome

This study was undertaken to test the effect of a teaching video on renal transplant recipient outcomes. Previous investigations of the efficacy of videos in educational programs identified benefits as (1) the ability to provide large amounts of consistent information in an interesting, nonthreatening way, (2) the opportunity to replay as needed, and (3) convenience.

A quasi-experimental, pretest/posttest design was used with a sample of 62 adult patients admitted to the study hospital's organ transplant unit. One group was taught in the traditional fashion, whereas the experimental group had unlimited access to the video. Patients unable to read English and those who did not have primary responsibility for their own care management after discharge were excluded.

The study found that use of a teaching video with patients undergoing renal transplantation significantly increased posttransplantation knowledge of care delivery regimens. The video maximized learning with greater retention of information provided during routine patient teaching efforts. Differences in long-term outcomes were less evident. There were no differences for hospital readmission rate or for frequency and type of postdischarge patient/family phone contact.

According to the author, this study demonstrates that videos can serve as an excellent adjunct to teaching for renal transplantation patients. There is a need for additional research to demonstrate the impact of this teaching method on long-term outcomes in patients with families.

Giacoma, T., Ingersoll, G., & Williams, M. (1999). Teaching video effect on renal transplant patient outcome. *American Nephrology Nurses's Association Journal, 26*(1), 29–41.

teaching also requires the nurse to function as the interdisciplinary team member who furnishes a link between the referral source and community-based setting. The nurse has the responsibility of being the client's advocate, providing a critical communication channel between community organizations and providers who are members of the team. Coordinating communication among many care providers ensures

COMMUNITY-BASED NURSING CARE GUIDELINES

Characteristics of Successful Discharge Teaching

- Use varied teaching techniques.
- Provide a follow-up visit.
- Plan telephone calls after discharge to review learning objectives.
- Provide hands-on practice before discharge.
- Structure home visit to reduce anxiety and enhance learning.
- Promote self-care.
- Provide link between acute care facility and community-based care.

TABLE 6–5 • Combating Barriers to Successful Home Teaching

Barriers	Sample Nursing Interventions
Home Environment	
Examples:	Involve client and family in all stages of planning.
Home setting is nonstructured.	Build trusting relationship with client and family,
Environment is the client's and	maintaining respect for family's culture and
family's home turf.	values.
Equipment and setting are	Adapt the home environment to facilitate learning
inadequate for teaching.	and compliance.
Nurse Caregiver	
Examples:	Approach the client with a nonjudgmental attitude.
Nurse has less control over the	Acquire specific knowledge and skill in community-
outcomes of the teaching.	based care.
Nurse may have inadequate	Plan and organize ahead and bring all supplies.
preparation for providing	Facilitate communication and documentation
teaching in the home.	among caregivers.
Nurse must bring all the teaching	Focus on enhancing client's self-care
supplies along to the home.	instead of providing care to the client.
Nurse must coordinate patient	
teaching among many providers.	
Nurse role shifts from patient care	
manager to health care facilitator.	
Client/Family/Recipient of Teaching	
Examples:	Carefully assess learning need, learning
Wide variation in family members'	readiness, and past learning experiences of all
ages and cognitive and develop-	recipients of teaching. Involve family and client
mental stages	in all stages of planning and teaching.
Lack of adherence unless client/	
family are involved in the teaching	
plan	

▶ Box 6–9. Facilitating Successful Teaching Through Ongoing Communication ◀

Encourage the client to schedule the follow-up telephone call or office visit. Have the client write down the name of the contact person at the clinic or pharmacy, or other appropriate caregiver.

Keep the health care provider informed regarding any progress, or lack of it, when a new medication or treatment is started.

Be sure to identify any unexpected effects of treatment or drug interactions, even if they appear to be minor.

Encourage clients to ask questions until they understand what they need to know. Emphasize that there are no "stupid questions" regarding a client's health.

In asking the questions, have the client insist on answers in "layman's terms" in the most basic form of language used to communicate with any health care provider.

Adapted from Long, C., Ismeurt, R., & White, P. (1999). Preventing drug interactions in the home: A five-step approach for client teaching. *Home Healthcare Nurse, 17*(2), 106–112.

consistency in teaching and reinforcement of learning and enhances continuity of care. Ongoing communication is the foundation of good teaching and the key to maintaining safe, effective care. Following the suggestions in Box 6–9 can foster communication and enhance continuity and learning (Long, Ismeurt, & White, 1999).

Frequently, clients and family caregivers may only need reinforcement that the client is progressing normally in the recovery process. In these situations the focus should include care for the caregiver as well as care for the client. Affirming the quality of care provided by the family caregiver by listening to the concerns and frustrations of the caregiver should be a priority of the nurse. Other interventions to combat barriers to successful home teaching are seen in Table 6–5.

An advantage to teaching in the home is the reduction of anxiety in the learner. One of the basic principles of teaching is that when anxiety is reduced, learning is enhanced. The client is on "home turf" and has more control of the environment and the situation, thus helping to lessen anxiety (Fig. 6–3). As part of the original and ongoing assessment process, the nurse assesses the learner's anxiety level. If the learner exhibits anxiety that is interrupting learning, the learning plan must be modified. It is also important to plan lessons that include "digestible" segments that build on information shared in previous teaching sessions.

A study examined the effect of home nursing visits on parental anxiety and cardiopulmonary resuscitation (CPR) knowledge retention with parents of apnea-monitored infants. The use of structured home nursing visits was evaluated for its effect on parental anxiety and their retention of CPR knowledge. One group of parents received at-home teaching sessions; the second group was taught in the inpatient setting. The results showed a greater decrease in anxiety scores and maintained or improved CPR scores for the group that was taught at home (Komelasky, 1990).

Successful teaching promotes self-care. Home nursing visits increase client and family compliance with both appointments and medication management. In the home, the nurse can vary the environment and timing of instruction. The caregiver also has an opportunity to discuss fears and stresses, and the nurse has an opportunity to assess the caregiver for cultural tendencies, past experiences, and coping ability (Komelasky, 1990).

Behaviorally oriented client education, which emphasizes a change of envi-

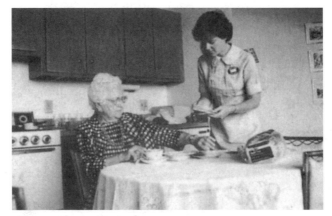

Figure 6–3. ▶ A teaching/learning experience in the home often is more successful because the client is in his or her own territory. The nurse is responsible for teaching and coordinating care.

ronment to facilitate client self-care, is the most successful method for improving the clinical course of chronic disease. In addition, behavioral education contributes to care's being more easily managed in the home. An example is rearranging furniture so that it is in the field of vision for a client with hemianopsia.

Although changing the environment can enhance self-care, this must be accomplished within the context of the client's and family's value system. When the nurse provides teaching in the context of their values and norms, learning is enhanced. Because care in the home is provided on the client's and family's "turf," it is particularly important to consider what the family values are when formulating a teaching plan.

Successful Teaching Techniques

Because of the increased workload of the nurse, decreasing length of stay in the acute care setting, and limited visits in home care, teaching time is limited. The nurse needs to be familiar with a variety of teaching techniques and be competent in choosing which technique is most suitable for the circumstance.

For example, demonstration of a new skill is used to change behavior, whereas videotapes are used to increase knowledge. Video use supplements one-on-one and group teaching. Videos can be viewed several times by anyone with access to a videotape player.

Many acute care settings use closed-circuit television for successful teaching programs and to reinforce learning. Before discharge, the client and family or caregiver may watch programs several times if reinforcement is necessary. The videotape can be used the same way in the home.

Learning is always enhanced by use of a variety of methods. Successful teaching strategies include showing as well as telling. Much teaching occurs while the nurse is providing client care—taking blood pressure or a temperature, giving a bath, examining a newborn or infant, weighing the client, and changing wound dressings. Client education seldom is the formal process one experiences in a classroom.

A variety of teaching methods and materials are available. Some of them are listed in Box 6–10. Choices depend on the developmental level of the client, the avail-

---

▶ **Box 6–10.** Sampling of Teaching Techniques ◀

One-on-one teaching
Group teaching
Self-evaluation/worksheet
Discussions/questions
Explanations/examples
Demonstrations/return demonstrations
Charts/graphs/diagrams
Pictures/photos/picture cards
Reading materials (pamphlets/books)
Role modeling/role playing
Audiovisuals (computer programs/movies/slides/TV/videotapes)
Equipment (such as catheters/tubing/port/monitors)
Models (such as fetus and uterine models/breast models)
Web page and Internet
Games
Health fairs

ability of materials, the setting for the educational opportunity, the time available for teaching, and the nurse's abilities to use various methods. In addition, teaching methods have to be acceptable and nonthreatening to the client and family or caregiver.

Actual equipment and objects can be used for effective teaching, including the catheter, tubing, port, monitor, or other devices. Picture cards can be made to illustrate each item in a procedure. Photos can be made of each key step or diagrams drawn for the cards. Quizzes can be developed with short statements related to the procedure in true or false categories. The nurse can design posters with information the client needs to learn. Worksheets can be developed to use with a videotape or audiotape.

A new teaching method for health education is the use of Web sites on the Internet. For example, one innovative program provides presurgical preparation for adolescent clients prior to tonsillectomy and adenoidectomy. Interactive content provides preparation without the client having to leave the home (O'Conner-Von, 2000). This method could be used for any type of teaching for clients who are computer literate and have access to a computer at home, school, or the public library.

Client teaching requires a therapeutic relationship, built on trust. Even Florence Nightingale recognized this. Furthermore, nurses may encourage clients to improve their health status, but the final choice is the client's. No matter how important the nurse feels certain actions are, the decision is the client's.

Teaching the Challenging Client

When the teaching plan is unsuccessful, special teaching strategies are used. Strategies include the use of good interpersonal communication, problem-solving, and contracting skills. Common reasons why clients do not follow treatment regimens are listed in Box 6–11. It is important to ascertain why the client is not following the prescribed treatment. The first problem-solving technique that can be used is to ask the client about his or her perception of progress made with the teaching plan. Once the etiology is identified, the nurse can tailor interventions accordingly. Etiology may stem from factors related to the client, home environment, or the teaching plan itself.

THE CLIENT

In some cases, client anxiety or fear may impede learning. Before any teaching occurs, the nurse must address the anxiety or fear of the learner. Learning needs

---

▶ **Box 6–11.** Common Reasons Why a
Client Does Not Follow the Treatment Plan ◀

Common Causes

- Lack of information
- Lack of skill
- Lack of valuing the treatment regimen
- Anxiety or fear

Barriers to Compliance

- Client factors
- Home environment
- Teaching plan

may come from lack of information. This learning need is easily met by identifying and providing information. Noncompliance may result from lack of skills. The nurse can encourage the client and provide opportunities to practice these skills, resulting in enhanced skill.

The nurse, however, may interpret a learning need as an impediment, when the client's behavior simply reflects the values and attitudes of the client and the client's community. If lack of adherence stems from the client's attitudes and values, the appropriate intervention is different from interventions used when it arises from lack of information. Lack of adherence will result if the client does not value the treatment. Consequently, the nurse must address this lack of valuing by attempting to modify the teaching regimen to better fit the client's value system. The revised learning plan that reflects the client's value system will differ based on whether it is lack of knowledge, skill, confidence, fear, or values. On the other hand, no individual is totally compliant. The nurse must use professional judgment to gauge what level of adherence to treatment is acceptable.

THE HOME ENVIRONMENT

Behaviorally oriented client education, which emphasizes the change of the environment in which the client does self-care, is often the most successful strategy. Changing the home environment is credited with improving the clinical course of clients instructed in the home. Careful assessment of the home environment allows the nurse to identify and modify problematic issues and enhance learning outcomes. These interventions may be as simple as providing better light for a teaching session by opening the drapes, moving a lamp, or replacing a burned-out light bulb.

THE TEACHING PLAN

Effective teaching requires sound interpersonal skills. First and foremost, a trusting relationship must be established among the nurse, client, and involved family members. As in all therapeutic relationships, the nurse in community-based care must avoid personal bias. When care is provided in the client's home, the nurse's nonjudgmental attitude is essential.

Contracting is important to effective teaching. The nurse and the client can set a contract at the first visit and each subsequent visit. Contracting can be done at the beginning of a therapeutic relationship through use of both formal and informal techniques. This may prevent some noncompliance from the onset. Most agencies have formal contracts such as a "Bill of Rights" or "Client Responsibilities." Review and implementation of the content of these standards on the first visit is one way to encourage compliance with all clients and their families.

The most logical resolution for clients who are not following treatment is to set up a mutual plan of action for adherence to the treatment plan. This can be accomplished through use of a learning contract, such as the one shown in Box 6–12. A learning contract may include a date, names of those involved, specific expected behaviors, date of achievement, action that will be taken if the contract is not followed, and the date and signatures of those involved. Informal and short-term contracting on each visit is beneficial and encourages compliance.

Clients and families who do not comply with the teaching regimen may be assisted through the establishment of a trusting relationship, formal and informal contracting, and a thorough assessment of the factors that contribute to noncompliance. If the nurse follows the principles of community-based nursing, learning will be enhanced.

▶ **Box 6–12.** Sample Learning Contract ◀

Steve Hunt agrees to monitor his blood sugar by using the One Touch monitor at 8:00 AM and 6:00 PM for 1 week from June 1 through June 8, 2002. If this contract is not abided by, Best Home Healthcare will discharge Steve Hunt back to Dr. Berger of Neighborhood Clinics. This discharge relieves Best Home Healthcare from any further responsibility for the care of Steve Hunt.

Signed _____

Date _____

Signed by Case Manager _____

Date _____

Teaching Related to Levels of Prevention

Teaching, whether it is in the acute care or community-based setting, occurs at all levels of prevention. An important goal of teaching is to prevent the initial occurrence of disease or injury through health promotion and prevention activities. Secondary prevention is teaching targeted toward early identification and intervention of a condition. The teaching of tertiary prevention focuses on restoration of health and facilitation of the individual's and family's skills for coping with an existing condition.

An important focus of teaching is the prevention of the initial occurrence of disease or injury through health promotion and prevention activities. A nurse teaching a nutrition class to parents and day care providers is an example of health promotion. A school nurse teaching parents about preventing childhood injuries is focusing on health protection. Teaching parents and day care providers about the importance of immunization is primary prevention, as is teaching about community resources that provide free or inexpensive immunization.

Teaching secondary prevention helps to point out the early identification and intervention of a condition. A home care nurse teaching the parents of a ventilator-dependent child about early signs of upper respiratory infection and when to contact the nurse on call is focusing on secondary prevention.

Most teaching in the home setting addresses tertiary prevention because most home care clients have chronic conditions. Tertiary prevention arises from teaching that attempts to restore health and facilitate coping skills (Fig. 6–4). The home care nurse may teach family members with a ventilator-dependent child the importance of handwashing in preventing the spread of pathogens and

COMMUNITY-BASED NURSING CARE GUIDELINES

Interventions Used With the Client Who Does Not Follow the Treatment Plan

- Establish a trusting relationship.
- Contract at each visit.
- Identify the etiology of the noncompliance.
- Use a learning contract for specific problems.

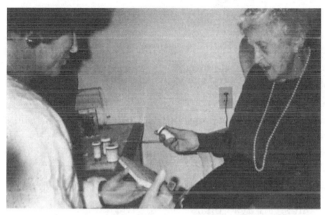

Figure 6-4. ▶ Tertiary prevention involves helping restore the client to health. On this visit, the nurse uses a weekly medication container to help an older woman with limited vision devise a plan for compliance in taking her medications.

upper respiratory infections. Older clients with a new diagnosis of diabetes require a great deal of instruction in changing the diet, handling syringes, giving themselves injections, and measuring their blood sugar. Teaching family or caregivers about community resources that are available for respite care facilitates coping skills and falls in the category of tertiary prevention.

Evaluation

The last phase of the teaching and learning process is evaluation. Both learning and teaching are evaluated to determine if the learning outcomes were met and if the teaching methods were effective. The plan is then modified as necessary.

Learning is evaluated by deciding if the learning outcomes were met. The following questions may be asked to assess the level of learning:

What additional data do I need to collect to evaluate the progress made toward the learning objectives?

What other learning needs apply to this client and family?

Were the objectives met? If not, why not?

How do I know that my client learned what I planned to teach?

Did the timing of the teaching impede or enhance learning?

Is the nurse, client, or family satisfied with the outcome? If not, what would provide satisfaction?

Second, evaluation of teaching appraises the efficacy of the teaching plan and methods. Evaluation of teaching considers the barriers to, and characteristics of, successful teaching. The nurse may ask:

Did the teaching focus on the most important problem for this family in relation to the potential of the client for self-care?

Was the plan collaborative?

Was there reinforcement?

Was the home environment appropriate? If not, how was it modified?

Was the equipment adequate?

Was the nurse prepared?

Did the nurse use a variety of teaching methods?

Did the learner have the opportunity for hands-on practice?

Was the visit structured to reduce anxiety and enhance learning?

Was the teaching plan realistic?

Were the learning objectives, teaching plan, and methods realistic and appropriate for this client and family?

Were the family strengths considered when determining the learning objectives and teaching methods?

If this session were to be repeated, which strategies or tools could be used?

Evaluation must always consider what the client and family believe they need to know as well as what the nurse considers essential. It is also important for the nurse to recognize when the learning needs of the client, family or caregiver are beyond the educational preparation of the nurse so that a referral to appropriate resources can be made.

Documentation

Documentation of teaching is essential (1) as a legal record, (2) as communication of teaching and learning to other health care professionals, and (3) for determination of eligibility for care needed and for reimbursement of care provided. The following parts of the teaching process should be documented:

▶ Assessment of the learner's readiness, need, and life experiences
▶ Identification of learning needs
▶ Identification of barriers to successful learning
▶ Plan for teaching and learning outcomes
▶ Content taught
▶ Teaching techniques used
▶ Evaluation of teaching and learning including learner response and recommendations for the next step

An additional component of documentation is confidentiality.

COMMUNITY-BASED NURSING CARE GUIDELINES

Confidentiality

- Maintain confidentiality in consultation, teaching, and writing.
- Ensure privacy before engaging in a discussion of content to be entered into the record.
- Release information only with written consent.
- Use professional judgment regarding confidentiality when the information may be harmful to the client's health or well-being.
- Use professional judgment when deciding how to maintain the privacy of a minor. Be aware of your state's legal ramifications of the parent's or guardian's right to know.

EXAMPLE OF A CLIENT SITUATION

Teaching in the Home Setting

Assessment

Kathy is the home care nurse assigned to care for Ina, a 76-year-old widow recently diagnosed with insulin-dependent diabetes. Friday, November 1, Ina visited the clinic with complaints of polyuria, polydipsia, and polyphagia. Her blood sugar was 456 mg/dL. The clinic educator saw her on November 1 and charted the following on the referral form:

Client stated, "I have not slept well for 2 weeks because I have to get up so often to go to the bathroom." After the initial teaching session, which covered the basics of the diabetic diet and the action of insulin, the client was unable to demonstrate retention of knowledge or skill from any of the topics covered.

Recommendation to home care: Client requires diabetic teaching in the areas of diabetic diet, drawing up of insulin and giving injections, and monitoring blood sugar. Client will receive insulin in the clinic until home visit on Tuesday to teach about injections.

Reimbursement: This client requires teaching to manage home treatment of insulin-dependent diabetes diagnosed on 11/1/02. This teaching meets the criteria of Section 205.13 of Medicare Guidelines for Coverage of Services Revision 222.

On Tuesday, November 5, Kathy visits Ina at home. Ina greets Kathy at the door with the statement, "When I was at the clinic on Friday I was so nervous about all of the things they were telling me, but I am more relaxed today. I talked to my friend Richard who is a diabetic and manages really well. When my granddaughter Karen was a little girl I gave her shots and got along just fine."

Ina's home is very dark so Kathy asks if she can open the drapes and move two chairs closer to the window before they start to talk. Kathy begins visiting with Ina and attempts to begin developing a trusting relationship. Kathy learns that Ina has some knowledge about diabetes from talking to her friend Richard and she has also asked her son Mark, who is a nurse, to pick up some pamphlets about diabetes at the hospital.

Ina states that she learns best by doing. She does not drive but states that her son will be able to pick up her medication and syringes, or she can take the bus to the pharmacy. Kathy notices a magnifying glass on the table and a large-print book on a bookshelf. Kathy asks Ina about her vision. She responds that she has had three cataract surgeries and has difficulty reading so she frequently uses the magnifying glass.

Kathy concludes that Ina sees a need to learn and is ready to learn. Kathy also believes that Ina's past experiences will enhance her learning, not impede it. Concerned about Ina's restricted vision, Kathy makes a note to continue to assess this aspect. At this point Kathy completes the Learning Assessment Guide, as shown in Box 6–13.

Identification of Learning Need

Kathy and Ina conclude that Ina's overall learning need is:

Risk for Injury *related to lack of knowledge regarding diabetic self-care*

For this visit Kathy concludes that the priority need is:

Risk for Injury *related to client's lack of knowledge and inability to manage diabetes for the next 24 hours until the home visit the next day, as manifested by visual impairment*

Planning

Kathy and Ina decide that the learning objectives for today will be:

1. Cognitive objective: Client will state when insulin is given and how much to draw up by the end of the visit on 11/5.
2. Psychomotor objective: Client will identify three sites for subcutaneous injection of insulin and demonstrate proper techniques for injection by the end of the visit on 11/5.
3. Affective objective: Client will state she is comfortable injecting insulin by the end of the visit on 11/5.

► **Box 6–13.** Sample Learning Assessment Guide ◄

Client name *Ina*

Health condition requiring health education *Insulin-dependent diabetes diagnosed on November 1, 2002.*

Primary caregiver *Home care nurse, client, and Mark*

Learner *Ina* _____ Relationship to client _____

Age *76* ___ Gender *Female* ___ Occupation *retired legal secretary*

Developmental Stages and Implications for Learner

   Psychosocial stage— *The client is in the integrity vs. ego despair stage. She describes her life as*
"I have been blessed, I have 10 wonderful children, 25 grand and 10 great-grandchildren. I loved my
work after my kids grew up. My husband and I had a good relationship."

   Cognitive stage— *No evidence of cognitive impairment*

   Language— *Speaks English, visual impairment, stated "I was writing a novel about Ireland until I started to*
have problems with my eyes."

How does the caregiver or client feel about the responsibilities of self-care

   States she is more relaxed than 11/1 when diagnosed.

Describe any disabilities or limitations of the learner (including sensory disabilities)

   Visual impairment and statement "I am afraid that I will not be able to see the numbers on the syringes."
   Disabilities—arthritis in left knee and left hip

Describe any preexisting health conditions of the learner

   Client has had multiple cataract surgery and has visual impairment.

List sociocultural factors that may impede learning *None*

(continued)

► **Box 6–13.** Sample Learning Assessment Guide *(Continued)* ◄

State learner behaviors that indicate motivation to learn

Client stated she was more relaxed about her diagnosis, asked her son to get information about diabetes,

contacted a friend with diabetes.

Can the learner read and comprehend at the reading level required by the task?

Yes, but may not have visual acuity to see the calibration on the syringe.

Does the learner show an ability to problem solve at a level that provides safe care in the home?

Client has managed health problems in her home with her granddaughter's illness 10 years ago.

Is the home environment conducive to the learning required by the care?

Home is very dark with poor lighting.

If not, what modifications are necessary? *Need better lighting in the kitchen.*

If the learner is not able to carry out the care, are other caregivers available for backup support?

Yes

If so, please name. *Mark (son), Karen (granddaughter), Richard (friend)*

Phone number *555-5555*

Address *3400 Belmont, White Kitty Lake*

What other support is available for the client and caregiver? *Client has ten children,*

three who live in the area. Client is active in her church, which has a parish nurse and a befriender program.

There is a support group for newly diagnosed diabetics, which meets at a hospital near client's home. Client lives

on the bus line with service to the clinic, hospital, and church.

Implementation

1. Cognitive objective: Client will state when insulin is given and how much to draw up by the end of the visit on 11/5.

Together Kathy and Ina review the written material on insulin, when it is given and how much to draw up. Kathy proceeds at a slow pace as she teaches, repeats the information frequently, and does not rush Ina. The teaching sheet is on white, nonglossy paper with bold, black print. After the teaching session, Ina states, "Insulin should be given before meals and as the schedule states. I am to give myself insulin according to the schedule." Kathy leaves a videotape that covers the information in the teaching session.

2. Psychomotor objective: Client will identify three sites for subcutaneous injection of insulin and demonstrate proper technique for injection by the end of the visit on 11/5.

Kathy demonstrates injecting the insulin into a model and identifies three sites for subcutaneous injection. Then Ina injects into the model. Kathy draws up the insulin as ordered before dinner and Ina injects herself at 5:00.

Evaluation

Learning objectives 1 and 2 met: Ina identifies three sites for injection and injects herself correctly. Teaching was focused on the most important problem for this client, the plan was collaborative, and reinforcement was provided with a videotape. The learner had the opportunity for hands-on practice and a variety of teaching methods were used.

Implementation

3. Affective objectives: Client will state she is comfortable injecting insulin by the end visit on 11/5.

Ina discusses her feelings with Kathy regarding the teaching session. Kathy asks her if she feels comfortable giving herself an injection and she says. "No, but I think it will come." Kathy leaves a short videotape on injecting insulin for Ina to review before the next visit.

Evaluation

Learning objectives not met at this time.

Teaching: Kathy encourages Ina by stating how well she has done the first time handling the syringe. Kathy tells Ina specifically what she did well, that she did not hesitate before putting the needle in, and she found a correct site and charted it accurately on the flow sheet. She adds this objective to the list of the next lesson's objectives.

Assessment and Planning for Next Teaching Session

Kathy noted Ina's problems with her eyesight in the initial assessment, suggesting that Ina may have difficulty drawing up insulin with a syringe. Kathy discusses her concern with Ina and asks to come back the next day. She also asks Ina if there is a friend or family member who might be available to assist with her care. Ina responds that her son Mark has indicated that he is willing to help with the injections. Kathy requests that Ina contact Mark and ask that he be present at the next home visit.

Identification of Learning Need

Together, Kathy and Ina decide on the learning need for the home visit the next day:

Risk for Injury related to client's lack of knowledge and inability to read the calibration on the syringe as manifested by client statement, "I have to use the magnifying glass to see print. I can't see the numbers on the syringes. Is it OK if I just estimate?"

Planning

Kathy and Ina decide that the learning objectives for tomorrow will be:

1. Cognitive objective: Client will state when insulin is given, how much to draw up, and how to use magni-guide syringe.
2. Psychomotor objective: Client will demonstrate how to draw up accurate amount of insulin with magni-guide syringe.
3. Affective objective: Client will state that she feels confident in her ability to draw up accurate amount of insulin.

As Kathy leaves Ina's home Ina hugs her and says, "Thanks for all your help today. You have helped me so much!"

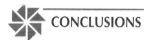

CONCLUSIONS

Because of circumstances in the current health care system, quality teaching has become essential. There are benefits to quality teaching in all settings. Good teaching improves client self-care and independence. Client, family, and staff satisfaction is improved if teaching results are positive. Another benefit to quality instruction is the more efficient use of resources.

Avoiding barriers and incorporating characteristics of successful teaching can enhance teaching in community-based nursing. Including learning theory in community-based teaching ensures quality instruction. Comprehensive assessment of the client and family safeguards accurate identification of learning needs. Collaborative planning preserves successful learning outcomes because clients and families are more likely to learn when they have participated in the planning. Following these principles protects the teaching process in community settings.

The first and most important goal of teaching in community-based care is to assist the client and family to achieve independence in self-care. Self-care is provided in the context of the values and resources of the client and family with a prevention focus. Continuity requires documentation and interdisciplinary communication, which augment teaching efficacy. Successful teaching in community-based care meets all of these goals.

References and Bibliography

————. (2000). Effective medication counseling: 26 steps. *Home Healthcare Nurse, 18*(3), 157–160.

Barry, C. (2000). Teaching the older client in the home: Assessment and adaptation. *Home Healthcare Nurse, 18*(6), 374–385.

Bennet, R., & Tandy, L. (1998). Postpartum home visits: Extending the continuum of care from hospital to home. *Home Healthcare Nurse, 16*(5), 295–303.

Beuscher, R. (1998). Community outreach: Foot care for the elderly—A winning proposition. *Home Healthcare Nurse, 16*(1), 27–44.

Biordi, D., & Theis, S. (1999). Work strategies of patients and families for care in the home. *Orthopaedic Nursing, 18*(2), 58–71.

Bowne, A. (1999). Using games to teach. *Journal of Emergency Nursing, 25*(5), 415–416.

Byrd, P., & Givens, K. (1996). Mutual goal setting with young women and a reduction in their extrinsic risk factors for osteoporosis. *Virginia Nurses Today, 4*(2), 28–29.

Carpenito, L. J. (2000). *Nursing diagnosis. Application to clinical practice* (8th ed.). Philadelphia: Lippincott Williams & Wilkins.

Cooper, J. (1999). Teaching patients in post-operative eyecare: The demands of day surgery. *Nursing Standard, 13*(32), 42–46.

Dunbar-Jacob, J. (1999). Five steps to better treatment adherence. *Nursing 99, 29*(11), 32hm14.

Giacoma, R., Ingersoll, G., & Williams, M. (1999). Teaching video effect on renal transplant patient outcomes. *ANNA Journal, 26*(1), 29–31.

Haynes, R, Montague, P., Oliver, T., Mckibbon, K., Brouwers, M., & Kanani, R. (2000). Interventions for helping patients to follow prescriptions for medications. *The Cochrane Library, 2*, 2000. Oxford: Update Software.

Jarvis, C. (1996). *Physical examination and health assessment* (2nd ed.). Philadelphia: Saunders.

Knox, A. B. (1985). *Helping adults learn—A planning guide: Implementation and conducting programs*. San Francisco: Jossey-Bass.

Komelasky, A. L. (1990). The effect of home nursing visits on parental anxiety and knowledge of parents of apnea monitored infants. *Journal of Pediatric Nursing, 5*(6), 387–392.

Kulbok, P., Gates, M., Vicenzi, A., & Schultz, P. (1999). Focus on community: Directions for nursing knowledge development. *Journal of Advanced Nursing, 29*(5), 1188–1196.

Leske, J., & Pelczynski, S. (1999). Caregiver satisfaction with preparation for discharge in a decreased-length-of-stay cardiac surgery program. *Journal of Cardiovascular Nursing, 14*(1), 35.

Lockhart, J., & Resick, L. (1997). Teaching cultural competence: The value of experiential learning and community resources. *Nurse Educator, 22*(3), 27–31.

London, F. (1999). *A nurse's guide to patient and family education*. Philadelphia: Lippincott Williams & Wilkins.

Long, C., Ismeurt, R., & White, P. (1999). Preventing drug interactions in the home: A five-step approach for client teaching. *Home Healthcare Nurse, 17*(2), 106–112.

Miller, C. (1999). *Nursing care of the older adult—Theory and practice* (3rd ed.). Philadelphia: Lippincott Williams & Wilkins.

O'Conner-Von, S. (2000). *Tonsils! Who needs them?* St. Paul, MN: Author.

Pillitteri, A. (1999). *Maternal and child health nursing: Care of the childbearing and childrearing family* (3rd ed.). Philadelphia: Lippincott Williams & Wilkins.

Rice, R. (1996). Patient education in the home. In R. Rice (Ed.). *Home health care nursing practice: Concepts and applications* (2nd ed.). St. Louis: Mosby–Year Book.

Riley, M., & Theilan, K. (1999). Attachment impacts a culturally diverse population in the homecare setting. *Journal of Intravenous Nursing, 22*(6), 325–330.

Rubin, R. (1961). Basic maternal behavior. *Nursing Outlook, 9,* 683–684.

Rutledge, D., & Donaldson, N. (1998). Improving readability of printed materials in patient care and health services. *Online Journal of Clinical Innovation, 1*(3), 1–27.

Stanley, M., & Beare, P. (1999). *Gerontological nursing: A health promotion/protection approach* (2nd ed.). Philadelphia: Davis.

Steps for effective medication counseling. (2000). *Home Healthcare Nurse, 18*(3), 157–160.

Stone, J., Wyman, J., & Salisbury, S. (1999). *Clinical gerontological nursing* (2nd ed.). Philadelphia: Saunders.

Taylor, C., Lillis, C., & LeMone, P. (1997). *Fundamentals of nursing: The art and science of nursing care*. Philadelphia: Lippincott-Raven.

U.S. Department of Health and Human Services. (2000). *Healthy people 2010: Understanding and improving health*. Washington, DC: U.S. Government Printing Office.

Weber, J. (1997). *Nurses' handbook of health assessment* (3rd ed.). Philadelphia: Lippincott-Raven.

Weissman, M., & Jasovsky, D. (1998). Discharge teaching for today's time. *RN, 61*(6), 38–43.

Whitehead, D. (1999). The application of health promotion in orthopaedic settings. *Journal of Orthopaedic Nursing, 3*(2), 101–107.

Wilson, A., & Robledo, L. (1999). Listening to Hispanic mothers: Guidelines for teaching. *Journal of the Society of Pediatric Nurses, 49*(3), 125–127.

LEARNING ACTIVITIES

LEARNING ACTIVITY 6-1

▶ **Client Care Study:** Teaching in Postpartum

Jennifer is a nurse working on a postpartum unit. She is caring for Joan, a 35-year-old primipara (NSVD), who delivered a boy yesterday and is going home at noon today. Joan states she has been working full-time since she graduated from law school. She is the youngest of three siblings. She and her husband Tim took prenatal classes, and she describes him as being very excited about the baby. Jennifer interviewed Joan and Tim to determine their learning needs. They both tell Jennifer that they are wondering about having their baby circumcised. They also wonder how they are going to take care of the surgery site after the procedure on their newborn. Joan had a sitz bath and pain medication 45 minutes ago. Both parents have good eye contact and relaxed postures as Jennifer interviewed them.

1. Determine the behaviors that show that Joan and Tim are ready to learn.
2. List the factors Jennifer should assess regarding Joan's and Tim's readiness to learn.
3. Recognize what indicates to Jennifer that Joan and Tim show a need to learn.
4. Examine Joan's and Tim's prior experience and knowledge base related to the topic.
5. Identify Joan and Tim's learning need in each domain: cognitive, affective, and psychomotor.
6. State one learning outcome for Joan and Tim for each learning need.
7. Discuss how the principles of community-based care apply to the learning needs of Joan and Tim.

LEARNING ACTIVITY 6-2

▶ **Practical Applications:** Applying Principles of Teaching and Learning

Hazel is a 65-year-old woman whose husband is blind and was recently diagnosed with early signs of dementia. Shannon is doing preadmission teaching with Hazel, who is scheduled for outpatient surgery tomorrow morning. Shannon knows it is important to assess Hazel's readiness to learn. If Hazel is thinking about her husband's care during the time she is preparing for surgery, she may not hear Shannon tell her that she should not drive or make important decisions for at least 24 hours after receiving general anesthesia

Explain how Shannon will assess Hazel's readiness to learn.

LEARNING ACTIVITY 6-3

▶ **Critical Thinking Exercise:** Self-Evaluation and Reflection

1. In your clinical journal, discuss a situation in your clinical experience in which you observed or were the caretaker for someone who had several teaching needs. Outline the process used to assess, plan, and teach the client and family members.
2. Using theory from this chapter, identify what was successful and what was not successful related to teaching and learning for this client and family.
3. What would you do differently next time? What did you learn about yourself and teaching clients and families from this experience?

Nursing Implications for Various Developmental Stages

Age	Physical Development	Language (Cognitive) Development (based on Piaget)	Psychosocial Development (based on Erikson)	Nurse's Approach to Assessment
Overview of birth to 1 y		*Sensorimotor stage of development*	*Development task: trust vs. mistrust.* Learns to trust and to anticipate satisfaction. Sends cues to mother/ caretaker. Begins understanding self as separate from others (body image).	Involve caretaker in assessment, eg, allow him or her to hold child in lap for parts of examination.
1–2 mo	Lifts chin and chest off bed. Holds extremities in flexion and moves at random; weak neck muscles. Activity varies between quiet sleep to drowsiness to alert activity.	Can discriminate between various sensations and prefers certain ones. Follows moving objects with eyes.	Begins to bond with mother during alert periods.	Conserve infant's body heat. Assess while asleep or quiet. Place infant on table or in caretaker's arms. Give bottle if awake.
3–4 mo	Head and back control developing. Holds rattle. Looks at own hands. Infant reflexes begin to disappear. Able to sit propped. Props self on forearm in prone position. Rolls from side to back and vice versa and from back to abdomen. Takes objects to mouth. Drools with eruption of lower teeth.	Responds to parent. Social smile. Begins to vocalize; coos, babbles. Locates sounds by turning head, looking.	Learns to signal displeasure. Shows excitement with whole body. Begins to discriminate strangers. Squeals.	Speak softly to infant. Use brightly colored toys, bells, rattles to elicit necessary responses and to distract. Assess ears, mouth, nose last. Assess lungs and heart when quiet.

(continued)

Age	Physical Development	Language (Cognitive) Development (based on Piaget)	Psychosocial Development (based on Erikson)	Nurse's Approach to Assessment
5–8 mo	Begins to develop teeth. Birth weight doubled. Grasps objects. Sits unsupported.	Begins to imitate sounds, two-syllable words (dada, mama). Responds to own name.	Increased fear of strangers. Definite likes/dislikes. Responds to "no."	Place on caretaker's lap (same as above).
9–12 mo	Birth weight tripled. Anterior fontanel nearly closed. Learns to pull in order to stand, creep, and crawl.	Says two words besides "dada, mama." Understands simple commands. Imitates animal sounds.	Looks for hidden objects. Unceasing determination to move about. Clings to mother. Shows emotion. Plays peek-a-boo and pat-a-cake.	
1–3 y	Begins to walk and run well. Drinks from cup, feeds self. Develops fine motor control. Climbs. Begin self-toileting. Kneels without support. Steady growth in height/weight. Adult height will be approximately double the height at age 2. Dresses self by age 3.	*Preoperational stage of development.* Has poor time sense. Increasing verbal ability. Formulates sentences of 4 to 5 words by age 3. Talks to self and others. Has misconceptions about cause and effect. Interested in pictures. *Fears:* • Loss/separation from parents —peak • Dark • Machines/ equipment • Intrusive procedures • Bedtime Speaks to dolls and animals. Increasing attention span. Knows own sex by age 3.	*Developmental task: autonomy vs. shame and doubt.* Establishes self-control, decision making, independence (autonomy). Extremely curious and prefers to do things himself. Demonstrates independence through negativism. Very egocentric; believes he or she controls the world. Attempts to please parents. Participates in parallel play; able to share some toys by age 3.	Be flexible. Begin assessment with play period to establish rapport. Be honest. Praise for cooperation. Begin slowly; speak to child. Involve caretaker/parent in holding on exam table. Let child hold security object. Allow child to play with stethoscope, tongue blade, flashlight before using on child if possible. Assess face, mouth, eyes, ears last. May need to restrain when lying prone. If resistant, save that part of the assessment for later.

(continued)

Age	Physical Development	Language (Cognitive) Development (based on Piaget)	Psychosocial Development (based on Erikson)	Nurse's Approach to Assessment
4–6 y	Growth slows. Loco-motion skills increase and co-ordination improves. Tricycle/bicycle riding. Throws ball but difficulty catching. Constantly active, increasing dexterity. Eruption of permanent teeth. Skips, hops, jumps rope.	*Preoperational/thought stage of development continues.* Language skills flourish. Generates many questions, eg, How, Why, What? Simple problem solving. Uses fantasy to understand and problem solve. *Fears* • Mutilation • Castration • Dark • Unknown • Inanimate • Unfamiliar objects Causality related to proximity of events. Enjoys mimicking and imitating adults.	*Developmental tasks: initiative vs. guilt.* Attempts to establish self like his or her parents, but independent. Explores environment on own initiative. Boasts, brags, has feelings of indestructibility. Family is primary social group. Peers increasingly important. Assumes sex roles. Aggressive, very curious. Enjoys activities such as sports, cooking, shopping. Cooperative play. Likes rules. May stretch the truth and tell large stories.	Establish rapport through talking and play. Introduce self to child. Have parent present but direct conversation to child. Games such as "follow the leader" and "Simon says" can be used to elicit necessary behaviors. Explain each assessment in simple language. Ask for child's help and use flattery. Use pictures, models, or items he or she can see or touch. Reserve genital examination for last; drape accordingly.
6–11 y	Moves constantly. Physical play prevalent; sports, swimming, skating, etc. Increased smoothness of movement. Grows at rate of 2 inches/7 lb a year. Eyes/hands well coordinated.	*Concrete operations stage of development.* Organized thought; memory concepts more complicated. Reads, reasons better. Focuses on concrete understanding. *Fears:* • Mutilation • Death • Immobility • Rejection • Failure	*Developmental task: industry vs. inferiority.* Learns to include values and skills of school, neighborhood, peers. Peer relationships important. Focuses more on reality, less on fantasy. Family is main base of security and identity. Sensitive to reactions of others. Seeks	Explain all procedures and impact on body. Encourage questioning and active participation in care. Be direct about explanation of procedures, based on what child will hear, see, smell,

(continued)

Age	Physical Development	Language (Cognitive) Development (based on Piaget)	Psychosocial Development (based on Erikson)	Nurse's Approach to Assessment
			approval and recognition. Enthusiastic, noisy, imaginative, desires to explore. Likes to complete a task. Enjoys helping others.	and feel. (In addition, explain body part involved, and use anatomical names and pictures to explain step by step.) Be honest. Reassure child that he or she is liked. Provide privacy. Involve parents, but give child choice as to whether parent will stay during exam. Reason and explain. Allow child some choice as to direction of assessment. May be able to proceed as if assessing adult. Praise cooperation.
12–18 y	Well developed. Rapid physical growth (early adolescence: maximum growth). Secondary sex characteristics.	*Formal operations stage of development.* Abstract reasoning, problem solving. Understanding of multiple cause-and-effect relationships. May plan for future career. *Fears:* • Mutilation • Disruption of body image • Rejection by peers	*Development task: identity vs. role confusion.* Predominant values are those of peer group. Early adolescence: outgoing and enthusiastic. Emotions are extreme, with mood swings. Seeking self-identity; sexual	Respect privacy. Accept expression of feelings. Direct discussions of care and condition to child. Ask for child's opinions and encourage questions. Allow input into decisions.

(continued)

Age	Physical Development	Language (Cognitive) Development (based on Piaget)	Psychosocial Development (based on Erikson)	Nurse's Approach to Assessment
			identity. Wants privacy and independence. Develops interests not shared with family. Concern with physical self. Explores adult roles.	Be flexible with routines. Explain all procedures/ treatments. Encourage continuance of peer relationships. Listen actively. Identify impact of illness on body image, future, and level of functioning. Correct misconceptions. Involve parent in assessment only if child requests presence.
19–30 y		*Formal operations*	*Developmental task: intimacy vs. isolation.* Intimate relationships are ultimate.	Involve significant other in care and consider how the client's condition affects the relationship.
30–60 y		*Formal operations*	*Developmental task: generativity vs. stagnation.* Concerned with parenthood, mentoring and guiding the next generation.	Work, family, and children are priorities. Teach with this concern in mind.
60 y to death		*Formal operations*	*Developmental task: integrity vs. despair.* Reviews life to bring life events into an integrated life theme.	Use life review to help client reduce anxiety and blocks to learning.

Used with permission from Weber, J. (1997). *Nurses' handbook of health assessment* (3rd ed.). Philadelphia: Lippincott-Raven.

Case Management

R O B E R T A   H U N T

▶ L E A R N I N G   O B J E C T I V E S ◀

- Define case management.
- Discuss the steps of case management as they relate to community-based nursing.
- Identify the relationship between case management and managed care.
- Discuss nursing skills and competencies needed in the nurse manager role in the community-based setting.
- Apply the five rights of delegation to a client situation.

▶ K E Y   T E R M S ◀

brokerage model
case finding
case management
collaboration
consultation
coordination

delegation
interdisciplinary team
    model
managed care
referral and follow-up
unlicensed assistive personnel

Significance of Case Management

Definitions and Models

Nursing Skills and Competencies in Case Management

Barriers to Successful Case Management

Elements of Successful Case Management

Conclusions

SIGNIFICANCE OF CASE MANAGEMENT

In this era of short length of stay in acute settings, where clients are discharged "quicker and sicker," case management has become an even more important aspect of community-based nursing care. However, it is not a new concept to nursing in community settings. The origins of this intervention were nurses who staffed settlement houses at the turn of the century. An article by Tahan (1998, p. 56) describes a system of cards used by nurses at the settlement houses, which stated that the duties of the staff were to " . . . list family needs, establish a mechanism for follow-up, facilitate the delivery of services and ensure that families were connected with appropriate resources."

This same focus on continuum of care was used to facilitate the return of discharged World War II to civilian life (Lyon, 1993). Other examples of this framework are seen in the management of client with long-term rehabilitation needs. The concept of case management as it is commonly thought of today springs from the insurance industry's interest in cost containment. Case management now is now common in a variety of settings and situations as more health care is provided in the community.

 DEFINITIONS AND MODELS

Case management, also known as care management or **care coordination,** is a complex concept with many definitions. This often leads to confusion about what is the correct or best definition. The Case Management Society of America (CMSA, 1994) defines case management as a "collaborative process which assesses, plans, implements, coordinates, monitors, and evaluates options and services to meet an individual's health needs through communications and available resources to promote quality, cost-effective outcomes." According to Mitchell and Reaghard (1996), the purpose of case management is to serve as a client advocate by enhanced coordination of services.

Although numerous definitions of case management exist, the goals typically aim to achieve a balance between quality and cost. These goals are to:

▶ Improve the quality of client care by emphasizing the importance of health restoration and maintenance and increased continuity of care
▶ Decrease the cost of care by empowering clients and their families to maximize self-care capabilities and prevent unnecessary or lengthy admissions
▶ Improve client nurse and physician satisfaction and professional development by promoting multidisciplinary collaborative practice and coordinated care (Lee, Mackenzie, Dudley-Brown, & Chin, 1998)

Note how closely these goals parallel those of community-based nursing, which are to facilitate continuity and self-care in the context of the clients, family, culture, and community by considering the principles of disease prevention, health promotion, and collaboration.

There are several case management models. Understanding these may help clarify why the case manager has one set of responsibilities in one situation and a different set in another. The **brokerage model** defines the role of the case manager as a coordinator of care mediating among all parties. The **interdisciplinary team model,** built on the concepts of collaboration, allows each professional on the team to offer his or her particular specialty. One member of the team is of-ten the primary or lead manger, usually depending on the needs of the client (Chan, Mackenzie, Tin-Fu, Leung, & Ka-yi, 2000).

In some models, unlicensed assistive personnel provide care, with the nurse acting as case manager. In this model, appropriate delegation is the key element. This text will primarily focus on the foundational models—the inter-disciplinary team model and model using the nurse as care manager of non-professional caregivers.

In some settings, a case manager's only role is to manage a number of cases, whereas in other settings the nurse has many roles, with case manager being one. For example, a nurse working in an emergency department (ED) may func-tion as a staff nurse and also call clients the day after their ED visit for follow-up. A home care nurse may be the client's case manager as well as the direct care provider and health educator. The ways this role is operationalized differ by ge-ographic areas, provider, payment restriction, and setting.

Thus, case management is a term with many definitions and implementation models. In community-based care, case management is the vehicle to care co-ordination and continuity of care. To accomplish this end, the nurse uses col-laboration, consultation, delegation, advocacy, and referral and follow-up. Case management in community-based settings reflects a commitment to facilitate self-care in the context of the client's family, culture, and community.

 ## NURSING SKILLS AND COMPETENCIES IN CASE MANAGEMENT

Case management follows several prescribed steps similar to the nursing process (Box 7–1). It is essential to assess the client's level of functioning to determine the resources and services necessary to maximize quality of life. The nurse involves the client and family in the design and implementation of the plan of care. Col-laboration plays a central role in coordinating the services as the nurse serves as client advocate, troubleshooting to resolve barriers. Last of all, progress toward achievement of outcomes is evaluated, revising the plan accordingly.

Case management has long been an important role for the nurse providing care in community settings. From old letters from Lillian Wald and Mary Brew-ster, nurses who worked in the settlement houses in New York City at the turn of the century, to nurses currently practicing, Betsy Rodgers explored what nurses who work in the community say about care coordination. She studied sto-ries of these case managers through old records and interviews with practicing nurses. The nurse–client relationship and outside connections were the central

---

▶ Box 7–1. Steps of Case Management ◀

1. Involve clients and families in assessing their level of functioning.
2. Determine the resources and services necessary to maximize quality of life.
3. Involve clients and families in identifying, exploring, and accessing available resources.
4. Have client and family identify the most appropriate referral for their needs.
5. Make the referral and supply service with needed information.
6. Act as an advocate or troubleshooter as necessary.
7. Evaluate progress toward the health outcomes and revise plan accordingly.

elements to successful care coordination (Rodgers, 2000). A summary of Rodgers's research is seen in Box 7–2.

Forming the Nurse–Client Relationship

According to Rodgers's research, several components work together to build the nurse–client relationship. The first is establishing a pact in which the relationship becomes the foundation of coordination (Fig. 7–1).

> ▶ I don't care what color you are, or where you come from or who you are or where you have been in your life, if you are my patient, I am going to do the very best that I can. I have a commitment. It's like when you walk into somebody's home and you form a bond with that person. It's like a pact that I'm going to be there for you until you die, and I'm going to take you through it, we're going to go through it together. (Rodgers, 2000, p. 303)

The second theme within the nurse–client relationship is talking and listening. Most basic to good therapeutic communication, sometimes just listening allows the nurse to assess the client's most immediate needs. Further, listening is often a powerful nursing intervention.

> ▶ Five years ago, my baby daughter died of SIDS. The nurse in the clinic just sat with me and let me cry. That was so helpful. I will always be thankful that she took the time to sit with me. (Julie, a nursing student)

Building trust is the third element found in Rodgers's research. Strategies to build trust are seen in Box 7–3.

Giving back control is the next step in forging the nurse–client relationship. From the first chapter this text has emphasized mutual care planning and self-care. The ultimate in successful nursing care is the plan that leads the client to independent self-care.

▶ Box 7–2. Essentials of Care Coordination ◀

Nurse–Client Relationship

Establishing a pact
Talking and listening
Building trust
Giving back control
Holding it together
Absent families

Outside Connections

Nurse knowing the community
Client advocacy
Going beyond the job description
Optimizing the client's environment

Adapted from Rodgers, B. (2000). Coordination of care: The lived experience of the visiting nurse. *Home Healthcare Nurse, 18*(3), 301–307.

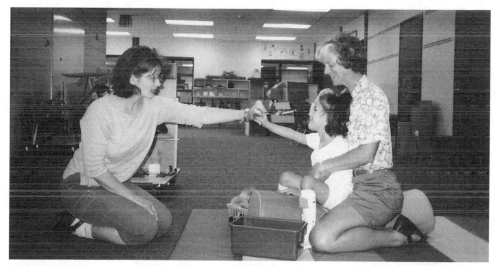

Figure 7–1. ▶ A strong and trusting nurse–client relationship is the foundation of coordinated care.

The fifth component of the nurse–client relationship found in Rodgers's research is holding it all together. This may seem like an almost impossible task for some of the complex individuals and families we care for in community settings.

▶ Jack is one of the more difficult clients I have ever cared for. He is 80 years old with very brittle diabetes. His wife died last year. She was the one who could drive, cook, and check his blood sugar. His daughter said she would help by dropping by with a meal every day. He has refused Meals On Wheels, says that welfare is for old people, and will only eat what his daughter brings for him. Now his daughter is in the hospital having a spinal fusion, so I don't think he is eating. I am trying to problem solve with him about alternatives, hoping we will be able to uncover an option he is comfortable with before he ends up back in the hospital. (Kathy, a home health care nurse)

The last theme in care coordination considers the nurse–client relationship when the family is absent. It is not uncommon for family members to become estranged from one another or unable or unwilling to assist one another during ill-

---

▶ Box 7–3. Trust-Building Strategies ◀

- Begin cultivating the client's trust with the first contact.
- Establish credibility with the client.
- Use an empathic, nonjudgmental approach.
- Guard the client's privacy.
- Expect testing behavior from clients.
- Learn to trust the client.
- Persevere with the nurse–client relationship.

Wendt, D. (1996). Building trust during the initial home visit. In R. Hunt (Ed.). *Readings in community based nursing* (pp. 154–160). Philadelphia: Lippincott Williams & Wilkins.

ness. In some situations, when an individual has a chronic illness over a long period of time, everyone is exhausted from managing the work of the illness. In others, there may be estrangement of many years.

> ▶ Earnest had no family or social support. Ernest had three children but they all live on the West Coast. Earnest and his wife separated 15 years ago, because of his substance abuse. When we called to see if she would be able to assist with his care, she really gave the nurse an ear full! His family has been totally unwilling to assist with his care. (Phyllis, a home care nurse)

Outside Connections: Working with Community Resources

The second pattern that emerged from Rodgers's research involves community connections essential to providing effective care management. The nurse must know the community and the resources available within that community. Often nurses in community settings act as client advocates or participate in activities that may not be in their job description. Several factors are essential for outside connections to result in care coordination.

The first factor is the nurse's knowledge about the community. To provide comprehensive, coordinated care, the nurse must know the client, the client's family and culture, and the broader community in which they live. To make appropriate referrals to ensure continuity, the nurse must know what services are available. For these outside connections to be accessed, the client and family first must know about the service and then must be willing to accept help.

> ▶ I had been making home visits to a client after the birth of her twins. She was about to be evicted from her home. Her relationship with the father of her babies was volatile. He was not living with her and not supportive. Every visit, she talked about the lack of progress she had made in finding a place to live. "Nobody will take someone with five kids," she would say over and over again. "I am going to be homeless with my kids," she exclaimed. In our community there is virtually no low-cost housing. We had explored every option available to her with no success. One day when I went to make my weekly home visit and weigh the twins, she didn't answer the door. I could hear the kids inside and knew she must be home. I knocked and waited. She finally opened the door. Both of her eyes were black and her face was bruised and swollen. She shamefully said, "He beat me up in front of the kids. I am never going to see him again, but I have no place to go." I knew about special housing available in our county for those experiencing domestic violence. I explained to her that she would have to go to a shelter for domestic abuse, but from there she could get into the housing program. Her mother helped her pack up her kids and she moved to the shelter the next day. (Mary, a senior nursing student)

Another element of community connections is client advocacy. **Client advocacy** is defined as intervening or acting on behalf of the client to provide the highest quality health care obtainable. Sometimes our health care system is characterized as uncaring, impersonal, and fragmented. Clients become frustrated, often feeling devalued and unable to cope with the system. A community-based nurse acts as an advocate for the client and family. Nurses have always been involved in promoting the health care needs of the client, acting as the client's spokesperson, and providing information to the client to help ensure uninterrupted care. In many situations, the client is very vulnerable, which often results in the nurse contacting a community service, other caregivers, or a physician on the client's behalf.

For example, a school nurse notices that a 13-year-old child often comes to the nurse's office complaining of a stomachache on Monday mornings. When the girl comes in for 3 weeks in a row, the nurse asks her, "Tell me about your weekend." The child starts crying and says, "My dad doesn't live with us any more. My mom drinks beer and yells at me." The nurse and the child discuss the child's feelings and fears about her family situation. Then the nurse explains to the child that with her permission, she would like to talk to the school counselor about their conversations, to learn about some groups that may help her. Second, the nurse tells the child that she would like to call her mom and talk to the two of them about her stomachaches. In this situation, the nurse is acting as an advocate for the child, with the goal of facilitating self-care in the context of the student's family. The nurse is collaborating with other professionals to enhance care.

The client advocate role involves informing clients about the nature of their health problems and the choices they have in seeking to resolve or alter their health care needs. This role is activated whenever clients are unable to take responsibility for their own health care, lack knowledge or skill, or do not have the financial or emotional basis from which to act. The advocacy role is also one of support after clients have been informed, have made choices, and need to implement these choices. Clients have an inherent right to make their own decisions and to take responsibility for those decisions. The nurse lends support and respect for clients whether or not the nurse agrees with their decisions (Arnold & Boggs, 1995).

To advocate for clients, the nurse must consider all aspects of the clients' lives. Advocacy is often used with vulnerable populations who have a weak voice within a system. Some people, because of age, cognitive abilities, lack of sophistication, or other factors need assistance in speaking for themselves. Clarification of a do-not-resuscitate order on behalf of an elderly client who is unaware of the need to explicitly state his preference is one example of a nurse acting as a client advocate.

Sometimes visiting nurses do things that are an extension of their usual role responsibilities, as found in Rodgers's research. For example, Celia is 62 years old, living home alone in her apartment. She is diabetic and also had surgery for breast cancer last month. She just started chemotherapy this week. She takes the bus to an outpatient clinic for her treatment, but she must pick up her insulin at a drugstore that is six blocks away and not on a bus line. She would like to get her medication at the pharmacy at the outpatient clinic, but her insurance company will pay only if she fills it at the drugstore. Her home health care nurse knows that the insurance company makes exceptions in some situations. She calls the customer relations representative at the insurance company and arranges for Celia to pick up her medication at the outpatient clinic.

Health is related to the environment, and sometimes our environment is detrimental to our health. Chapter 6 discussed the benefits of altering the environment to enhance learning. The same is true with case management because the nurse may use interventions that indirectly affect the client's or family's health. For example, with the client's consent, the nurse arranges for the home health aide to dispose of piles of old magazines and papers. This eliminates a fire hazard, prevents a potential fall, and may improve the client's psychological status by making the environment more pleasant.

Intervention Strategies

Several intervention strategies, which have not been discussed, may enhance case management. They include case finding, referral and follow-up, collaboration, consultation, and delegation.

COMMUNITY-BASED NURSING CARE GUIDELINES

Steps in the Referral Process

1. Establish the need for referral.
2. Set objectives for the referral.
3. Explore the resources that are available.
4. Have the client make decisions concerning the referral.
5. Make the referral to the selected service.
6. Supply the agency with needed information.
7. Support the client and family in pursuing the referral.

Case Finding

Case finding is a set of activities used by the nurse working in community settings that identify clients who are not currently receiving health care but could benefit from such care. The nurse, of all members of the interdisciplinary team, usually has the most contact with the client and family. This allows the nurse to assess and identify client service needs that, if addressed, would enhance care coordination or case management. In some cases, this may be a simple process, with the nurse making one contact or giving the client one suggested referral. Case finding happens in every setting where care is provided, and it requires an open attitude and skillful assessment by the nurse.

Referral and Follow-up

Referral and follow-up is the process by which nurses in all settings assist individuals and families to identify and access community resources to prevent, promote, or maintain health. To be skilled in this competency, the nurse must know the community and the resources available in that community. Obviously, just knowing what resources are present in the community is only the first step. For example, when caring for a client who has just had a knee replacement, the nurse learns that the client lives alone and does not have friends or family living nearby. It will be difficult for the client to cook for several weeks. Giving the client the telephone number for Meals On Wheels is one nursing intervention. The client is concerned about getting to the grocery store. There is a grocery delivery service, which has a reduced rate for senior citizens. A second intervention is giving the client the name and telephone number of the service. Chapter 8, Continuity of Care, provides a more in-depth discussion of the referral process.

Collaboration

Frequently a client requires services from many different disciplines. The case manager often initiates referrals and requests these services. Some of the various professionals the nurse will work with are physicians, social workers, nutritionists, physical and occupational therapists, and pharmacists. One of the many roles the case manager must assume is that of collaborator. **Collaboration** means working jointly with others in a common endeavor—to cooperate as partners (Spradley & Allender, 1996). It takes team effort to care for a client well, and the team leader is often the nurse. The following steps of coordinating multiple disciplines must be taken by the nurse to facilitate continuity of care:

▶ Notify all disciplines involved when there is a change in the client's health.

▶ Coordinate visits with the client to avoid two professionals visiting at the same time and tiring the client.

▶ Integrate services to provide maximum benefit to the client; for example, have the physical therapist measure blood pressure when at the home to ambulate the client.

▶ Problem solve jointly with other team members and include the client when appropriate.

The role of the case manager is often viewed as that of gatekeeper. Often the manager is a broker for services. For example, a community-based nurse who served worker's compensation clients described her role as "interpreting the insurance company's medical information and working with health care providers to find the most efficient means of helping people return to the workplace" (Margaret, an occupational health nurse). Other nurse case managers describe their role as "assessing and evaluating delivery systems and benefit criteria . . . making sure that resources are available . . . stretching the dollar . . . client advocacy . . . and making sure the client and family are fully involved in the decision and care."

Consultation

Consultation is an interactive problem-solving process between the nurse and the client. From a list of alternative options generated by the nurse and client, the client selects those most appropriate for the situation. The case manager uses basic steps in the consultation intervention (Box 7–4).

Delegation

Delegation is a key intervention in successful case management. **Delegation** is a management principle used to obtain desired results through the work of others

---

▶ Box 7–4. Steps in Consultation for the Case Manager ◀

1. Establish a trusting relationship with the client and family.
2. Clarify the client's perception of the problem, the causes, and anticipated results.
3. Assess all issues in a mutual process with the client.
   • Determine the impact the issue has on the client's experience.
   • Identify everyone involved in the issue and how they are affected.
   • Determine how the client and family's attitudes, beliefs, and behaviors may be contributing to the issues.
   • Explore environmental aspects.
   • Identify strengths and barriers for the client and family.
   • Anticipate what may be gained or lost by solving or addressing the issue.
   • Consider how a solution might affect the client and family.
4. Through mutual planning the nurse and client:
   • Identify the desired outcome
   • Consider the advantages and disadvantages of each
   • Support the client as they choose the preferred option
5. Determine support essential to facilitate implementing the plan.
6. Evaluate the process and outcome.

Adapted from Minnesota Department of Health, Section of Public Health Nursing. (2000). *Public health nursing interventions II. Basic steps to the consultation intervention.* Minneapolis: Author.

and is a legal concept used to empower one person to act for another (National Council of State Boards of Nursing [NCSBN], 1997). **Unlicensed assistive personnel** (UAP) are any unlicensed workers, regardless of title, to whom nursing tasks are delegated (NCSBN, 1997). As more UAP are providing care to individuals in community settings, the issues related to delegation have becomes central to the case manager.

According to the NCSBN (1997), all decisions related to delegation of nursing activities must be based on the fundamental principle of public protection. Licensed nurses have ultimate accountability for the management and provision of nursing care, including all delegated decisions and tasks. This accountability is outlined in the Five Rights of Delegation, shown in Box 7–5.

Managed Care Skills

Managed care is an organized system of health care that carefully plans and monitors the use of health care services so that standards are met while costs are minimized (Ludwig-Beymer, 1999). Many health maintenance organizations (HMOs) and insurance companies use managed care. Preferred provider organizations (PPOs) are another form of a managed care organization. An increasing segment of the population receives health care through managed care. Skills needed for nurses to work effectively in a managed care environment are listed in Box 7–6.

Often a nurse is the person responsible for evaluating what care is necessary. Sometimes this puts the nurse in the difficult position of seeing firsthand the needs of the client, but discovering that coverage limitations of the managed care contract prohibit the provision of the needed care. Sometimes, this is the point where the nurse acts as an advocate for the client to secure the service.

Documentation

Documentation of care management is essential as a legal document, as means of communication to other health care professions and UAP, and for determination of eligibility of care.

BARRIERS TO SUCCESSFUL CASE MANAGEMENT

There are countless barriers to successful case management, all contributing to lack of continuity for the client and family. One barrier is the lack of a consistent definition of case management. With so many definitions, case management is not a concept that is easily understood or operationalized. Because it is not easily understood, nurses may not know where their job responsibilities begin and end related to case management. There are numerous models of case management, adding to the confusion about who does what for the client and when is it done.

A second barrier to case management is lack of time. Each year, with cost-containment concerns dictating who gets what care, nurses in all settings are pressed to care for more clients with more complex needs. "The problem is that it's hard for case managers to focus on the tasks of the day and get patients through episodes of care if they're also trying to run teams and coordinate data" (Moore, 1999, p. 28). In these situations, only the most essential and immediate aspects of care are addressed.

Lack of preparation for the case manager role is another barrier. There is little literature on how to best prepare nurses for this role. Often, case manage-

▶ Box 7–5. The Five Rights of Delegation ◀

1. Right task
Is this a task that may be delegated?

- Depending on the state, assessment may or may not be delegated to others.
- Does the task require extensive training to reliably, consistently, and safely perform it? If so, it should not be delegated.
- Does the task require alteration based on the client response during the task? If so, this need for professional judgement deems that the task should not be delegated.

2. Right circumstances
Are the care settings, available resources, and other relevant factors conducive to ensuring client safety?

- Is there potential for harm to the client?
- Is the complexity of the nursing activity low?
- Are the required problem solving and innovation minimal?
- Is the outcome of the task predictable?
- Is there ample opportunity for patient interaction?
- Is a registered nurse (RN) available to adequately supervise?

3. Right person
Is the right person delegating the right task to the right person to be performed with the right client?

- An RN may delegate all functions to another RN as long as that individual agrees.
- Others to whom an RN delegates should have reasonable knowledge, training, and experience to ensure consistent and safe performance of the task.
- Likewise, an RN should not accept the responsibility for carrying out tasks for which he or she has not had the proper training or experience to ensure safe and effective care.
- The client's stability and/or response to the task must be predictable and not require professional judgment in order for the administrator to respond effectively.

4. Right direction/communication
Are expectations clearly and concisely stated, including objectives, limits, and expectations?

- If the task is new to the RN or developmental in nature, or the description requires complex or multiple steps, the task is probably not delegable.

5. Right supervision

- Is the supervising RN accessible for answering questions and directly supervising?
- Are appropriate monitoring, evaluation, and feedback ensured? As a rule, the more complex the task, the less experienced the delegatee, and/or the more unstable/unresponsive the client, the more physically close the supervising RN should be.

Adapted from Minnesota Department of Health, Section of Public Health Nursing. (2000). *Public health nursing interventions II. The five rights of delegation.* Minneapolis: Author.

Adapted from National Council of State Boards of Nursing. (1997). *The delegation resource folder.* Web site address: http://www.ncsbn.org.

> ▶ **Box 7–6.** Skills Needed by Nurses in a Managed Care Environment ◀
>
> - Negotiation skills
> - Delegation skills
> - Ability to analyze care in terms of cost and benefit
> - Ability to understand the process of care provision across the continuum
> - Ability to look at and predict outcomes
> - Ability to collect and evaluate outcome data
> - Business understanding, or ability to understand and use financial data
> - Advocacy skills
> - Assessment skills
> - Ethical decision-making skills
> - Collaboration skills
>
> ---
>
> Kersbergen, A. (2000). Managed care shifts health care from an altruistic model to a business framework. *Nursing and Health Care Perspectives, 21*(2), 81–83.

ment is a minor aspect of theory content and absent altogether from clinical experiences in nursing programs.

ELEMENTS OF SUCCESSFUL CASE MANAGEMENT

Successful case management requires the nurse to function as an interdisciplinary team member who furnishes the link between the referral source and the client. An ED in Alabama is using case managers in a multidisciplinary team with clients with asthma. Use of a standardized care plan and follow-up telephone call has resulted in a decreased length of stay and fewer repeat visits by clients receiving the case management care (Zimmermann, 1998). In addition, staff consults the emergency department case manager when patterns of frequent visits result from nonadherence with treatment or drug-seeking behavior.

Another ED works to manage care at both admission and discharge. At admission, for clients who are denied care at that facility but must go to another for the presenting condition, the nurse provides the client with information that lists treatments sites, reinforces the information, and verifies that the clients knows the location. At discharge, the case manager provides for client needs, whether a home health referral or follow-up physician referral. This model has improved customer relations as well as appropriate utilization of community services (Zimmerman & Pierce, 1998).

Successful case management programs demonstrate that with nursing leadership, client outcomes and quality of care can be enhanced by following the basic interventions of case management. Research Box 7–1 presents an example of nursing research related to interdisciplinary case management.

Case Management and Self-Care

The community-based nurse must be able to understand what promotes and what inhibits the abilities of others. This is evident when the nurse recognizes the ability of a client to irrigate and dress his or her own wound. Using this as a starting point, the nurse coaches and encourages the client to take charge of his or her own care. The nurse also uses the techniques of establishing trust, mak-

RESEARCH RELATED TO COMMUNITY-BASED NURSING CARE

Research Box 7–1 ▶ The Impact of Interdisciplinary Case Management on Client Outcomes

The purpose of this study was to describe the use of interdisciplinary case management with underserved, minority clients. The Omaha System, a model for organizing, documenting, and evaluating the outcomes of community-based care, was used. The two study sites were a community health center and an alternative high school. The study subjects were high-risk women, eligible to participate in the interdisciplinary case management program. Students and faculty from nursing, pharmacy, public health, social work, and medicine were on the interdisciplinary team.

Case management activities began with an intake summary. Each subsequent encounter was documented using the Omaha system of documentation. Weekly case management conferences were held with all members of the team attending. Each member of the team took a turn at facilitating the weekly conference. During this conference, problems were identified and solutions sought through discussion with each team member sharing his or her discipline perspective. Outcomes of each conference included a plan for the next encounter with an identified team member to address the problems and issues identified by the conference. Sometimes the students made team visits; other times only one discipline made the next home visit.

Important findings of this study were that this interdisciplinary case management program appears to have had a substantial impact on outcomes in this underserved, minority population. The greatest impact was on client knowledge, specifically, in the psychosocial domain, growth and development and emotional stability as well as improved communication with community resources.

Slack, M., & McEwen, M. (1999). The impact of interdisciplinary case management on client outcomes. *Family Community Health, 22*(3), 30–48.

ing appropriate referrals, advocating, consulting, and collaborating to facilitate self-care.

Case Management and Prevention

Significant economic changes in health care have dramatically altered the role of the nurse. Large areas of responsibility are delegated to nurses' aides, who, on the average, have 6 weeks or less of training. Nursing care in the acute and long-term care settings and in home health care is being assigned to less-prepared providers, families, and UAP.

The case management model of care delivery places a large burden on the RN who works in community-based care. People living with a chronic condition often require a great deal of assistance with health promotion to help maximize the quality of their lives. Because chronic diseases are the major cause of morbidity and mortality in developed countries, nurses are increasingly involved with illness prevention and health promotion.

Case Management in the Context of Community

Community-based nursing occurs within the context of the client's community. The nurse is responsible for identifying resources and identifying constraints or limitations for care that exist in the community. This can occur when the nurse states clearly and coherently to the client the purpose of the nursing care and how all the care needs will be met with organizational and community resources. For example, a 76-year-old client living in a rural community was originally treated for metastatic cancer of the prostate in a large, urban medical center 175 miles away from his home. Now he needs 6 weeks of daily radiation treatments for his metastasis. The nurse recognizes a problem with the client's being so far away from his original primary care institution and arranges treatment at a hospital 40 miles from the client's home. When arranging care, the nurse coordinates care between the two facilities so continuity is not lost and the client is ensured the best care possible within the constraints of his community.

Case Management and Continuity of Care

Collaboration and acting as an advocate on behalf of the client are important aspects of ensuring continuity of care. Using an analytical approach to make referrals and follow up on client progress is another strategy to promote continuity.

EXAMPLE OF A CLIENT SITUATION

Case Management

Steve, age 40, and Barb, age 37, are a young couple with three children: Brook, 15, Jane, 13, and Jack, 11. Both parents are professionals. Steve works at the Veterans Administration, where he is in charge of the information systems, and Barb is a professor at a small liberal arts college. Because Steve has a family history of colon cancer (his paternal grandfather died of colon cancer at age 41, his father and uncle had surgery for colon cancer at ages 65 and 60, respectively), he was advised to have a colonoscopy at age 40. One month after his 40th birthday, he schedules a test. He has no symptoms. He is diagnosed with colon cancer 3 days after the test, on Christmas Eve day. Because of the size of the tumor, Steve's physician recommends he have the surgery at a large medical center 200 miles from Steve's home. Two days after Christmas he has a colon resection without a colostomy at Methodist Hospital. At that time it is determined that the cancer is between class D and class C according to the Duke classification system (or stage 4 with the other commonly used classification). Although he was a candidate for a colostomy, he and Barb decided they wanted to try the more conservative approach, with the option of a colostomy later, if necessary.

Barb has been with Steve throughout his hospital stay while their three children have been home, 200 miles away, staying with Barb's elderly mother. It is 14 days after the operation, and he is to return home the day after tomorrow. He will begin chemotherapy at the rural hospital close to his home next week.

- You are a staff nurse caring for Steve in the hospital. What strategies to manage care would you use, starting from the first day?
  The first step in care management is establishing a relationship with the client and family by listening and talking. By doing this you hope to build trust.

By now you would have established a very open relationship with Barb and Steve. You ask Barb and Steve how they anticipate that the homecoming will go when they arrive home. Barb says, "We have both really missed the kids. I really want to have a normal life again. Sleep in my own bed and make breakfast for everyone. Just normal stuff."

Steve says, "I can't wait to get out of here. But I am worried about the chemo. We had one conversation with the nurse at the clinic and she said that we have to have the chemo in the morning. I have most of my meetings at work in the morning and would rather do the chemo in the afternoon."

- How could you, as a staff nurse, respond to this comment?
  To help give some control back to the client you might encourage him to call the clinic that day and explore whether chemotherapy could be scheduled at a time more convenient for his work schedule.

You are working in a clinic as an oncology nurse providing chemotherapy where Steve will be receiving his treatment. This is the third week of his treatment, and you have established a relationship with both Barb and Steve. After beginning administration of his chemotherapy, you asked them how things are going. Barb tells you, "Awful. Brook was picked up for shoplifting and her grades are dropping in school." You note that Steve is unusually quiet and does not make eye contact with you. You ask, "Steve, you look down today. Are you doing OK?"

"It feels like it is all coming apart. I can't keep up at work, the kids are having trouble . . ." Steve shares.

"He won't listen to me about resting. And he's throwing up all the time. That medication you gave him doesn't work." Barb reports.

- What are some interventions you could use at this point in your care of Steve and his family?
  Possible interventions include:

  Using the steps of the referral process to find some community resources to support the family with the issues the family is facing, including the daughter's shoplifting and falling grades.
  Advocating for the client by calling the physician to identify additional antiemetics that may be helpful in controlling the nausea and vomiting.
  Contacting a social worker (with the family's knowledge) to begin to collaborate and problem solve regarding the family's issues and stress

Ten months later, Steve has completed chemotherapy and radiation therapy. Because of the intensity of the radiology treatment, he has developed interrupted bowel function. He has been to the clinic and the emergency department several times in the past weeks with severe cramps. You receive a call late in the afternoon from Barb. She states that the medication given at the last clinic visit is not helping, that Steve has been throwing up all day, has severe abdominal cramps and a temperature of 103°. You tell them to go to the local emergency department.

At the ED, Steve is diagnosed with a bladder and kidney infection and bowel obstruction, and is admitted to the hospital. A complete work-up is performed while he is in the hospital, and liver cancer is discovered throughout his liver, with lesions in the brain as well. He is discharged home unable to eat, with a central line and hyperal for total parenteral nutrition.

You are Steve's home care nurse. On the first home visit his functional capacity for activities of daily living is clearly impaired. He is homebound and needs a home health care aid to help him bathe and shave. Barb is working two jobs to try to make ends meet. The plan is for the home health aid to come every other day, with you coming once a day to start the hyperal. Two months later, at one of your visits, Steven says, "The home aide says he can do the hyperal and clean the site on the days when he is here. Then you don't have to come every day."

- Can you delegate the administration of hyperal to the home health aide?
  According to the Five Rights of Delegation from the NCSBN (Box 7–5), this task may not be delegated for the following reasons:

  Assessment may be needed.
  The task requires extensive training.

The task requires professional judgement regarding client response.
There is potential for harm.
The RN would not be immediately available for assistance or direct supervision.

Steve's condition continues to deteriorate over the next month. As you are getting ready to leave after a visit, Barb asks you, "Do you think we should be making plans for Steve's death?"

- You conclude that Barb and Steve may be ready to talk about hospice care. How do you proceed?
  Using the steps for consultation in Box 7–4, you determine the family's needs. Through mutual problem solving you determine if and when the family is ready to meet with the hospice nurse. At that time you contact her for the family and arrange for her to visit.

 CONCLUSIONS

Although case management is a role that is over 100 years old for nurses, the model has evolved. Nurses on all levels are care managers for some parts of their jobs. Themes from the care manager role include establishing trust, giving control, helping families hold it all together, advocacy, taking care of the environment and dealing with absent families. Interventions commonly used in case management are case finding, referral and follow-up, collaboration, consultation, and delegation. These interventions are particularly applicable in the changing managed care environment. The care manager in community-based settings always encourages self-care with a preventive focus that is provided within the context of the client's community while following the principles of collaboration to achieve continuity.

What's on the Web

Case Management Society of America
8201 Cantrell Road, Suite 230
Little Rock, AR 72227
Telephone: (501) 225-2229
Fax: (501) 221-9068

Internet address: http://www.cmsa.org

This site offers educational opportunities, both CEUs and case management credential courses. It also provides extensive information on case management.

Case Management Resource Guide

Internet address: http://www.cmrg.com

This site has a comprehensive on-line directory of health care organization. It also contains an extensive case manager resource guide.

National Council of State Boards of Nursing
Delegation Resource Folder

Internet address: http://www.ncsbn.org/files/delegation.asp

The NCSBN has produced an excellent resource on the topic of delegation, which serves as the major reference for information on delegation. The Council's material is contained in the delegation resource folder and can be downloaded from the Council's Web site.

There is great overlap between case management and continuity of care; Chapter 8 has additional resources.

References and Bibliography

Advocacy in action. (1999). *RN, 62*(7), 26hf2.

American Nurses Association. (1988). *Nursing case management.* Kansas City, MO: Author.

Arnold, E., & Boggs, K. (1995). *Interpersonal relationships: Professional communication skills for nurses* (2nd ed.). Philadelphia: Saunders.

Burke, S. (1999). Creating competency for home healthcare: Case management manual. *Home Healthcare Nurse Manager, 3*(6), 2–5.

Campinha-Bacote, J., & Campinha-Bacote, D. (1999). A framework for providing culturally competent health care services in managed care organizations. *Journal of Transcultural Nursing, 10*(4), 290–291.

Case Management Society of America. (1998). Center for Case Management Accountability (CCMA). http://www.cmsa.org.

Chan, S., Mackenzie, A., Tin-Fu, D., Leung, J., & Ka-yi, B. (2000). An evaluation of the implementation of case management in the community psychiatric nursing service. *Journal of Advanced Nursing, 31*(1), 144–156.

Dunbar, S., Jacobson, L., & Deaton. C. (1998). Heart failure: Strategies to enhance patient self-management. *AACN, 9*(2), 244–256.

Fletcher, I., & Coffman, S. (1999). Care management in the nursing curriculum. *Journal of Nursing Education, 38*(8), 371–372.

Getty, C., & Knab, S. (1998). Capacity for self-care of persons with mental illnesses living in community residences and the ability of their surrogate families to perform health care functions. *Issues in Mental Health Nursing, 19*, 53–70.

Howe, R. (1999). Case management in managed care: Past, present and future. *The Case Manager, 10*(5), 38–48.

Kersbergen, A. (2000). Managed care shifts health care from an altruistic model to a business framework. *Nursing and Health Care Perspectives, 21*(2), 81–83.

Lee, D., Mackenzie, A., Dudley-Brown, S., & Chin, T. (1998). Case management: A review of the definitions and practice. *Journal of Advanced Nursing, 27*, 933–939.

Ludwig Beymer, P. (1999). Transcultural nursing's role in a managed care environment. *Journal of Transcultural Nursing, 10*(4), 286–287.

Lyon, J. (1993). Modules of nursing care delivery and case management: Clarification of terms. *Nursing Economics, 11*(3), 163–178.

McClaran, J., Franco, E., Lam, Z., & Snell, L. (1999). Can case management be taught in a multidisciplinary forum? *Journal of Continuing Education in the Health Professions, 19*(3), 181–191.

McKenna, M. (1999). Let us try to keep culturally competent care in managed care. *Journal of Transcultural Nursing, 10*(3), 293–293.

McKay, T. (1999). Managed care: A turning point for nursing. *Journal of Transcultural Nursing, 10*(4), 292.

Minnesota Department of Health, Section of Public Health Nursing. (2000). *Public health nursing interventions II.* Minneapolis: Author.

Mitchell, A., & Reaghard, D. (1996). Managed care and psychiatric-mental health nursing services: Implications for practice. *Issues in Mental Health Nursing, 17*(1), 1–9. (Cinahl link).

Moore, A. (1999). Hospitals shift responsibility for cross-continuum care. *RN, 62*(9), 28nm4–28nm6.

National Council of State Boards of Nursing. (1997). *The delegation resource folder.* Available on-line at: http://www.ncsbn.org/files/delegation.asp.

Nolan, M., Harris, A., Kufta, A., Opfer, N., & Tunner, H. (1998). Preparing nurses for the acute care case manager role: Educational needs identified by existing case managers. *Journal of Continuing Education in Nursing, 29*(3), 130–134.

Reed, B. (1999). Desperately seeking continuity. *The Practicing Midwife, 2*(9), 46.

Rodgers, B. (2000). Coordination of care: The lived experience of the visiting nurse. *Home Healthcare Nurse, 18*(3), 301–307.

Schmidt, S. Guo, L., Scheer, S., Boydston, J., Pelino, C., & Berger, S. (1999). Epidemiological determination of community-based nursing case management for stroke. *Journal of Nursing Administration, 29*(6), 40–47.

Sokol, D. (1999). John needed all I could give. *RN, 62*(11), 44–47.

Slack, M., & McEwen, M. (1999). The impact of interdisciplinary case management of client outcomes. *Family Community Health, 22*(3), 30–48.

Spradley, B. W., & Allender, J. A. (1996). *Community health nursing: Concepts and practice* (4th ed.). Philadelphia: Lippincott-Raven.

Standards of practice for case management. (1995). Little Rock, AR: Case Management Society of American (CMSA) Publications.

Tahan, H. (1998). Case management: A heritage more than a century old. *Nursing Case Management, 3*(2), 55–69.

Tholcken, M., Lehna, C., & Robinson, S. (1999). Children with disabilities: Teaching baccalaureate nursing students community-based case management. *Journal of Care Management, 5*(4), 32–39.

Walsh, K. (1999). ED case managers: One large teaching hospital's experience. *Journal of Emergency Nursing, 25*(10), 17–20.

Wayman, C. (1999). Hospital-based nursing case management: Role clarification. *Nursing Case Management, 4*(5), 236–241.

What preparation do case managers really need? (1999). *Case Management Advisor, 10*(7), 112–113.

Zerull, L. (1999). Community nurse case management: Evolving over time to meet new demands. *Community Health, 22*(3),12–29.

Zimmerman, P., & Pierce, B. (1998). Case managers. *Journal of Emergency Nursing, 24*(6), 589–591.

LEARNING ACTIVITIES

LEARNING ACTIVITY 7-1

▶ **Client Care Study:** Effective Case Management

You are a home health care nurse responsible for the care of 15 clients. It's Monday morning, and you are reviewing your phone messages as well as looking over the charts of the clients you are scheduled to visit in the next 2 days. How will you rearrange home visits for the next 2 days based on the following information?

SCHEDULED VISITS FOR MONDAY AFTERNOON AND TUESDAY
MONDAY
1:00 Mr. Carmody—routine visit to monitor symptoms of congestive heart failure

2:30 Mrs. Gothie—routine follow-up visit after hip replacement and discharge from acute care last Wednesday, and your last visit was Friday

4:00 Mrs. Violet—monthly blood draw for lithium levels

TUESDAY

9:00 Mr. Heaney   scheduled to discharged from the hospital Monday night after open heart surgery; assessment visit and blood draw

10:30 Mr. Sund—follow-up visit for knee replacement surgery; discharged from the hospital last Thursday, and your last visit was Friday

1:00 Mr. Vang—reinforcement teaching for care of a leg wound

2:30 Mrs. O'Conner—follow-up visit for assessment after scheduled discharge from the hospital on Monday evening; administration of IV antibiotic medication

PHONE MESSAGES ON MONDAY AT 8:00 AM

Mr. Vang called you this morning and said that he ran out of dressings on Friday. He was very upset and stated that the sore on his leg looked more red and there was some sticky green stuff dripping off of it.

Mrs. Sund called and said her husband had so much pain in his knee over the weekend that he could not sleep. She said he also has pain in the back of his calf, it is red, and it hurts if he flexes his foot.

LEARNING ACTIVITY 7-2

▶ **Critical Thinking Exercise:** Self-Evaluation

In your clinical journal, describe a situation you have observed in clinical where a client experienced difficulty due to lack of effective case management. If you were the nurse in charge, what would you have done differently?

In your clinical journal, describe a situation you have observed in clinical where a client received effective case management. What made the care effective?

In your clinical journal, describe a situation where you observed or initiated two of the following intervention strategies. Discuss what happened.

Referral and follow-up

Consultation

Collaboration

Advocacy

Delegation

CHAPTER 8

Continuity of Care

ROBERTA HUNT

Nurses have been involved in **continuity of care** since the late 1880s. In 1906, both Massachusetts General Hospital in Boston and Bellevue Hospital in New York City designated a nurse to tend to the needs of those patients about to be discharged. Recently, interest in discharge planning was renewed with the concern about escalating medical costs. Currently, nurses are involved with continuity of care more than ever, as health care reform continues. Future reforms center around the use of inpatient facilities for briefer, more intense care; cost-containment efforts to deliver care at the lowest cost with more efficiency; expanded community-based care; and an emphasis on primary, preventive care delivered with a continuum of care. Nursing will focus on quality of care issues and development of skills in community-based care.

Ongoing health care planning and referral are described as a bridge between one health care setting and another environment. A comprehensive plan of care and effective referrals are essential elements for continuity of care. Collaboration is important as the multidisciplinary team works together to promote quality health care by maximizing the client and family's attainment of optimum functioning and self-care. The nurse is often the primary player in ascertaining the quality of the health plan.

Both discharge planning and continuity of care rely on community resources. A community with many resources can help support the client and family through a recovery period or can help families in their health promotion. The community with few resources will be inefficient in its support of its citizens who require assistance with health care needs.

In this chapter, continuity of care is presented as facilitating entrance, exit, and transfer within the health care system. Examples are given to show how coordination of services is used in continuity. The concepts of community resources and referral are discussed. Two types of resources are explained. Steps in the referral process are outlined, along with information about financing referrals. The chapter ends with a section on skills and competencies the nurse needs to improve continuity of care, a discussion of barriers to continuity, and examples of programs successful in enhancing continuity.

 ## SIGNIFICANCE OF CONTINUITY OF CARE

Continuity of care has been described as the coordination of activities involving clients, providers, and payers to promote the delivery of health care. This is the process by which a client's ongoing health care needs are assessed, planned for, coordinated, and met without disruption. Some may view it as a method to control health care costs. Clients may view it as promoting their right to make choices about health care services.

Regardless of how it is perceived, continuity of care requires a strong organizational structure to prevent the client from getting "lost" in the system. Nurses must provide a leadership role in determining how and where the best care can be provided for a client and then ensuring that the client receives that care. The nurse accomplishes this by thoroughly assessing the client's needs, participating in multidisciplinary planning and intervention, and using appropriate resources, follow-up, and evaluation. Successful attainment of continuity of care is essential to ensure quality health care and is promoted through successful planning and effective referral.

 ## ENTERING AND EXITING THE HEALTH CARE SYSTEM

Principles of continuity apply to transitions of care between any community settings. "Discharge from a community-based healthcare setting needs the same, or possibly greater, level of attention than from acute care facilities" (Craven & Hirnle, 2000, p. 344). If discharge instructions for a client in ambulatory surgery are clearly explained, then successful follow-up, fewer complications, and good recovery are more likely. Likewise, if the nurse in the clinic provides the client with a clear, succinct explanation for care at home, recovery will be enhanced. If the home health care nurse of a pediatric client communicates with the school nurse about daily treatment needs, continuity will be enhanced and complications and added costs avoided.

Unlike the past, when clients typically went from an acute care setting to home, clients today enter the health care system in various ways. They may be referred from a clinic visit to home care, from school to a physician's office, from home care to an acute care setting, or from adult day care to an extended care facility. Figure 8–1 illustrates the flow of continuity of care.

Clients may be transferred several times from one community-based setting to another. For example, Juan falls in the bathroom in his home and breaks his hip. He enters the system through the emergency department and is transferred to the operating room and then to the orthopedic unit in the hospital. After discharge from the hospital, he stays in a transitional facility for follow-up physical therapy and skilled nursing care. Then he is moved to assisted living for 4 months. After being transferred to three different services in the hospital and being discharged from four different agencies, he is back in his own home 6 months after the fall.

Admission

Admission occurs when an individual enters the health care system. Each new setting involves a new admission, with continuity serving as a bridge between the new setting and the previous setting. No matter what the setting, the client and family enter with apprehension. Each new facility or agency presents strange surroundings and new people. Anxiety levels may be high. In addition to concern over the client's present condition and the future outcome, the client and family may feel overwhelmed by new people and new equipment. What may be a routine admission to the nurse is seldom routine for a client. The nurse's confidence, competence, and concern are essential in putting the client and family at ease. The nurse's attitude may exert great influence on the further course of care.

Apprehension may be lessened by the following nursing actions:

▶ Establishing rapport
▶ Indicating sincere concern for the client and family
▶ Defining the purpose and expectations of this admission

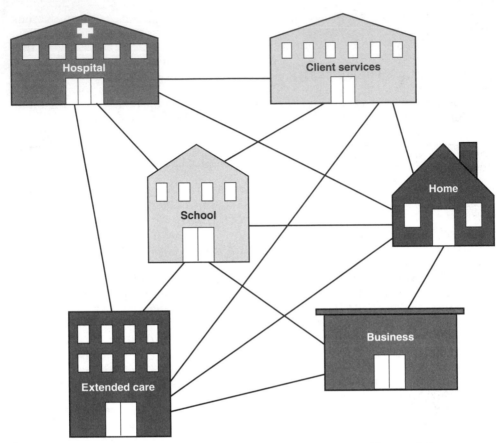

Figure 8–1. ► Continuity of care in community-based nursing is like a web between and among settings.

> ► Aiding the client in understanding how to participate as fully as possible in care-related decisions
> ► Clarifying the nursing role in relation to the client's health care needs
> ► Including the family in explanations, unless the client indicates otherwise
> ► Explaining equipment and procedures
> ► Explaining equipment to be used when calling for assistance
> ► Documenting the procedure

Admission procedures are somewhat similar for entering any system. Examples of admission procedures in various health care facilities are summarized in Table 8–1.

An admission form is always completed on entry into any health care service. Depending on the client's condition and the reason for admission, the form may be short or rather long. Insurance information, consent forms, and other forms are included in the admission paperwork.

During admission it is reassuring if the nurse explains to the client and family how they can participate in decision-making and care planning. The nurse may say, "The nutritionist will be here to talk to you this afternoon. He will discuss your food preferences. Unless the physician or nurse tells you differently,

TABLE 8–1 • Overview of Admission to Various Health Care Facilities

Facility	Possible Admission Procedures
Acute care setting	Introduction; orientation to room and equipment; complete nursing history, vital signs, and other physical assessment
Emergency department	Introduction; ABCs (airway, breathing, and circulation); vital signs; focused assessment for acute problems; orientation to surroundings
Clinic or physician's office	Introduction; explore reason for seeking medical care and focused assessment of that problem; vital signs
Nursing home	Introduction; review of written or verbal report from transferring agency; nursing history and assessment focusing on functional abilities; orientation to new surroundings
Hospice	Introduction; review of referral; nursing history and assessment focusing on pain control, functional abilities, coping, and support; wishes concerning terminal care and death (eg, living will); orientation to procedures and care
Psychiatric facility	Introduction; mental health evaluation, including history, mood state, suicide risk, use of drugs, support system
Home visit	Introduction; review of referral and client's medical and nursing problems, home environment, caretaker and family support, community resources

Craven, R. F., & Hirnle, C. J. (2000). *Fundamentals of nursing: Human health and function.* (3rd ed.). Philadelphia: Lippincott Williams & Wilkins.

you may also eat any food brought from home. Perhaps your spouse will want to cook your favorite dish."

Admission may be as anxiety-provoking for the family as for the client. The nurse supports the family by giving the location of waiting rooms, restrooms, public telephones, the nurse's station or offices, and other areas of interest, such as vending machines or cafeterias. If the client is being admitted for day surgery, the nurse may explain where the family can wait, who will bring a report, and when. In many cases, comforting the family is as important as calming the client.

Transferring

Sometimes the term *discharge* is used when a client is being **transferred**. A client typically is transferred within the same institution, most often from the emergency department to the acute care setting or intensive care unit. Another type of transfer is when the client leaves the emergency department by ambulance to be transferred to another acute care facility or transitional hospital. For example, Nhu is an 80-year-old woman who is admitted to the emergency department after a fall at her daughter's home. After examination, it is discovered that she has shattered her hip and requires extensive surgery to repair the fractures. The physicians recommend transfer to a large medical center that specializes in orthopedic repair of complex hip fractures. Nhu is transferred by ambulance to the medical center. In community-based health care, clients may be transferred from one setting to another.

With transfer, specific information must accompany the client. In a general transfer, the packet includes the following:

- ▶ Physician transfer orders
- ▶ Chest radiograph (preferably within 39 days)
- ▶ Medical history and physical examination results
- ▶ Laboratory results
- ▶ Electrocardiogram (ECG) results
- ▶ Urinalysis results
- ▶ Preadmission screening (PAS), preadmission screening and annual resident review (PASAAR) forms
- ▶ Assessment from nursing, physical therapy, occupational therapy, speech therapy (as needed)
- ▶ Social service assessment
- ▶ Do-not-resuscitate (DNR) forms (if appropriate), living wills, medical power of attorney
- ▶ Copies of important information such as results of computed tomographic (CT) scans, echocardiograms, Dopplers, magnetic resonance imaging (MRI) scans, miscellaneous cardiodiagnostic tests as appropriate (Powell, 2000, p. 404)

DISCHARGE PLANNING

Discharge planning is an accepted nursing intervention aimed at the prevention of problems after discharge (Mistiaen, Duijnhouwer, Prins-Hoekstra, Ros, & Blaylock, 1999). Discharge planning ensures continuity of care by a systematic process of coordinating various aspects of care at the time the client is discharged from a facility or program. This planning involves many individuals who make assessments, collaborate with the client and family, plan, and then communicate the critical information to the organization or individual who will next assume responsibility for the client's health care needs after discharge. The process, when it works well, is dynamic, interactive, and client-centered.

The inception of Medicare in 1966 promoted discharge planning as an essential component of client care. Social Security legislation in the 1960s and 1970s provided coverage for hospital, physician, and other health care costs. Discharge planning became a central event as a method to reduce costs, lower hospital readmission rates, and provide the client with posthospital care options. The concept of discharge planning beginning with admission to a hospital or ambulatory care setting became even more critical with the advent of the diagnosis-related group system.

Discharge planning is not limited to the physical transfer of the client, nor does it focus only on physical needs. It is much more. It is a process of early assessment of anticipated, individual client needs. It centers on a concern for the total well-being of the client and family, and it involves the client, family, and all caregivers in interactive communication during the entire planning process. It also requires ongoing interdisciplinary collaboration between many health care providers. This results in mutual agreement and appropriate options for meeting health care needs through a thorough and up-to-date review of all of the resource alternatives.

Ongoing nursing assessment of future client needs is mandated by accreditation agencies. The Joint Commission on the Accreditation of Healthcare Organizations (JCAHO) requires that the discharge plan should be initiated at admission as part of the nursing care plan (JCAHO, 1996).

Discharge planning creates bridges between settings, as shown in Figure

8–1. If the discharge plan is carefully thought out and based on collaboration among the nurse, physician, other health care providers, the client, and family, then the bridge will be strong and the transition between settings smooth. On the other hand, if the discharge plan is nonexistent or haphazardly thrown together, the transition will be bumpy with resulting complications, rehospitalizations, or unnecessary stress, all interrupting the client's recovery. Consequently, poor continuity of care has the potential to result in disaster for the client and increased cost for the health care system.

The Discharge Planning Process

Discharge planning is similar to the nursing process. Discharge planning begins with the initial assessment at the first encounter. Nurses need to know the client's plans for managing care and what the expectations are. Planning and setting goals focus on both client and family needs. Written and verbal instructions about the medication regimen, treatment, and follow-up must be provided to the client. The client also needs to be educated about any signs and symptoms that may indicate problems or complications with the condition and who to contact if this should occur. At this point, the client must have the opportunity to verbalize and discuss any concerns or questions regarding care and recovery. The intervention phase of the nursing process involves identifying needed resources and making appropriate referrals. Important telephone numbers, names, and community services should be given in writing to the client and family and explained thoroughly.

Steps of the Discharge Planning Process

Steps of the discharge planning process are as follows:

1. *Identify client discharge needs.* The nurse is often the first link in the discharge planning process. In some settings, social workers may have the primary responsibility for discharge planning; however, nurses are frequently charged with the responsibility of coordinating and communicating the discharge plan. This may involve the nurse asking questions, making sure the client is satisfied with the information given, and questioning any inconsistencies. Without clear verbal and written communication among all participants, the plan may be unsuccessful.

   The nurse must concentrate on careful assessment of the client, identifying needs as early as possible. As soon as a client is admitted, the nurse assesses for discharge needs. With each client encounter, the nurse discusses the discharge and asks the following questions: "When you are discharged . . ."

   How are you going to manage at home?
   Considering the treatments ordered for you, what are you going to need to manage at home?
   What help do you need?
   What help do you have at home now?

   The nurse is in the best possible position to clearly identify the client's needs. The nurse provides direct care and treatment for the client, which allows for the observation of responses to care. Nurses have contact around the clock in an acute care setting. The information gained about the client's ability to provide self-care after discharge is critical to planning for discharge. Assessing needs, communicating with others, and involving the client and family on an ongoing basis contribute to a realistic strategy.

2. *Anticipate changes in client needs and plan how they will be met.* Nurses have an ongoing relationship with the client, family, or caregivers. Frequent communication with the client gives the nurse the opportunity to learn about client and family interaction and communication. If the client has special care needs after discharge, the trusting relationship established between nurse and client is essential to the next step of client and family teaching. The nurse can also anticipate the needs of the client and family at home because the nurse has observed their interactions and sometimes has even observed these interactions within the home. The nurse can provide answers to the following questions:

> Will the family need changes in routine?
> Will the family be able to provide all of the care needed?
> Do they need home health care assistance?
> What are the family's resources and limitations?

3. *Ensure continuity of care and progress toward health and quality of life.* Once client needs are identified and plans are made to meet these needs, nurses promote continuity of care through coordination of services for the client and communication among health care team members. A discharge plan is not complete without considering community resources and subsequent referrals based on client needs and resources. Today, because of the costs of health care, the discharge plan is driven more often by resources than by needs. Referrals must consider client resources (eg, insurance coverage, financial status) as well as community resources. The availability of services within the geographic area can also limit access to resources. For instance, there may or may not be a hospital, nursing home, or home health care agency in the client's community.

 ## COORDINATION OF SERVICES

Successful continuity of care depends on the coordination of interdisciplinary sources of care and support. **Coordinated care** includes assisting with financial arrangements, contacting vendors and arranging for equipment, making referrals to home health care agencies, making appointments with health care providers, predischarge teaching, and follow-up to arrange additional referrals as indicated. Figure 8–2 illustrates differences between coordinated care and unorganized care.

Continuity of care is promoted by appropriate use of resources and effective referrals. Resources are defined as the available means for accomplishing a task, including staff and budget as well as physical space and equipment. Referrals are the actual exchange of information and constitute the formal links between the client, the health care setting, and the community or home. The information exchanged is the sum of assessment, nursing diagnosis, and planning. The intervention phase of the nursing process includes identifying resources and making referrals.

Client and Community Resources

Because of current health care costs, the health plan is often driven by the client's financial resources rather than by need. An example is a client who needs home visits for assistance with activities of daily living (ADL), meal preparation, house-

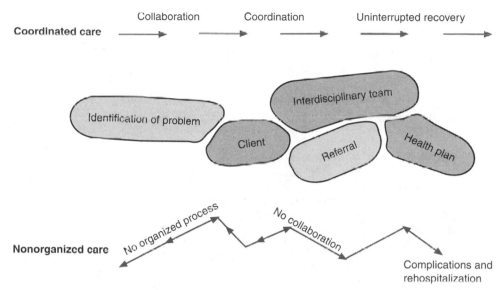

Figure 8–2. ▶ There are major differences between coordinated care and unorganized care.

hold chores, transportation, and physical therapy. The client's insurance pays only for physical therapy. This requires that the nurse, client and client's support person, physician, and multidisciplinary team (social worker, physical therapist, etc.) set priorities based on what the client can afford and explore alternative ways to meet the additional needs. Alternatives might be Meals On Wheels, volunteer transportation, family participation, church visitation, and so forth. Referrals must consider the client's resources as well as the community's resources.

To facilitate continuity of care when referring clients to an acute care setting, home, or community, the nurse must be aware of the various types of individuals and organizations available as community resources. Box 8–1 lists resources that can be used for the ill or older population of the community. Resources include physicians, hospital centers, clinics and nursing centers, specialized care centers, and long-term care facilities. School nurses and occupational nurses are resources, as are various agencies and organizations. Resources may include a range of health-related services, from drug and alcohol treatment programs to safety education to prevent rollerblading injuries. Each resource exists to provide services to meet particular needs. The nurse must know what these resources are and their eligibility requirements.

Community resources can be characterized as either health care providers or supportive care providers. Health care providers include all health care settings, health departments, community service agencies, and private practice physicians. Support care providers include psychological services, churches, and self-help groups.

Health Care Providers

Health maintenance, health promotion, and health prevention are universal needs. Health care providers include, but are not limited to, physicians, dentists, ophthalmologists, therapists (such as occupational and physical), alternative care practitioners (such as chiropractors and acupuncturists), home health care

▶ **Box 8–1.** Community Resources for Older and Ill Clients ◀

Transportation Difficulty

- Carpools with neighbors, families of other older people, fellow volunteers or workers
- City provisions for older people: reduced bus fares, taxi scrip, "Trans-Aide"
- Volunteer services: Red Cross, Salvation Army, church organizations for emergency or occasional transportation

Living Alone and Fearful of Accidents Within the Home

- Telephone checkup services through local hospitals or friends, neighbors, or relatives
- Postal alert: register with local senior center; sticker on mailbox alerts letter carrier to check for accumulation of mail
- Newspaper delivery: parents of the delivery person can be given an emergency phone number if newspapers accumulate
- Neighbors can check pattern of lights on/off

Personal Care Assistance Needed

- Private pay for hourly services: home aides from private agencies listed in the telephone book
- Visiting Nurse Association: services include aide services with nurses are used
- Medicaid/Medicare: provisions for home aides are limited to strict eligibility requirements, but such care is provided in certain situations
- Student help: posting notices on bulletin boards at nursing schools can yield inexpensive helpers
- Home sharing: sharing the home with another person who is willing to provide this kind of assistance in exchange for room and board

Occasional Nursing Care or Physical Therapy Needed

- Visiting nurse: services provided through Medicare or Medicaid or sliding scale fees; must be ordered by a physician
- Home health services: private providers listed in phone book; also nonprofit providers, Medicare and Medicaid reimbursement for authorized services

Problems Involving Shopping, Cooking, and Planning Nutritional Diets

- Home-delivered meals: Meals On Wheels delivers frozen meals once a week, sliding fees
- Nutrition sites: meals served at senior centers, churches, schools, and other locations
- Cooperatives: arrangements with neighbors to exchange a service for meals, food shopping, and so on

Insufficient Activity and Social Contacts

- Senior centers: provide social opportunities, classes, volunteer opportunities, and outings
- Church-sponsored clubs: social activities, volunteer opportunities, and outings
- Support groups: for widows, stroke victims, and general support
- Adult day care: provides social interaction, classes, discussion groups, outings, and exercise

(continued)

> ► **Box 8–1.** Community Resources for Older
> and Ill Clients (*Continued*) ◄

Problems With Housework

- Homemaker services for those meeting income eligibility criteria
- Service exchanges with neighbors and friends (ie, babysitting exchanged for housework help)
- Home helpers: hired through agencies or through employment listings at senior centers, schools, etc.
- Home sharing: renting out a room or portion of the home, reduced rent for help with housework

Problems Related to Finances

- Power of attorney given to a friend or relative for handling financial matters
- Joint checking account with friend or relative for ease in paying bills
- Volunteer assistance available from the American Red Cross, Salvation Army, church groups, senior centers, other organizations

Legal Assistance

- Senior citizens' legal services
- Lawyer referral service offered by the county bar association
- City/county aging programs, hot lines for information and assistance in phone book

Adapted from Hooyman, N. (1983). Social support networks in services for the elderly. In J. K. Whittaker, & J. Garbarino (Eds.). *Social support networks: Informal helping in the human services* (pp. 145–146). New York: Aldine de Gruyter Publishing Company. Copyright 1983, James K. Whittaker and James Garbarino.

agencies, outpatient clinics, diagnostic screening programs, and health education programs. Such diverse providers and programs can be funded by the government and may include private offices, neighborhood centers, and schools, to name only a few. Table 8–2 gives examples of roles of some health care providers. Community services share one thing in common—they provide service to the public to meet the health care needs of clients and families in the community.

Supportive Care Providers

Supportive care providers, or support services, are services that help people avoid problems or solve problems that interfere with their self-care and well-being. The primary service offered is not necessarily health-related. This category of service may be more difficult to find and identify than services directly related to health care needs. Other resources on the health care team may be able to assist with a support need. The hospital social worker, for example, will be knowledgeable about financial aid, legal service, recreation, housing, protective service, day care, peer support groups, community education, and food services. Support services are not always obvious to clients or their families, but acquiring information about them is an important piece of continuing care.

When the nurse looks for information before making a referral to an agency or service with which the nurse is not familiar, specific questions should be asked in relation to the services required:

TABLE 8–2 • Health Care Providers Used in Discharge Referrals

Health Care Provider	Role
Home health nurse	Provides assessments, direct care, client teaching and support, coordinates services, evaluates outcomes
Home health aide	Provides hygiene care, cooking, supervision, and companionship
Social worker	Assists in finding and connecting with community resources or financial resources, provides counseling and support
Physical therapist	Assists with restoring mobility, strengthens muscle groups, teaches ambulation with new devices
Occupational therapist	Helps clients adjust to limitations by teaching new vocational skills or better ways to perform activities of daily living
Nutritionist	Teaches clients about meal planning and diet restrictions
Speech therapist	Assists clients to communicate better and works with clients who have swallowing problems
Respiratory therapist	Provides home follow-up for clients with respiratory problems including assessment, oxygen administration, and home ventilator care

Craven, R. F., & Hirnle, C. J. (2000). *Fundamentals of nursing: Human health and function* (3rd ed., p. 348). Philadelphia: Lippincott Williams & Wilkins.

Can you adequately serve this client? Do you work with individuals? Families? Is your agency culturally competent and sensitive to diversity?

What are the eligibility requirements for your services? How does a client or family contact you? When can my client get an appointment?

What is the cost of the service? What financial arrangements can be made? Do you accept payment from the client's third-party payer?

Where are you located? Are you near public transportation? Is parking available? What about accessibility for the disabled? Do you travel to the area where the client lives?

What else do I need to know about your agency?

Referrals

The purpose of a **referral** to another organization or provider is to ensure that appropriate and timely information is communicated so that the client's needs are met and care is coordinated effectively. During the referral, information about the client's medical condition, care needs, and social environment is exchanged, and a formal relationship is established between the discharging and care-providing organizations. The acute care nurse will refer primarily to health care resources. The community-based nurse will not only initiate referrals to other support services but will also receive referrals from other community providers.

Characteristics of an effective referral include the following:

▶ *Merit and reliability are evident.* Merit comes from a careful assessment of the client's needs and resources; reliability derives from a follow-up evaluation of the community resources.

▶ *The referral is practical and timely.* A nurse making a referral must consider the client's ability to pay, the client's time and personal responsibilities, and whether or not the client is willing and able to address a health care need.

▶ *The referral is individualized.* What works for one client may not work for another. Differences in individual needs, resources, family, and culture and support systems must be recognized, respected, and communicated to ensure appropriate planning and intervention.

▶ *The referral is coordinated and mutually agreed on.* Are services being duplicated? Have the client and family been involved in initiating the referral? Is the referral clear and mutually agreed on?

All of these are essential elements for success of the plan of care and the client's return to the optimum level of health. Keep in mind that clients have the right to say no to any referral or recommendation about their health care.

The ideal circumstance is to have the client and family participate in the referral process so they are involved in decision-making and can choose providers or organizations they prefer. The nurse, however, may be in the best position to determine needs. For example, Suzie, a juvenile diabetic, is having trouble regulating her glucose levels. She asks you, "What *can* I eat?" Her mother says, "Sometimes I'm confused about what she can eat." Her father states, "We've been having problems with our car lately. We can't drive all the way across town to talk to someone about this." The nurse makes a referral to a dietitian located near the family's home to help determine the source of the glucose level variances and to initiate nutritional planning with Suzie and her family. Often there are multiple referrals to make for a client, and the nurse acts as coordinator between members of this expanding team.

Sometimes it is necessary to have different service providers collaborate and coordinate for a client's care to continue uninterrupted. For example, physical therapy for an older client with arthritis may be most effective in the afternoon, when the nurse is scheduled to visit. After discussing this with the client and the physical therapist, the nurse changes her visits for medication instruction to the morning so the client's need can be met.

Steps in the Referral Process

The following are the steps in making an effective referral:

1. *The health care team establishes the need.* The need is identified based on the clinical assessment by the physician, information provided or questions asked by the client, and a thorough assessment by all team members, including the nurse.
2. *The nurse sets objectives for the referral.* The client or family's needs from community resources are identified as the nurse assists the client to understand what is needed and the available resource options. The nurse does not assume that the client knows what he or she wants because the client may not know the range of options. By establishing a trusting relationship with the client and family, the nurse will be better able to identify the objectives.
3. *The nurse continuously explores for available resources.* Appropriate continuing care relies on nurses' having detailed, current knowledge about the community's resources. The nurse should collect data over time concerning community organizations and agencies. Reference books on community resources are available through organizations such as the United Way. It is important to know what these service organizations can provide as well as specific services, location, telephone number, contact person, eligibility requirements, and referral procedures. Current and reliable knowledge about what resources exist in the community is essential to assist the client or family in learning about and identifying appropriate organizations to provide care.
4. *The client makes the decision about the referral.* The nurse acts as a teacher to facilitate a decision by the client and family. This involves helping the client identify a need and accept help. The nurse's manner should reassure the client that the client is in control and making decisions and that these decisions will

be respected. The client's feelings about the need for the referral will invariably affect the outcome.

5. *The nurse makes the referral to the selected service.* A variety of formats can be used when making a referral. Not all standard forms are suited for every need and every client. The nurse can adapt or modify a form to communicate complete, appropriate information.

6. *The nurse supplies the agency with needed information.* Basic client information must be communicated along with the following:
   ▶ Health care needs: medical diagnosis, nursing problems, limitations or barriers to health, special procedures/treatments, continuing care objectives, a client's perception of the prognosis, attitudes toward continuing care
   ▶ Personal information: the client's level of knowledge about the medical condition and prognosis, the client's emotional and physical response to treatment, attitudes, beliefs, and values that affect care, level of support from family, important features of the living situation

7. *The nurse supports the client and family in pursuing the referral.* For example, Amy is a 14-year-old Native American girl admitted to the acute care setting with type 1 diabetes mellitus. She is afraid and does not want to face the realities of her new diagnosis. She tells the physician, "I don't want anything to do with this diet and stuff! I just want to go home, hang out with my friends, and eat what I want." The physician asks the nurse to explore this statement and Amy's general feelings about her diagnosis. Amy, her mother and father, and the nurse sit down in the conference area. As the discussion proceeds, the nurse discovers that Amy is afraid that she won't ever be able to eat out with her friends. Amy's mother says, "She loves fry bread, but she can't ever eat that again, right? What am I supposed to cook for her, anyway?"

   At this point, the nurse suggests the diabetes education classes at the hospital clinic. Amy's father responds, "I don't want to go back to that clinic where there are only white people." The nurse makes several telephone calls trying to identify a resource for a teenager with a new diagnosis of diabetes who follows a traditional Native American diet and whose family prefers a caretaker who is Native American. The nurse identifies the International Diabetes Clinic, which has a clientele and staff of many different nationalities. He also learns that there is a support group for Native American teens with diabetes at the American Indian Center near the family's home.

   The nurse makes a home visit to Amy's home. He gives Amy and her parents a pamphlet about managing diabetes and discusses setting an appointment with the International Diabetes Clinic. The nurse tells Amy about the support group at the neighborhood American Indian Center. He gives Amy the name of the nurse at the American Indian Center and encourages her to call and check out the support group.

Financing Referrals

Because of rising health care costs, health care organizations must now find additional funds in the form of voluntary donations and state and federal programs. The same is true for many individuals who join health maintenance organizations or rely on government-funded health care such as Medicare and Medicaid. Insurance plans, health maintenance organizations, and governmental-funded programs provide a variety of coverage plans. Many do not cover preventive care, psychiatric treatment, outpatient support services, or medications. Most limit the amount of service for which payment is made (eg, the number of home health care visits).

Nurses must assist clients in learning about their insurance coverage and in creating a plan of care that the payer will cover. Most health care plans employ case managers who understand health care needs and subsequently make decisions, based on diagnosis and need, about services that will be authorized for payment. Sometimes the authorization or denial of authorization is in conflict with decisions made by the health care team. This may require the interdisciplinary team to revise the plan, based not necessarily on what is felt to be best for the client but on what the client's financial resources and insurance coverage will pay. For example, insurance companies will not pay for home health care that consists solely of a home health aide making daily visits for the client's personal care. The client must need the skilled services of a registered nurse or physical or occupational therapist before the payer will pay for personal care needs. If the client cannot pay out-of-pocket for personal care, the team must reevaluate the client to determine if there are skilled nursing needs that could qualify the client for authorization of payment by the insurance carrier. The nurse is an important player when resource availability is dictated not necessarily by need but by payment source.

NURSING SKILLS AND COMPETENCIES IN CONTINUITY OF CARE

To enhance continuity, the nurse must develop nursing expertise in anticipating the needs of clients and their families. Continuity of care also requires collaboration skills such as knowledge of the workings of other departments within the system (eg, physical therapy, social services, transportation, pharmacy, home

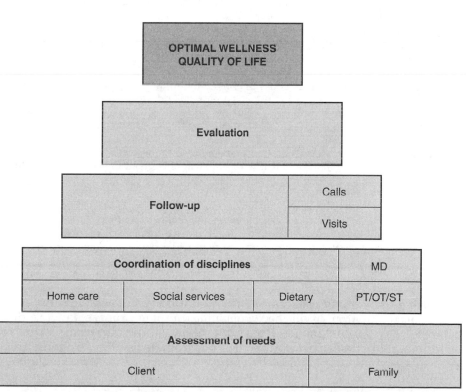

Figure 8–3. ▶ Building blocks of a well-organized discharge planning process.

health care). Discharge planning is the primary role for nurses related to continuity of care in community-based care. In some areas of the country, this person is titled continuity of care nurse, discharge planning nurse, or case manager. Primary competencies include manager, teacher, and communicator. There is no universal level of educational preparation required for any of these roles.

A significant correlation exists between the degree of structure provided in the plan and the client's return to health. Success is more likely if the discharge plan is viewed as methodical placing of building blocks, as illustrated in Figure 8–3.

EXAMPLE OF A CLIENT SITUATION

Building Block Phases in Client Care

Margret Carolan is a 72-year-old retired woman who lives alone, has no family, but has supportive friends from her church. She does not drive because of her poor vision. She has a history of type 2 diabetes mellitus and congestive heart failure. Currently, she takes insulin, ASA, propranolol, K-Dur, and Lasix every day. Three months ago, Ms. Carolan was seen in the emergency department for a transient ischemic attack. She is in the acute phase of recovery (see Fig. 8–4) when she is admitted to ambulatory surgery for arthroscopic surgery on her left knee under general anesthesia. She is instructed to be non–weight-bearing on her operative knee for 24 hours and to arrange for physical therapy twice a week for 1 month.

Ms. Carolan's Blaylock Discharge Planning and Assessment Score is 11 (see Fig. 8–5). She is alert and oriented and depends on assistance for her transportation needs. Her history indicates that because she has complex problems, careful discharge planning is required. The team collects further data on her health, her personal situation including her environment, any teaching she may require for ongoing care, her financial status, and support needs she may require at home.

Ms. Carolan enters the transitional phase of recovery (see Fig. 8–4). Her discharge plan includes teaching her the following: weight-bearing instructions for the first 24 hours, signs and symptoms of infection, wound care, analgesic use, dosage of insulin, and possible changes that may occur in her need for an increased or decreased dosage. Referrals for postdischarge physical therapy are made and transportation to and from the outpatient therapy clinic is arranged. No identified needs for home health care are apparent at this time. If complications arise, a home health care agency will be contacted.

When Ms. Carolan leaves the surgery center she is in the continuing care phase of her recovery. At this point the nurse may lose contact with the client. Other members of the multidisciplinary team assume responsibility for the client's ongoing needs and implementation of the discharge plan.

When Mrs. Carolan returns to the orthopedic clinic a month after surgery, she is assessed by a physician and nurse practitioner. They find her completely recovered from her surgery and refer her back to her primary clinic. No more specialist visits are necessary. The orthopedic surgeon sends a report to her primary provider stating all goals were met.

Using the nursing process to ensure continuity follows the same steps as any clinical situation. In discharge planning, nursing process parallels defined phases. These are outlined in Figure 8–4. Although the nurse is a key player in determining continuity of care in transitions from one setting to another, a comprehensive plan must involve the entire multidisciplinary team, including the client and the family. A health care plan is not complete without considering community resources and referrals to meet the client's needs.

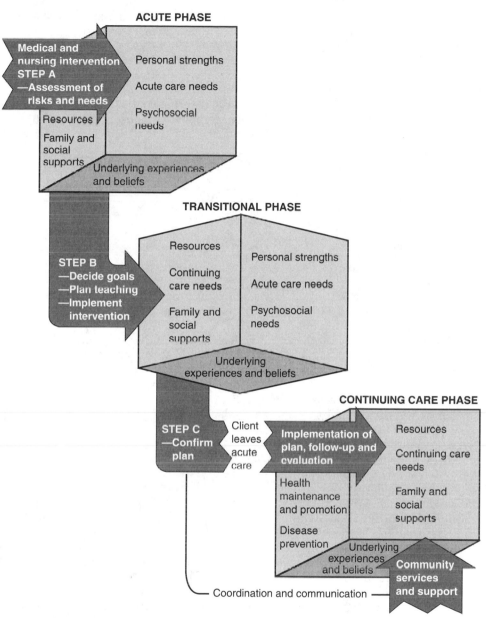

ACUTE PHASE

Medical and nursing intervention
STEP A
—Assessment of risks and needs

Personal strengths

Acute care needs

Psychosocial needs

Resources

Family and social supports

Underlying experiences and beliefs

TRANSITIONAL PHASE

STEP B
—Decide goals
—Plan teaching
—Implement intervention

Resources

Continuing care needs

Family and social supports

Personal strengths

Acute care needs

Psychosocial needs

Underlying experiences and beliefs

CONTINUING CARE PHASE

STEP C
—Confirm plan

Client leaves acute care

Implementation of plan, follow-up and evaluation

Resources

Continuing care needs

Health maintenance and promotion

Family and social supports

Disease prevention

Underlying experiences and beliefs

Community services and support

Coordination and communication

Figure 8–4. ▶ Rorden and Taft's model of the phases of the discharge planning process. Rorden, J. W., & Taft, E. (1990). *Discharge planning guide for nurses* (p. 26). Philadelphia: Saunders.

Assessment

Assessment of client needs must begin on admission to the facility or shortly thereafter. It can also begin at a preadmission point. The nurse uses his or her skills to identify and anticipate the client's specific needs and the services that will be needed after discharge. Assessments may be conducted by different disciplines (eg, the nurse, someone from the financial department, a physician, and a social worker) when the client enters the health care environment. The initial assessment identifies acute problems and needs. It must include a discussion with the client and family about what they perceive their health care needs to be.

Discharge planning assessment begins at admission. Ongoing assessment monitors the client's response to treatment; seeks the client's and family's input regarding their desires, needs, and resources; and initiates the coordination of the multidisciplinary team. The essential elements of a discharge planning assessment for a client include the following:

▶ Health data
▶ Client and family knowledge
▶ Personal data
▶ Financial and support needs
▶ Environmental data

Discharge planning assessment can be conducted by using a high-risk screening tool, such as the Blaylock Risk Assessment Screening Score (BRASS) index. This may be used by the nurse at the bedside to gather comprehensive initial and ongoing data. The aim of the BRASS index is to identify, after hospital admission, elderly clients who are at risk for prolonged hospital stay. Early identification of people who will have intense discharge needs may prevent or reduce postdischarge problems.

The index is shown in Figure 8–5. It contains 10 items, each judged by a nurse, using normal diagnostic procedures and questions at admission. The nurse goes through the questions, giving the client a score for every section. The Risk Factor Index at the bottom of the page indicates the client's need for discharge planning and resource planning. Research Box 8–1 presents for recent research on the BRASS index.

A second assessment tool designed to enhance continuity of care is the Nursing Continuing Care Needs (NCCN) assessment tool. This form is a valid, sensitive, specific, and feasible tool first developed by the Health Care Financing Administration. A revised version is used extensively at Mayo Clinics. The NCCN serves a valuable purpose before a client is discharged in enhancing communication between hospital nurses and any receiving care providers. Further, it contributes to efficient assessment and communication of discharge planning needs. An outline of the NCCN tool is shown in Box 8–2.

Assessments also are used to determine continuing care needs. When assessing the need for ongoing care, the client, family, culture, and environment are all viewed as a unit of care. The nurse cannot collect all of the data. Information about the client's home environment may require a home visit by social services, for example. The interdisciplinary team collects information about the client's health, personal circumstances, home, community, environment, and background, as well as current conditions and any financial or support services. The elements of health planning are valuable in providing a general source of information about the client, family, and environment. Some clients are at higher risk and need immediate intervention by specific supportive services.

A thorough collection of information is needed to plan effectively for continuity of care, but it is not always easily obtained. The client's successful recovery and return to optimal health often depend on collecting the right information during the assessment phase of planning. Nurses need to have multiple skills to facilitate this collection of information and plan adequately.

Blaylock Discharge Planning Risk Assessment Screen

Circle all that apply and total. Refer to the Risk Factor Index*

Age
- 0 = 55 years or less
- 1 = 56 to 64 years
- (2) = 65 to 79 years
- 3 = 80 + years

Living Situation/Social Support
- 0 = Lives only with spouse
- 1 = Lives with family
- 2 = Lives alone with family support
- (3) = Lives alone with friends' support
- 4 = Lives alone with no support
- 5 = Nursing home/residential care

Functional Status
- 0 = Independent in activities of daily living and instrumental activities of daily living

Dependent in:
- 1 = Eating/feeding
- 1 = Bathing/grooming
- 1 = Toileting
- 1 = Transferring
- 1 = Incontinent of bowel function
- 1 = Incontinent of bladder function
- 1 = Meal preparation
- 1 = Responsible for own medication administration
- 1 = Handling own finances
- 1 = Grocery shopping
- (1) = Transportation

Cognition
- (0) = Oriented
- 1 = Disoriented to some spheres some of the time†
- 2 = Disoriented to some spheres all of the time
- 3 = Disoriented to all spheres some of the time
- 4 = Disoriented to all spheres all of the time
- 5 = Comatose

Behavior Pattern
- (0) = Appropriate
- 1 = Wandering
- 1 = Agitated
- 1 = Confused
- 1 = Other

Mobility
- 0 = Ambulatory
- (1) = Ambulatory with mechanical assistance
- 2 = Ambulatory with human assistance
- 3 = Nonambulatory

Sensory Deficits
- 0 = None
- (1) = Visual or hearing deficits
- 2 = Visual and hearing deficits

Number of Previous Admissions/Emergency Room Visits
- 0 = None in the last 3 months
- (1) = One in the last 3 months
- 2 = Two in the last 3 months
- 3 = More than two in the last 3 months

Number of Active Medical Problems
- (0) = Three medical problems
- 1 = Three to five medical problems
- 2 = More than five medical problems

Number of Drugs
- 0 = Fewer than three drugs
- 1 = Three to five drugs
- (2) = More than five drugs

Total Score: __11__

*Risk Factor Index: Score of 10 = at risk for home care resources; score of 11 to 19 = at risk for extended discharge planning; score greater than 20 = at risk for placement other than home. If the patient's score is 10 or greater, refer the patient to the discharge planning coordinator or discharge planning team.
†Sphere = person, place, time, and self.
Copyright 1991 Ann Blaylock

Figure 8–5. ▶ Sample of the Blaylock Discharge Planning Risk Assessment Screen.

RESEARCH IN COMMUNITY-BASED NURSING CARE

Research Box 8–1 ▶ Predictive Validity of the Blaylock Risk Assessment Screening Score

Discharge planning is one of the most important nursing interventions related to ensuring continuity. The Blaylock Risk Assessment Screening Score (BRASS) index is a risk screening instrument that can be used at admission to identify clients in need of discharge planning. This research tested the predictive validity of the BRASS index in screening patients with postdischarge problems.

Five hundred and three elderly clients were screened at admission with the BRASS index. It was found that the higher the BRASS scores the greater the difficulty after discharge in all domains. This study found that the BRASS index is a good predictor for identifying clients who are not candidates for discharge to home. It also accurately predicts clients who will have problems after discharge.

Mistiaen, P., Duijnhouwer, E., Prins-Hoekstra, A., Ros, W., & Blaylock, A. (1999). Predictive validity of the BRASS index in screening patients with post-discharge problems. *Journal of Advanced Nursing, 30*(5), 1050–1056.

Nursing Diagnosis

The nurse needs to be skillful in identifying the client's strengths and needs so that efficient care may be given. Nursing diagnoses will help other nurses streamline their care. For instance, if the visiting nurse sees that the previous visiting nurse has noted *Parental Role Conflict,* the second nurse will be ready to pick up on communications occurring within the home. *Risk for Loneliness* would be a clue the clinic nurse could state to direct follow-up. In an ongoing manner, this information is shared with all pertinent members of the health care team.

Planning

The goal of health planning is to assist the client and family in the achievement of an optimal level of wellness (Fig. 8–6). The key to successful planning is the exchange of information between the client, present caregivers (eg, nurse, physician, social worker, respiratory therapist, physical therapist, occupational therapist, nutritionist, psychologist, or speech therapist) and those responsible for the continuing care (eg, family, support services, and individuals or care-givers). Planning for the client involves:

▶ Recognizing and using the resources of the family
▶ Educating the family about the options available and encouraging their participation in the decision-making process
▶ Assisting the client and family to feel they have control over their own welfare and assisting them to identify resources that could help them in this process

Sociocultural factors can influence the planning phase. It is important for the nurse to identify and acknowledge issues that may influence the plan. These may include beliefs about the causes of illness and death and dying, language, nutrition practices, healing practices, and sexual orientation.

▶ Box 8–2. Domains and Subcategories of the Nursing
Continuing Care Needs Assessment Instrument (NCCN) ◀

Cognitive/Behavioral/Emotional Status

Anticipated level of consciousness on discharge
Cognition
Comprehension
Expression
Usual mode of communication
Emotional/behavioral factors

Health Status

Perception of prognosis
Current health problems
Risk factors

Functional Status

Activities of daily living
Instrumental activities of daily living

Finances

Resources

Environmental Factors in Postdischarge Care

Barriers
Need for assistive devices

Anticipated Skilled Care Requirements for Discharge

Skin: pressure ulcer
Skin: wound care
Nutrition
Hydration
Respiratory
Cardiovascular
Elimination
Neuromusculoskeletal
Speech and language
Counseling
Patient/family education
Administration of medications
Coordination of care needed

Meeting Continuing Care Needs

Summary of continuing care needs
Resource availability
Resource provider

Adapted from Holland, D., Hansen, D., Matt-Hensrud, M., Severson, M., & Wenniger, C. (1999).
Continuity of care: A nursing needs assessment instrument. *Geriatric Nursing, 19*(6), 331–334.

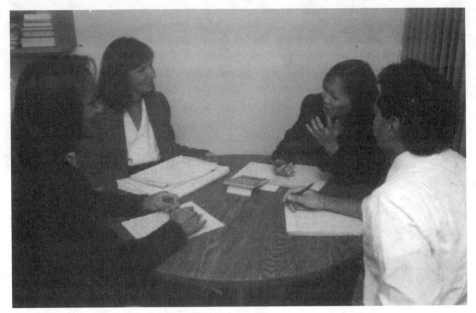

Figure 8–6. ▶ The key to successful planning is the exchange of information among those concerned about the client's care.

During the planning phase, the client and the multidisciplinary team develop realistic expected outcomes. Frequent communication and coordination among the multidisciplinary team, client, and client's family facilitates reaching realistic expected outcomes in a well-designed discharge plan. This is accomplished through:

▶ Consulting between the physician and the social worker or discharge planner
▶ Determining the client's prognosis
▶ Setting priorities
▶ Designing realistic time frames
▶ Determining responsibility
▶ Analyzing alternative resources for appropriateness and availability
▶ Exploring financial resources and burdens
▶ Involving and educating the family
▶ Setting appropriate and realistic expected outcomes
▶ Coordinating community resources

Expected outcomes help the multidisciplinary team know what is expected of the client. When these outcomes have been agreed on by the client and family, all participants know what the goals are and can evaluate whether they have been obtained.

Implementation

Nursing interventions focus on assisting the client to achieve the highest possible level of functioning and wellness. Interventions involve coordinating multidisciplinary plans, teaching the client and family, using appropriate community resources through referrals, case management, and dispelling the client's or family's apprehension about continuing care needs.

Discharge plan interventions such as health education, referral to community resources, and ordering equipment for the home depend on the nurse's being competent to assess the client's ability to manage daily activities in the home, judge the client's and family's compliance with the therapeutic regimen, assess the client's knowledge of self-care, and coordinate the team members.

Because the plan involves a multidisciplinary team, it is critical for the plan to be structured and organized. However, it must also be flexible enough to allow for change as the client progresses toward health. The team begins activities that lead toward the achievement of expected outcomes. Revisions to the plan must be made as indicated.

As the client moves from one care setting or care provider to another, careful planning of intervention strategies must consider how the changes affect the client and the family. Probably clients and families will feel anxious about the change. This is especially true if they have been hurried through an acute care setting or if discharge plans were discussed only on admission when their acute condition prohibited them from fully participating. From the time of admission on, the nurse will need to work with the client and family to reinforce the importance of early discharge planning for the client to achieve maximum quality of health. Being sensitive to the client's needs while planning care will help to reduce anxiety and increase the client's participation and acceptance of care transitions.

A variety of intervention skills promote recovery and increase the effectiveness of the plan of care. Teaching skills are important and may include both prevention and promotion strategies (Fig. 8–7). Teaching and demonstrations are integral to some types of ongoing care. They may need to be repeated because of the client and family's anxiety or inability to learn quickly. The nurse must use effective interpersonal skills when communicating with other organizations or individuals who will provide continuing care to the client. Proper im-

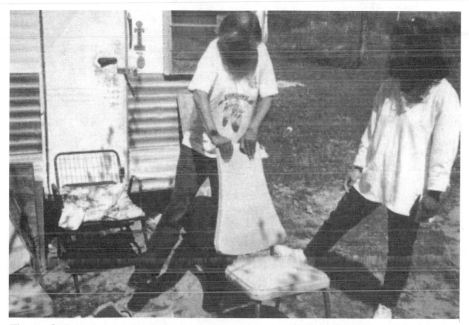

Figure 8–7. ▶ A community-based nurse teaches a Native American elder range-of-motion exercises outside his rural home. She is providing prevention and promotion strategies in her continuity of care of her client.

plementation of the plan ensures that duplication of services does not occur and that confusion or conflicts that arise are promptly handled.

Evaluation

Evaluation is the measurement of the outcomes or results of implementing the plan for continuity. This involves gathering data on the client's response to interventions. Data can be collected from the client, family, physician, and referral sources. The major purpose of evaluation is to see if expected outcomes were reached. Evaluation is ongoing; reviews are made to determine if needs were met and problems resolved, and if the plan needs to be revised. Evaluation continues as the client moves from one setting to another.

In evaluating the effectiveness of continuity of care, it is essential to consider:

▶ Whether or not the health planning was initiated when the client first obtained health care services
▶ If discharge planning was discussed with the client and family at the beginning of care
▶ Whether the client and family participated in early planning for ongoing care
▶ If there was interdisciplinary planning with all involved professionals
▶ If the care being provided to the client is empathic, based on mutual trust and cultural sensitivity
▶ If the client and family believe they had all the information they needed
▶ Whether the client felt prepared for self-care at home
▶ Whether the client and family believe they had the resources needed for self-care
▶ If there is new information that suggests the plan should be revised

The nurse is responsible for monitoring and documenting the client's response to care. Evaluation is effective only if there is a plan with expected outcomes or goals established by the interdisciplinary team. The evaluation process is more meaningful if the expected outcomes are written in a clear, measurable way.

Judgment skills are necessary when comparing real outcomes with expected outcomes. If the client's behavior matches the desired outcomes, the goal has been met. If the goals are not met, then the nurse must examine the reasons for the shortfall.

Unmet goals may be due to inadequate data collection, incorrect identification of need, unrealistic planning, or poor implementation (Spradley & Allender, 1996). The client's living situation or physical condition may have changed. New, previously unidentified needs may require additional care or services. Some services may no longer be necessary, or the client may be ready for discharge. Whatever the conclusion, after evaluation the appropriate members of the interdisciplinary team must reassess and plan for the continuing needs of the client.

Documentation

The nurse is always responsible for documenting the client's response to care. Concise and reliable documentation that reflects both progress and response to treatment builds a clear outline for subsequent evaluation. Documentation of all teaching performed is critical to team communication. What was taught, what return demonstrations were completed, and what written materials were given to the client should be included.

A written discharge plan is one method used for communication and coordination among team members. Collection and evaluation of data for the purpose of discharge planning are done in varying degrees of formality (interviews, physical examinations, questionnaires, etc), but communication is better served if the recording of such data is kept formal and organized. Use of well-constructed and consistently used discharge planning documents becomes vital to the success of coordination of disciplines and, therefore, to effective planning. Essential for successful implementation of the discharge plan is documentation that includes the client's response to interventions in the plan, continued assessment for changes in client needs, the client's desires and goals, and evidence of continued collaboration of all involved disciplines.

Documentation has a valuable role in the evaluation of discharge planning, using record audits as in quality improvement programs. The retrospective review of client records to determine compliance with standards of quality care has an advantage in that an audit deals with "hard" data. A client record either has a discharge plan documented or it does not; either discharge teaching was documented or it was not. A review of records is the most straightforward way of determining whether procedures have been done.

 BARRIERS TO SUCCESSFUL CONTINUITY OF CARE

Each client situation is unique. The nurse must be aware of *barriers* that may adversely affect continuity. These blocks may result from social factors, resource limitations, family matters, communication difficulties, or cultural differences. For example, a center for diabetic education may have materials printed in English only, thereby creating a communication and cultural barrier. When individuals cannot fully understand the material, a communication barrier is created. The health care system itself poses many barriers to continuity of care.

Social Factors

Reimbursement
Because health care policy is driven by cost, client-centered choices and quality of care are often denied. Rules for health care reimbursement and qualifications for access and use of services often create a lopsided service system with gaps in care. In some instances, the lack of payment for services creates a barrier to the health care system itself, which purportedly is the client's advocate. The health care worker may be left feeling apathetic toward planning and referral when services are available only when there is a source of payment. Problem-solving must occur to remove or work with these constraints.

Attitude of Health Care Worker
The health care worker's attitudes and biases can affect whether the client and family will use available resources. Clients are quick to sense bias and judgment. For example, a prenatal clinic for low-income women may have no place for small children to wait while their mothers are examined. In fact, the mothers are discouraged from bringing their children to the clinic when they have appointments. The women sense this judgment, but most of them cannot afford child care. Consequently, they do not follow through on essential prenatal care, resulting in interrupted continuity.

Client Motivation
The client may not follow through on a suggested referral if there are more pressing matters at hand. When people are ill, they are often concerned only with

meeting basic needs and not with meeting more involved goals, such as belonging or self-esteem. Consequently, when clients are asked to make decisions about their higher needs, their motivation may be diminished because all their energy is going toward getting their basic health care needs met. Client priorities can explain why preventive health care services, for instance, may not be considered a priority when the client has difficulty just feeding and clothing the family. The nurse must be aware of the client's priorities. The nurse must first assist with meeting the needs the client sees as a priority before progressing.

Lack of Knowledge

When clients do not understand the need for a service, they may avoid using that service. Understanding the reason for a referral to an outside organization, as well as understanding the consequences of not following through, increases the likelihood of clients using the service. This can be true in the case of prenatal care for the adolescent who is pregnant for the first time. She may know she "should" go to the clinic for checkups during pregnancy, but she may not know why. If the adolescent understands the purpose of prenatal care and the consequences of not receiving care, she is more likely to follow up with a referral to the antenatal clinic.

Family Factors

Both involvement in decisions about care after discharge and receiving relevant self-care information are rated as very important to clients and families being discharged from one setting to another (Clare, 1999). Family involvement may either enhance or interrupt continuity. Whatever the contributing factor affecting family involvement, be it family stress, family functioning, or financial resources, it is up to the nurse to solve problems and address these issues with input from the family.

Family Stress

Coping can be especially difficult for the client and family in the acute care phase of treatment when they are asked to begin planning for posthospital care. They may be just beginning to recognize and respond to the severity of the condition and subsequent need for treatment. The client and family are in the throes of a health crisis, while the health care team is attempting to educate, assess, and plan for continuing care needs. The nurse must assess the client's level of stress before involving that client and family in discharge planning and then must proceed accordingly.

Family Functioning

Sometimes delays in care are at the request of the family because of work schedule, other responsibilities, or illness. For example, a test or procedure may be delayed or scheduled on a day when a family member is able to be present. The nurse should evaluate, as much as possible, the home environment and relationships among family members. This can be accomplished by talking to the client, building a level of trust, and then assessing the level of family functioning. Every family operates differently; consequently, every family handles situations in different ways. It is up to the nurse to be aware of the client's needs and choices and to be prepared to advocate for the client when conflict arises.

A supportive family provides an environment conducive to healing and is more likely to help the client recover. An unsupportive family, on the other hand, can be an obstacle. For example, suppose a gay man who is positive for human immunodeficiency virus has a biologic family that is ashamed of and judgmental about his lifestyle. This conflict of values may stop him from seeking out and using appropriate community resources because he may feel that everyone will make the same judgments.

Financial Resources

Health care services are costly in the United States, and not everyone has health insurance. Consequently, many people do not seek health care services because they cannot afford them. This is often the case with the "working poor" who are underinsured or uninsured, or those who are on medical assistance and may not qualify for needed services. The nurse must be aware of the client's financial and insurance resources before making a referral. Financial reality creates a challenge for the nurse. At times it is difficult to find services in the community that will fill a client's needs when financial resources are inadequate.

Communication Barriers

Poor communication about recovery information is often attributed to language problems and hearing limitations. In general, health care providers expect client compliance, respect, and cooperation. Communication barriers can occur when the client does not speak English. They also occur when there is a cultural difference significant enough to prohibit communication (eg, reading and comprehension) or to create a venue where misunderstandings may occur as a result of, for example, the age of the client, sexual orientation, or use of nonverbal communication. A client may be offended and not listen to instructions or refuse referrals to community providers if the nurse does not practice culturally sensitive communication techniques. Increasing age brings hearing limitations, impaired eyesight, and memory loss, which can interfere with communication and retention of information.

Cross-Cultural Barriers

The biggest barrier, although not the most obvious, is the cross-cultural barrier that may exist between the provider and client. It may be difficult for the nurse to withhold judgment and accept the client or family of another culture. In the opinion of the nurse, clients from a different culture may ask "too many" questions, exhibit defensive behavior or a lack of deference to the recognized authority figure (eg, nurses and other health care providers), or have different perceptions of their role in the discharge planning and referral process.

Health care providers may have different cultural backgrounds, ethnicity, race, age, sexual orientation, gender, and experience in health care practices. The use of culture-specific behaviors positively influences the health care provided and, subsequently, the outcomes. The nurse learns culture-specific behaviors by building knowledge about cultural beliefs related to causes of illness and treatment of disease.

Ethnic and cultural values are pervasive in a person's life, and it is important for the nurse to identify them as they relate to health care practices. The nurse must constantly discriminate between the health care practices of the dominant culture and those of the client's cultural group.

Every culture has beliefs and values about health care practices. Cultural beliefs about the cause of illness, what heals an illness, and what are preventive measures vary widely across cultures. Some cultures do not practice preventive measures; the nurse may receive resistance to community referrals if they are focused on prevention practices. Decision-making processes also vary greatly, depending on culture and ethnicity. Indeed, it would behoove the nurse to ask the client if anyone besides the client should be involved in the decision-making and planning for discharge. Many cultures have hierarchies in families that must be honored in decision-making. It is critical to the client's recovery that the nurse acknowledges the existence of health care belief systems other than the Western medical model.

For example, harmonious relationships are a dominant cultural value for many Asians. Thus, these clients may always agree with the nurse or provide answers they think the nurse expects because they see the nurse as an authority figure. The nurse should phrase questions and explain situations in a way that avoids suggesting an expected response.

Nonverbal communication cues include facial expression, gestures, body posture, tone of voice, eye contact, touch, and use of personal space. These communication behaviors vary widely across cultures. Eye contact is one of the most variable behaviors. Many Native American, Arab, and Appalachian clients may consider direct eye contact impolite or aggressive. Views of physical contact can differ as well; patting the head of a Thai child is a sign of disrespect because the head is regarded as an area of strength.

Keep in mind that effective nursing care avoids using cultural, ethnic, or racial stereotypes to create assumptions about the client's preferences and subsequent care. Each cross-cultural client must be recognized as an individual.

Health Care System Barriers

Sometimes systems within the health care setting create barriers to successful continuity. The primary health care team may unintentionally interrupt continuity in several different ways. First, insufficient staff may create delays. Lack of time to address continuity needs is another barrier to continuity (Pichitpornchai, Street, & Boontong, 1999). Third, if staff communication is poor, delays may result.

Caregivers and services outside of the primary health care team may create delays. For example, laboratory test results may not be ready on time, or trans-

COMMUNITY-BASED NURSING CARE GUIDELINES

Strategies to Reduce Cultural Barriers in Discharge Planning

- Encourage nurses and health care workers to speak the language or provide competent interpreters for the population being served.
- Encourage health care workers to be sensitive to the background and previous health care experiences of the target group.
- Listen attentively; be aware of any impairment to communication.
- Elicit information about preferences and health care beliefs and include them in the plan of care.
- Actively inquire about significant others and available support.
- Inquire about the home environment.

port may not be provided during prescribed timelines. These delays are often not within the control of the primary health care team (Perlmutter, Suico, Krauss, & Auld, 1998). Sometimes a lack of services may create lack of continuity (Pichitpornchai et al., 1999).

Other barriers to continuity relate to discharge planning, such as failure to obtained skilled nursing care or visiting nurse service placement or approval in time for discharge. Sometimes delays arise from the nurse's inability to locate family members responsible for discharge (Perlmutter et al., 1998).

Medical equipment essential for home monitoring must be ordered in a timely fashion to avoid delays. There are often policies regarding discharge of a client who is dependent on high-technology monitoring devices. For example, an infant discharged with an apnea-bradycardia monitor may have to be free of apnea and bradycardia episodes for 48 hours before the infant can be discharged. (Perlmutter et al., 1998).

Barriers to Using Community Resources

Previous Experiences

If a client has not had a good experience with a referral in the past, he or she may be hesitant to use this type of service again. The same is true for a client's perception of a particular agency or organization. The nurse must acknowledge the client's feelings and opinions about past experiences. Talking with and listening to the client will help the nurse work with the client to get the best results from a referral to a community provider. The nurse may find that the client lacked information about the organization and a different approach is all that is necessary. Perhaps the client's complaints about the organization are justified, in which case it may be in the client's best interest to find an alternative provider.

Accessibility

A major barrier to using health care services is accessibility. Many communities do not have public transportation. Hospitals, clinics, and other health care services are closing, especially in rural areas, and many rural communities are being left with no local health care services. This requires clients to travel long distances to reach health care services. A city-dwelling client who uses public transportation instead of owning a car may have difficulty getting to a suburban clinic. The nurse must get information from the client about access to transportation before making a referral. This is especially important with low-income clients, urban clients, and those living in rural areas.

 ## ELEMENTS OF SUCCESSFUL CONTINUITY OF CARE

As with all nursing care, it probably goes without saying that it is always best to begin with the simplest interventions. These include building a trusting relationship and using therapeutic communication as the client and family are interviewed. All of the interventions discussed in Chapter 7 apply: care coordination, collaboration, delegation, and referral and follow-up. Much can be learned from successful programs designed to enhance continuity. Some very simple interventions emerge.

A home-based program enhances successful continuity of care for clients with chronic congestive heart failure (CHF), according to a study by Stewart,

Marley, and Horowitz (1999). Because hospital admissions among clients with CHF are a major contributor to health care costs, this study investigated the impact of a comprehensive home assessment by a cardiac nurse on CHF readmission rates over a 6-month period. Both study groups received the usual discharge planning, but only one group received home visit where the visiting cardiac nurse completed a comprehensive assessment 7 to 10 days after discharge. Another home visit was made only if the client had two or more unplanned readmissions within the 6-month period. Overall, there were fewer exacerbations of the condition and unplanned hospital readmissions with the group receiving the home visit.

Hip fractures represent a major health problem with the older population. This condition frequently results in care in several settings (eg, the hospital, transitional/subacute hospital, and assisted living or long-term care facility). Robinson (1999) studied factors that promote function and enable a successful transition to home for elderly recovering from a hip fracture. Several things can be learned from this study. First, discharge planning and follow-up should receive greater attention, with identification of resources at admission. Second, telephone reminders from the physical therapist after discharge result in the clients' continuing to exercise. This study reinforces the importance of nurse in-

RESEARCH IN COMMUNITY-BASED NURSING CARE

Research Box 8–2 ▶ Information Needs of Elderly Postsurgical Cancer Patients During the Transition From Hospital to Home

The purpose of this study was to describe information needs of elderly postsurgical cancer clients. The 148 clients surgically treated for a new diagnosis of cancer were randomly assigned to the treatment group and their responses were compared to a similar control group. The experimental group received a home care intervention consisting of three home visits and five telephone contacts from an advanced practice nurse.

Both groups received information during hospitalization and discharge with written instruction. It was found that the experimental group still needed information on multiple topics. The teaching needs identified as important by the clients and families included the topics of outlining the clinical course of the illness, community resources, events to report, and pain management.

The study concluded that the learning needs of elderly postsurgical cancer clients during the transition from hospital to home are complex and cannot be adequately addressed during hospitalization. Despite the teaching and written information received during usual discharge planning, these clients needed ongoing contact with nurses. Further, a nurse case manager model using a combination of home and telephone contacts may be a cost-effective option for providing continuity. Forty percent of the teaching completed in this study was done on the telephone. Further research is needed to determine the best methods for enhancing continuity between hospital and home for postsurgical clients.

Hughes, L., Hodgson, N., Muller, P., Robinson, L., & McCorkle, R. (2000). Information needs of elderly postsurgical cancer patients during the transition from hospital to home. *Journal of Nursing Scholarship, 32*(1), 25–30.

RESEARCH RELATED TO COMMUNITY-BASED NURSING CARE

Research Box 8–3 ▶ Postpartum Home Visits: Extending the Continuum of Care From Hospital to Home

The postpartum period is a time of great vulnerability for families. Often new parents are dealing with physical and psychosocial changes with little preparation. Home health visits can bridge the gap of continuity between hospital, clinic, and home. This study identifies typical postpartum needs and describes the related interventions of home health care nurses.

The sample population included 385 low-risk women who were postpartum and received home visits for 1 year. The top maternal psychosocial problems were, in order of significance, postpartum blues or depression, fatigue, lack of social support, and ineffective parenting. Breast-feeding issues, sore nipples, episiotomy/incision, and hemorrhoids were the top physical problems identified in the home visits. The top newborn problems were jaundice, feeding problems, weight problems, and dehydration.

This study suggests that families need an extensive amount of education in the immediate postpartum period. Further, this investigation found an increased number of emotional problems for young mothers, and more physical and psychosocial problems with single/divorced mothers than married mothers. According to the author, nurses must rise to the challenge of providing the full continuum of care to the postpartum family.

Bennett, R., & Tandy, L. (1998). Postpartum home visits: Extending the continuum of care from hospital to home. *Home Healthcare Nurse, 16*(5), 295–303.

volvement, even with the simplest intervention of a follow-up telephone call to enhance self-care. Research Boxes 8–2 and 8–3 offer more examples of successful programs to enhance continuity of care.

CONCLUSIONS

This chapter has taken a broad look at continuity of care. Essential to quality health care is a strong, ongoing health care plan that includes appropriate use of resources and effective referrals. Discharge planning has been described as a significant process that ensures continuity of care by coordinating various aspects of a client's care beginning with admission through transition from one health care setting to another. Planning for discharge begins with entrance into the health care system. Coordination of activities involving the clients, providers, and payers is essential in providing continued care. Identification of current and future needs leads to implementation of the referral process and continued care. The discharge planning process resembles the nursing process; therefore, the nurse is in an advantageous position to manage effective planning and continued care. Barriers to effective discharge planning include social, family, communication, system, and community resources issues. In evaluating the effectiveness of continuity of care, one must consider whether planning was initiated when the client entered the system, whether the client and family were part of the planning, and whether the plan was well coordinated with all members of the team.

What's on the Web

American Association for Continuity of Care
P. O. Box 7073
North Brunswick, NJ 08902
Telephone: (800) 816-1575
Fax: (301) 352-7686

Internet address: http://www.continuityofcare.com

This site has extensive information about the organization and pertinent issues. It also provides many links to other professional organizations related to continuity care.

Continuity Care Inc.
980 Palmerston Avenue
Winnipeg, Manitoba, Canada R3G 1J9
Telephone/Fax: (204) 779-1679

Internet address: http://www.mbnet.mb.ca/crm/lifestyl/advoc/contcare/index.html

This Canadian organization was established to assist families in planning with a family member with a disability.

There is great overlap between continuity of care and case management; see Chapter 7 for additional resources.

References and Bibliography

Bennett, R., & Tandy, L. (1998). Postpartum home visits: Extending the continuum of care from hospital to home. *Home Healthcare Nurse, 16*(5), 295–303.

Blaylock, A., & Cason, C. L. (1992). Discharge planning: Predicting patient's needs. *Journal of Gerontological Nursing, 18*(7), 5–10.

Blazys, D. (1999). Discharge planning. *Journal of Emergency Nursing, 25*(5), 386–387.

Chiverton, P., Tortoretti, D., LeForest, M., & Walder, P. (1999). Bridging the gap between psychiatric hospitalization and community care: Cost and quality outcomes. *Journal of the American Psychiatric Nurses Association, 5*(2), 46–53.

Clare, J., & Hofmeyer, A. (1999). Discharge planning continuity of care for aged people; Indicators of satisfaction and implications for practice. *Australian Journal of Advanced Nursing, 16*(1), 7–13.

Coulee, S., Bergen, A., Young K., & Kavanagh, A. (2000). A taxonomy of needs assessment, elicited from a multiple case study of community nursing education and practice. *Journal of Advanced Nursing, 31*(1), 126–134.

Craven, R. F., & Hirnle, C. J. (2000). Fundamentals of nursing: Human health and function (3rd ed.). Philadelphia: Lippincott Williams & Wilkins.

Dukkers, D., Ros, W., & Berns, M. (1999). Transition of care: An evaluation of the role of the discharge liaison nurse in the Netherlands. *Journal of Advanced Nursing, 30*(5), 1186–1194.

Hall, M., & Lawrence, L. (1998). *Ambulatory surgery in the United States, 1996. Advance data* (p. 300). Washington, DC: U.S. Department of Health and Human Services.

Holland, D., Hansen, D., Matt-Hensrud, M., Severson, M., & Wenninger, C. (1999). Continuity of care: A nursing needs assessment instrument. *Geriatric Nursing, 19*(6), 331–334.

Hughes, L., Hodgson, N., Muller, P., Robinson, L., & McCorkle, R. (2000). Information needs of elderly postsurgical cancer patients during the transition from hospital to home. *Journal of Nursing Scholarship, 32*(1), 25–30.

Johansson, B., Berglund, G., Glimelius, B., Holmberg, L., & Sjoden, P. (1999). Intensified primary care: A randomized study of home care nurse contacts. *Journal of Advanced Nursing, 30*(5), 1137–1146.

Joint Commission on Accreditation of Healthcare Organizations. (1996). *Accreditation manual for hospitals.* Chicago: Author.

Kauffmann, E., Harrison, M. B., Burke, S. O., & Wong, C. (1998). Stress-point intervention for parents of children hospitalized with chronic conditions. *Pediatric Nursing, 24*(4), 362–366.

Mistiaen, P., Duijnhouwer, E., Prins-Hoekstra, A., Ros, W., & Blaylock, A. (1999). Predictive validity of the BRASS index in screening patients with post-discharge problems. *Journal of Advanced Nursing, 30*(5), 1050–1056.

Perlmutter, D., Suico, C., Krauss, A., & Auld, P. (1998). A program to reduce discharge delays in a neonatal intensive care unit. *American Journal of Managed Care, 4*(4), 548–552.

Pichitpornchai, W., Street, A., & Boontong, T. (1999). Discharge planning and transitional care: Issues in Thai nursing. *International Journal of Nursing Studies, 36*(5), 355–362.

Powell, S. (2000). *Case management: A practical guide to success in managed care* (2nd ed.). Philadelphia: Lippincott Williams & Wilkins.

Robinson, S. (1999). Transitions in the lives of elderly women who have sustained hip fractures. *Journal of Advanced Nursing, 30*(6), 1341–1348.

Rorden, J. W., & Taft, E. (1990). *Discharge planning guide for nurses.* Philadelphia: Saunders.

Sparbel, K., & Anderson, M. (2000). Integrated literature review of continuity of care: Part 1, conceptual issues. *Journal of Nursing Scholarship, 32*(1), 17–24.

Spradley, B. W., & Allender, J. A. (1996). *Community health nursing: Concepts and practice* (4th ed.). Philadelphia: Lippincott-Raven.

Stewart, S., Marley, J., & Horowitz, J. (1999). Effects of multidisciplinary, home-based intervention on unplanned readmission and survival among patients with chronic congestive heart failure; a randomized controlled study. *Lancet, 354*(9184), 1077–1083.

Ware, N., Tugenberg, T., Dickey, B., & McHorney, C. (1999). An ethnographic study of the meaning of continuity of care in mental health services. *Psychiatric Services, 50*(3), 395–400.

Yarmo, D., Scanlan, N., Edge, V., & Getson, J. (1998). Embracing the continuum of care: An Australian private hospital's experience. *Journal of Case Management, 7*(3), 127–134.

LEARNING ACTIVITIES

LEARNING ACTIVITY 8-1

▶ **Client Care Study:** Continuity of Care After Surgery

Mr. Heaney, a 66-year-old man, is admitted for a total knee replacement. He has had continuous pain in his left knee for the past 2 years secondary to osteoarthritis. His wife of 45 years died just 2 months ago, and he has remained alone in their two-story home. Only one of their six children lives in the metropolitan area. On postoperative day 1 he begins physical therapy. His left leg is in a continuous passive motion device when he is in bed. The plan is to discharge him POD 2 with outpatient physical therapy, the use of the continuous passive motion at home, and continuation of oral analgesics for pain. He appears to be slightly confused during the discharge planning conference when the discussion about his continuing care is discussed.

1. Describe your role as the primary nurse in Mr. Heaney's discharge planning.
2. Explain why you are in an effective position to coordinate continuity of care.

3. Identify the risks Mr. Heaney may have after discharge. Use the Blaylock Discharge Assessment Risk Planning Screen (see Fig. 8–5) to assess for risks.
4. Propose recommendations for his living situation and home care.
5. List agencies/facilities or individuals you would recommend for Mr. Heaney's continuing care and give your reasons.

LEARNING ACTIVITY 8-2

▶ **Critical Thinking Exercise:** Self-Evaluation

In your clinical journal, describe a situation you observed where a client or family experienced difficulty because of poor continuity. If you were the nurse in charge, what would you have done differently?

In your clinical journal, relate a situation where you observed a client who received effective continuity of care. What made the care effective?

List any barriers you have noticed that have interrupted continuity for a client you have cared for in clinical. Discuss what happened and what you would do differently. Identify any systems issues that you think did not address the barriers (ie, chart forms such as discharge forms, admission forms, unit policies).

Community-Based Nursing Across the Life Span

In Chapter 2, you learned that although the U.S. health care system is the most expensive in the world, the United States lags behind other nations in key health indicators. This unit uses the recommendations from *Healthy People 2010* to outline the role that the nurse must play in improving the nation's health.

Each chapter begins with a discussion of the goals of *Healthy People 2010* as well as the major causes of mortality and morbidity for each age group. Nursing assessments and interventions follow. Chapter 9 discusses health promotion and disease prevention for maternal/infant, child, and adolescent populations. Chapter 10 outlines health promotion and disease prevention for adults, and Chapter 11 focuses on elderly adults.

The content in each chapter is also organized around the leading causes of mortality for each group. Disease prevention and health promotion strategies that address these causes are highlighted. Based on numerous sources, these strategies are intended for the practicing nurse to use with clients for teaching about health promotion and disease prevention. Unit III also contains numerous Web site and organization addresses as well as resources related to health promotion and disease prevention for clients across the life span.

Health Promotion and Disease Prevention for Maternal/Infant Populations, Children, and Adolescents

R O B E R T A   H U N T

►L E A R N I N G   O B J E C T I V E S ◄

- Identify the major causes of death for maternal/infant populations, children, and adolescents.

- Discuss the major diseases and threats to health for maternal/infant populations, children, and adolescents.

- Summarize the major health issues for maternal/infant populations, children, and adolescents.

- Identify nursing roles at each level of prevention for major health issues.

- Compose a list of nursing interventions for the major health issues for maternal/infant populations, children, and adolescents.

- Determine health needs for maternal/infant populations, children, and adolescents for which a nurse could be an advocate.

►K E Y   T E R M S ◄

Denver Developmental Screening
  Test (DDST)
fetal alcohol syndrome (FAS)
infant mortality rate
lead poisoning

low birth weight (LBW)
mortality
morbidity
neural tube defects (NTD)
sudden infant death syndrome (SIDS)

Significance of Health Promotion and Disease Prevention

Maternal/Infant Populations

SIGNIFICANCE OF HEALTH PROMOTION AND DISEASE PREVENTION

Crucial issues of health and health care are different today from what they were in the early part of the 20th century. Public health efforts have increased the life span of the average person, thanks to the development of effective medication, particularly antibiotics, and universal access to clean water, sanitation, and immunizations. Our focus as health care providers has changed from combating infectious diseases to addressing chronic conditions and unintentional injuries.

Health promotion is typically defined as a primary disease prevention strategy. It is commonly interchanged with terms such as health education and disease prevention. Often health promotion is discussed as the epitome of empowerment, in that it is a process that enables people to use health as a resource for their life. Health promotion is most often discussed as a strategy for an already healthy individual or population, but it applies to those with health conditions as well. Disease prevention is just as it states, preventing a disease from occurring. It also includes injury prevention, which will be discussed a great deal in this and the following three chapters.

Recommendations from *Healthy People 2010* form the foundation for all health promotion and disease prevention nursing actions. These recommendations are based on the primary causes of death, or **mortality,** rates and the rates of illness or injury, or **morbidity,** rates. *Healthy People 2010* is based on mortality and morbidity statistics that represent the primary causes of death and illnesses and injury experienced by the people living in the United States.

Most diseases and deaths result from preventable causes. The negative impact of many conditions can be minimized by early identification and interventions. This chapter addresses health promotion and disease prevention for pregnant women, infants, children, and adolescents.

MATERNAL/INFANT POPULATIONS

Florence Nightingale wrote in 1894 that "money would be better spent in maintaining health in infancy and childhood than in building hospitals to cure disease" (Monteiro, 1985, p. 185). The same philosophy holds true today. The health of infants and children has further-reaching implications than that of other population groups. "The health of mothers, infants and children is of critical importance, both as a reflection of the current health status of a large segment of the U.S. population and as a predictor of the health of the next generations" (U.S. Department of Health and Human Services [DHHS], 2000b, p. 16–3). The *Healthy People 2010* objectives for maternal and infant health are listed in Box 9–1.

Infant death is a critical indicator of the health of a population because it reflects the overall state of maternal health, as well as the quality and access of pri-

> ▶ **Box 9–1.** *Healthy People 2010* Objectives
> for Maternal and Infant Health ◀
>
> Reduce fetal and infant deaths.
> Increase proportion of pregnant women who receive early and adequate prenatal
> care.
> Increase the proportion of pregnant women who attend a series of prepared
> childbirth classes.
> Reduce preterm births.
> Reduce the occurrence of spina bifida and other neural tube defects.
> Increase abstinence from alcohol, cigarettes, and illicit drugs among pregnant
> women.
> Increase the percentage of healthy full-term infants who are put down to sleep on
> their backs.
> Increase the proportion of mothers who breast-feed their babies.
>
> ———————————
>
> U.S. Department of Health and Human Services. (2000). Maternal infant, and child health. In
> *Healthy people 2010. National health promotion, and disease prevention objectives.*
> Washington, DC: U.S. Government Printing Office.

mary health available to pregnant women and infants. The **infant mortality rate** is the number of infants (ages birth to 1 year) who die out of every 1,000 live births. Although the 1980s and 1990s saw steady declines in the infant mortality rate in the United States, it remains among the highest in the industrialized world.

Prenatal Care

The United States is the only industrialized nation in which not all pregnant women receive prenatal care. In the United States, the percentage of mothers receiving early prenatal care in the first trimester of pregnancy varies substantially among racial and ethnic groups, from 68% for Native American mothers to 90% for Cuban mothers. Overall, only 75% of all women receive adequate prenatal care. This number varies by age as well; the percentage is higher with increasing maternal age, whereas fewer than 50% of pregnant women aged 15 years and younger receive adequate care.

Every nurse in every setting should always encourage pregnant women to begin prenatal care in the first trimester. One very effective intervention is through home visits where nurses can provide prenatal care and lower the probability of low-birth-weight infants, thus helping to lower the infant mortality rate (Box 9–2). Some of the topics that are important for the nurse to assess and intervene accordingly in home visits to pregnant women are those that *Healthy People 2010* has deemed the leading causes of low-birth-weight infants, preterm births, infant mortality, and congenital anomalies.

Low Birth Weight

Low birth weight (LBW), or weight less than 2,500 g or 5.5 lb, is the leading cause of preventable neonatal death. This is included under disorders related to premature birth in Table 9–1. Approximately 7.5% of babies are LBW infants (Centers for Disease Control and Prevention [CDC], 2000a). This figure continues to rise. LBW is associated with long-term disabilities, such as cerebral palsy, autism, mental retardation, vision and hearing impairment, and other develop-

▶ Box 9–2. A Home Visiting Program: Minnesota Healthy Beginnings ◀

In many parts of the United States, home visits are offered to pregnant women and those with an infant, but most often the family must fall within certain income levels or be identified as high risk. Home visiting programs offer public health nurse assessment, ongoing visits by trained home visitors, and coordination of family services. This in turn reduces preterm births, increases the proportion of pregnant women who receive early and adequate prenatal care, and increases the proportion who know about and attend childbirth classes.

In some counties in Minnesota, all parents with a new baby are offered home visits by a nurse at no cost to the family. This program was established by the Minnesota legislature to promote strong families and healthy child development. In the planning phase of the program, focus groups were held with pregnant women and with fathers and mothers of babies younger than 1 year to determine the best approach for promoting acceptance of a home visit. When asked to describe the ideal home visit and home visitor, families reported activities and personal characteristics of the home visitor that would contribute to the decision to accept a home visit.

Intermediate outcomes for the participants of a home visiting program for pregnant women and new parents include the following:

- Enhances positive parenting
    Enriches the home environment
    Promotes a safe home environment
    Well-child visits kept up-to-date
    Provides an informal support and linkage to community resources
- Produces thriving infants
    Development as expected for age
    Immunizations kept up-to-date for age

Long-term effects of a home visiting program include the following:

- Enhances prenatal care
- Child maltreatment rates decrease
- Immunization rates increase
- Early childhood screening rates increase

There are many advantages to large-scale home visiting programs. First, investing in families strengthens the entire community. Second, offering information, support, and links to community resources to all families is a community responsibility. All families with new babies can benefit from reassurance that they are doing a good job caring for their new member. Last, offering information, support, and links to community resources to all families is a valuable use of public funds. Although home visiting has been discussed as a strategy for pregnant women, the value of home visiting to all families with children under 3 years of age is well documented. It is a nursing intervention that allows the nurse to implement disease prevention and health promotion strategies within a trusting relationship.

Promoting Minnesota Healthy Beginnings. (1999). *Findings from focus groups with expecting moms and new parents.* Minnesota Department of Health, Division of Family Health, Minnesota Healthy Beginnings.

TABLE 9-1 • Leading Causes of Death by Age Group, United States, 1997

Age	Cause of Death	Number of Deaths
Younger than 1 y	Birth defects	6,178
	Disorders related to premature birth	3,925
	Sudden infant death syndrome	2,991
1–4 y	Unintentional injuries	2,005
	Birth defects	589
	Cancer	438
5–14 y	Unintentional injuries	3,371
	Cancer	1,030
	Homicide	457
15–24 y	Unintentional injuries	13,367
	Homicide	8,146
	Suicide	4,186

U.S. Department of Health and Human Services. (2000b). Maternal infant, and child health. In *Healthy people 2010. National health promotion disease prevention objectives.* Washington, DC: U.S. Government Printing Office.

mental disabilities. LBW is also the main reason premature infants require care in neonatal intensive care units. It does not take a complicated cost analysis to conclude that it is much more expensive to care for a newborn in an intensive care unit then it would have been to provide prenatal care for the infant's mother. In 1988, the cost of a normal, healthy delivery averaged $1,900, whereas hospital costs for LBW infants averaged $6,200 (DHHS, 2000b). The primary intervention to prevent LBW is early initiation of prenatal care.

Neural Tube Defects

Approximately 50% of all **neural tube defects** (**NTDs**) may be prevented with adequate consumption of folic acid in the first trimester of pregnancy. Currently, the U.S. Public Health Service recommends that all women of childbearing age consume 400 μg folic acid daily. For women who are planning a pregnancy, 4,000 μg is recommended.

Cigarette Smoking

Cigarette smoking by the mother during pregnancy is a common cause of LBW infants. Between 20% and 33% of women smoke during pregnancy. Up to 25% of women who smoke before pregnancy stop before their first antenatal visit. However, the rest continue to smoke throughout the pregnancy (DHHS, 2000b). Smoking cessation programs have been shown to be effective in reducing smoking, increasing mean birth weight, and reducing LBW. It is imperative that nurses use smoking cessation programs to help their clients quit, especially when the client is pregnant (Lumley, Oliver, & Waters, 1999). Smoking cessation programs can be found on the Internet through Healthfinder (http://www.healthfinder.gov).

Alcohol and Drug Use

Moderate to heavy alcohol use by women during pregnancy has been associated with many severe adverse effects, including **fetal alcohol syndrome** (**FAS**) and other developmental delays. It is the nurse's responsibility to discuss alcohol and drug use with the client in an open and nonjudgmental manner. Currently, it is recommended that women do not consume alcohol during pregnancy.

COMMUNITY-BASED TEACHING

Help for Smokers: Ideas to Help You Quit

Want to Quit?

You promised yourself that you would finally quit smoking. It isn't easy giving up something that is so much a part of what you do every day. But you are not alone. Over 1 million people each year decide to quit and are successful.

Tried Quitting Before?

Maybe once, maybe more . . .
   You started out feeling the time was right, but for whatever reason, you're smoking again. Now, you're asking yourself whether it's worth it to try quitting again. You bet it is! Some smokers try a number of times before they quit for good. Studies show that each time you try to quit, the more likely you will be to eventually succeed. With each try, you are better able to know what helps and what hurts. Any attempt to quit is a step in a healthier direction.

Pregnant?

There's no better time to quit. And for two very good reasons:
• You
• Your baby
   Even if someone you know smoked during pregnancy and had a problem-free delivery, smoking puts your baby's health at risk. Quitting at any time during pregnancy is still the best chance for you and your baby to get a fresh start.
   It is also important to remember that infants and children exposed to second-hand smoke are more likely to develop health problems such as chronic ear infections and asthma. Helping to eliminate these health risks is another good reason to quit.

How Do I Start?

Make a Plan
• You may want to consult a health care professional to choose a quit smoking plan that is best for you.
• Set a quit date and stick to it.
• Get the support and understanding of your family, friends, and coworkers.
• Get rid of all tobacco products and ashtrays.

Get Support and Encouragement
Research funded by the Agency for Healthcare Research and Quality (AHRQ) shows that the more support you have, the greater your chance for success. Join a quit smoking program or start your own quit smoking group. Check with your health care professional, local hospitals, the American Cancer Society, American Lung Association, or American Heart Association for schedules for existing groups.

Learn How to Handle the Urge to Smoke
Be aware of things that may cause you to smoke, such as:
• Other smokers
• Stress
• Depression
• Alcohol

(*continued*)

COMMUNITY-BASED TEACHING (Continued)

What Works?

Current Treatments
There are no magic solutions for quitting smoking. But, if you are ready to quit, effective treatments are available that can help reduce the urge to smoke. Studies show that almost everyone can benefit from these nicotine replacement and non-nicotine therapies.

Nicotine Replacement Therapy
- Nicotine patch
- Nicotine gum
- Nicotine nasal spray (available only by prescription)
- Nicotine inhaler (available only by prescription)

Non-Nicotine Therapy
- Bupropion (available only by prescription)
You can get these through your pharmacy or health care provider.

More Resources

Additional free materials on quitting smoking from the U.S. Public Health Service can be requested:
Publications Clearinghouse
P. O. Box 8547
Silver Spring, MD 20907-8547
Or call toll-free in the United States at (800) 358-9295.
Also, you can access and download materials from the Surgeon General's Web site at http://www.surgeongeneral.gov/tobacco/default.htm.

Reproduced from *Help for smokers: Ideas to help you quit.* Based on the U.S. Public Health Service Tobacco Cessation Guideline, released June 2000. Agency for Healthcare Research and Quality, Rockville, MD. Available at: http://www.ahrq.gov/consumer/helpsmok.htm.

Newborn Care

The *Child Health Guide: Put Prevention into Practice* is an excellent tool for monitoring infant and child health. It is available on-line at http://www.ahcpr.gov/ppip/ppchild.htm, or a free copy can be ordered by calling (800) 358-9295. It provides parents with explanations of child preventive care and a convenient place to keep records of health care visits, growth, and immunizations. It recommends checkups at 3 weeks; 2, 4, 6, 9, 12, 15, and 18 months; and 2, 3, 4, 5, 6, 8, 10, 12, 14, 16, and 18 years with a pediatric nurse practitioner or physician. Bright Futures: Guidelines for Health Supervision of Infants, Children, and Adolescents, 2nd edition, can be downloaded from the Bright Futures Web site (http://www.brightfutures.org). It contains health supervision guidelines and information, including developmental charts for children aged newborns through adolescents.

An example of research relating to newborn care is shown in Research Box 9–1.

RESEARCH RELATED TO COMMUNITY-BASED NURSING CARE

Research Box 9–1 ▶ Massage as an Intervention for Preterm/Low-Birth-Weight Infants

Infant massage has been associated with improved sleep and contentment with both preterm and term infants. This integrative review discussed studies over the past 10 years that examined the impact of massage on preterm infants. One study compared preterm/LBW infants who received massage interventions to a comparable group who did not receive massage. It found that the group receiving massage gained more weight per day than control infants. Massage interventions decreased length of stay by 4.6 days. Those infants in the massage group improved performance slightly on the Brazelton scale for habituation, motor maturity, and range of state. No evidence of an effect of gentle still touch on neonatal morbidity score, days on oxygen, blood transfusions, activity, or behavioral distress cues was found. No adverse effects of touch or massage were reported in any study.

The nursing literature strongly advocates massage interventions in the care of preterm/LBW infants.

Vickers, A., Ohlsson, A., Lacy, J. B., & Horsley, A. (1999). Massage for promoting growth and development of preterm and/or low birthweight infants. *Cochrane Database System Review, 2,* CD000390.

Screening

All newborns should have blood tests in the hospital for phenylketonuria (PKU), thyroid disease, and sickle cell disease. The current recommendation is that all newborns should be screened for hearing impairment before they leave the hospital (CDC, 2000a). The parents should ask the nurse practitioner or physician if they are unsure whether these tests were done for their infant.

All infants' growth should be monitored and plotted on a growth chart outlines the developmental status of the infant. Charts are available from the U.S. DHHS at http://www.cdc.gov/growthcharts. To reduce mortality and morbidity, both the parent and the nurse must be diligent in following preventive measures for normal-risk infants. In all community-based settings, the nurse can assist the parent in following basic prevention recommendations for children. Clinical Preventive Services for Normal-Risk Children outlines current recommendations (Figure 9–1).

Immunizations

Fifty years ago, many children died from what today are preventable childhood diseases. Smallpox has been eradicated, poliomyelitis has been eliminated from the Western hemisphere, and the number of measles cases in the United States is at a record low. All of this progress has been made possible by immunizations. However, only if the number of vaccinated children and adults remains high will immunization programs continue to be effective.

Immunizations are considered primary prevention because they prevent the occurrence of a disease. It is imperative that all children be immunized according to recommended standards. Immunizations should begin at birth and

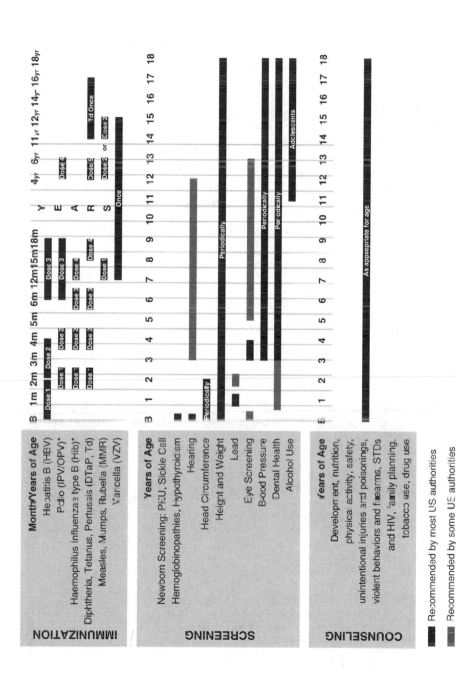

Figure 9–1. ▲ Clinical preventive services for normal-risk children. Source: Agency for Healthcare Research and Quality. (2000). *Child health guide: Put prevention into practice.* Rockville, MD. Available at: http://www.ahcpr.gov/ppip/ppchild.htm.

continue as recommended in Figure 9–1. Once a year, consult Every Child by Two at (202) 783-7034 (http://www.ecbt.org) for updates.

Nutrition

Breast-feeding is widely acknowledged to be the most complete form of nutrition for infants. The range of benefits includes health, growth, immunity, and development. Breast-fed infants have decreased rates of diarrhea, respiratory infections, and ear infections (Wright, Bauer, Naylor, Sutcliffe, & Clark, 1998). Breast-feeding improves maternal health by reducing postpartum bleeding, promotes return to prepregnancy weight, and reduces the risks of breast cancer and osteoporosis long after the postpartum period. The American Academy of Pediatrics (AAP) considers breast-feeding to be the ideal method of feeding and nurturing infants.

As with any teaching, consider the developmental stage, cognitive abilities, and culture of the client when initiating breast-feeding teaching. Teen-aged mothers are more interested in knowing that breast-feeding is easy, saves time, and will enhance weight loss so they can fit into their jeans sooner. Older mothers are typically more interested in the long-term benefits to their babies. The La Leche League is a wonderful resource for information on breast-feeding (http://www.lalecheleague.org). Encouraging new mothers to breast-feed is a simple intervention that can have a strong and lasting effect on the health of the mother and baby, second only to early prenatal care.

Safety

Because more children die of unintentional injuries than any other cause, it is important to counsel parents on home safety. The primary issue related to safety of the infant is sleep positioning. Parents should put newborns to sleep

COMMUNITY-BASED TEACHING

Guidelines for a Healthy Diet for the Infant to 2-Year-Old

- Breast milk is the single best food for infants from birth to 6 months of age. It provides good nutrition and protects against infection.
- Breast-feeding should continue for at least the first year, if possible.
- If breast-feeding is not possible or not desired, iron-enriched formula (not cow's milk) should be used during the first 12 months of life. Whole cow's milk can be used to replace formula or breast milk after 12 months of age.
- Breast-fed babies (particularly dark-skinned infants) who do not get regular exposure to sunlight may need to receive vitamin D supplements.
- Begin suitable solid foods at 4 to 6 months of age. Most experts recommend iron-enriched infant rice cereal as the first food.
- Start new foods one at a time to make it easier to identify problem foods. For example, wait 1 week before adding each new cereal, vegetable, or other food.
- Use iron-rich foods, such as iron-enriched cereals, other grains, and meats.
- Do not give honey to infants during the first 12 months of life.
- Do not limit fat during the first 2 years of life.

Agency for Healthcare Research and Quality. (2000). *Child health guide: Put prevention into practice.* Rockville, MD. Available at: http://www.ahcpr.gov/ppip/ppchild.htm.

COMMUNITY-BASED TEACHING

Safety Guidelines for Infants and Young Children

- Use a car safety seat at all times until your child weighs at least 40 lb.
- Car seats must be properly secured in the back seat, preferably in the middle.
- Keep medication, cleaning solutions, and other dangerous substances in childproof containers, locked up and out of reach of children.
- Use safety gates across stairways (top and bottom) and guards on windows above the first floor.
- Keep hot water heater temperatures below 120°F.
- Keep unused electrical outlets covered with plastic guards.
- Provide constant supervision for babies using a baby walker. Block the access to stairways and to objects that can fall (such as lamps) or cause burns (such as stoves).
- Keep objects and foods that cause choking away from your child, such as coins, balloons, small toy parts, hot dogs (unmashed), peanuts, and hard candies.
- Use fences that go all the way around pools and keep gates to pools locked.

Agency for Healthcare Research and Quality. (2000). *Child health guide: Put prevention into practice.* Rockville, MD. Available at: http://www.ahcpr. gov/ppip/ppchild.htm.

on their backs. This position dramatically reduces deaths from **sudden infant death syndrome (SIDS)**, a leading cause of death in infants. More information for parents on reducing the risk of SIDS is available from the National Institute of Child Health and Human Development, at http://www.nicdh.nih.gov/side/reduce_risk.htm.

PRESCHOOL-AGED CHILDREN

Healthy People 2010 objectives for child health are listed in Box 9–3. The leading cause of death in children of all ages is injury. Among children ages 1 to 4 years, the leading injury-related causes of death are motor vehicle crashes, drowning, and fires and burns. These deaths are, for the most part, preventable.

Screening

In all community-based settings, the nurse can assist the parent in following basic prevention recommendations for children to reduce mortality and morbidity. Clinical Preventive Services for Normal-Risk Children outlines current recommendations (see Fig. 9–1). All young children's growth should be monitored and plotted on a growth chart.

Preschool screening, which typically includes vision, hearing, height and weight, immunization status, and developmental screening, is an important preventive intervention. The cost of preschool screening is minimal when compared with the cost of undetected deficits that result in hardship and monetary costs to the child, parents, and society. The earlier a condition is identified, the greater the chances of lessening or eliminating the long-term effects (Sullivan, 1998).

▶ **Box 9–3.** *Healthy People 2010* Objectives for Child Health ◀

Reduce the rate of child deaths (ages 1–4 years).
Reduce or eliminate indigenous cases of vaccine-preventable disease.
Reduce iron deficiency among young children and females of childbearing age.
Increase the proportion of persons aged 2 years and older who consume at least two daily servings of fruit.
Increase the proportion of persons aged 2 years and older who consume at least three daily servings of vegetables.
Reduce the proportion of children and adolescents who have dental caries in their primary or permanent teeth.
Increase the proportion of children and adolescents who view television 2 hours or less per day.
Increase the proportion of the nation's public and private schools that provide access to their physical activity spaces and facilities for all persons outside of normal school hours (before and after the school day, on weekends, and during summer and other vacations).
Increase the proportion of preschool children aged 5 years and under who receive vision and hearing screening.

U.S. Department of Health and Human Services. (2000). Maternal, infant, and child health. In *Healthy people 2010. National health promotion disease prevention objectives.* Washington, DC: U.S. Government Printing Office.

The most widely used tool to assess development is the **Denver Developmental Screening Test (DDST)**. It is used to screen children from 1 month to 6 years, covering the topics of gross motor skills, fine motor skills, language development, and personal/social development. This easy-to-administer screening tool has the potential to identify developmental issues early for prompt intervention. The AAP states that early identification leads to more effective therapy for children with developmental disabilities (AAP, 1995). The DDST is an excellent example of secondary prevention.

Periodic screening benefits all children. Most screening programs are developed and run by nurses in community-based settings.

See Box 9–4 for an overview of poverty and its effect on child health.

Lead Screening

Lead has been present in our environment since industrialization. Children are particularly sensitive to the toxic effects of lead. Most often, **lead poisoning** is silent, with the individual having no symptoms until systemic damage has occurred. Decreased stature or growth, decreased intelligence, impaired neurobehavioral development, and adverse effects on the central nervous system, kidneys, and hematopoietic system are some of the common consequences of lead poisoning.

Lead poisoning is widespread. The last year that estimates were available, it was estimated that between 3 and 4 million children, or 17% of children, had lead blood levels above safe levels. About 74% of occupied, privately owned housing built before 1980 contains lead-based paint. In general, screening and assessment for lead poisoning should focus on children younger than 24 months and should begin at 12 months, because these ages are the most vulnerable (DHHS, 1991). Assessment of high-dose lead exposure should take place at birth.

► **Box 9–4.** Poverty and Child Health ◄

Poverty has both immediate and long-term negative effects on children and adolescents. Twenty percent of children live in poverty. This figure has remained virtually the same since 1980. More children who are living in poverty are younger than 6 years than any other age group. Most children in poverty are white, but the proportion of African American and Hispanic children in poverty is higher—11% of white children, 37% of African American children, and 36% of Hispanic children live in poverty.

Child health varies by family income. As family income increases, the percentage of children in very good or excellent health increases. Children in families in poverty have significantly higher rates of activity limitation than do children in more affluent families. The proportion of adolescents from poor households who are overweight is almost twice that of adolescents from middle- and high-income homes. Children in families with incomes below the poverty level are less likely to have received the combined required immunizations than children with family incomes at or above the poverty line. Children living in families who are poor are more likely to have difficulty in school and to become teen parents. Not surprisingly, children living in poverty are less likely to have any source of health insurance, and thus have restricted access to health care. In 1997, 14% of children younger than 18 years had no health insurance coverage.

Federal Interagency Forum on Child and Family Statistics. (1999). *America's children: Key national indicators of well being.* Federal Interagency Forum on Child and Family Statistics. Washington, DC: U.S. Government Printing Office.

Vision and Hearing Screening

Vision and hearing screening should be performed at 3 or 4 years of age and repeated once a year. New recommendations are to screen newborns for hearing right after birth (CDC, 2000a). If warning signs of visual or hearing impairment are present (Box 9–5), screening should be done earlier or more frequently than recommended.

COMMUNITY-BASED TEACHING

Lead Assessment for Parents

Use a check to mark "yes" answers to the questions below. Any "yes" answers may mean that your child needs lead tests earlier and more often than other children.

_____Lived in or regularly visited a house built before 1950 (this could include a day care center, preschool, the home of a babysitter or relative, etc)

_____Lived in or regularly visited a house built before 1978 (the year lead-based paint was banned for residential use) with recent, ongoing, or planned renovation or remodeling

_____Had a brother or sister, housemate, or playmate followed or treated for lead poisoning

Agency for Healthcare Research and Quality. (2000). *Child health guide: Put prevention into practice.* Rockville, MD. Available at: http://www.ahcpr.gov/ppip/ppchild.htm.

> ► **Box 9–5.** Vision and Hearing Impairment Warning Signs ◄

Vision

- Eyes turning inward or outward
- Squinting
- Headaches
- Not doing as well in school work as before
- Blurred or double vision

Hearing

- Poor response to noise or voice
- Slow language and speech development
- Abnormal sounding speech

Agency for Healthcare Research and Quality. (2000). *Child health guide: Put prevention into practice.* Rockville, MD. Available at: http://www.ahcpr.gov/ppip/ppchild.htm.

Immunizations

Immunizations are important preventive health measures for the preschool child. The schedule is found in Figure 9–1.

Nutrition

Nutritional status should be assessed. Infants and toddlers should be tested for anemia starting at 9 months of age. Hematocrit and hemoglobin screening should take place by 9 months if any of the following factors are present:

- ► Low socioeconomic status
- ► Birth weight less than 1,500 g
- ► Whole milk given before 6 months of age (not recommended)
- ► Low-iron formula given (not recommended)
- ► Low intake of iron-rich foods (not recommended)

Safety

Injury is the leading cause of death in young children, with automobile crashes the leading cause. In most states, the law requires that infants and children

COMMUNITY-BASED TEACHING

Guidelines for a Healthy Diet for Children 2 Years and Older

- Provide a variety of foods, including plenty of fruits, vegetables, and whole grains.
- Use salt and sugar in moderation.
- Encourage a diet low in fat, saturated fat, and cholesterol.
- Help your child maintain a healthy weight by providing proper food and encouraging regular exercise.

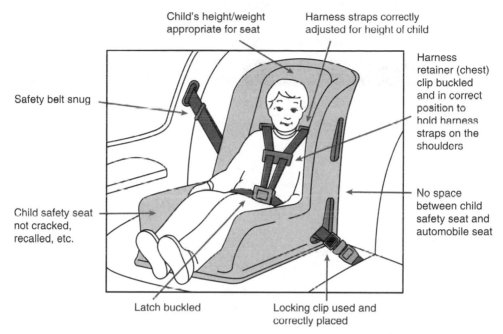

Child's height/weight appropriate for seat

Harness straps correctly adjusted for height of child

Harness retainer (chest) clip buckled and in correct position to hold harness straps on the shoulders

Safety belt snug

No space between child safety seat and automobile seat

Child safety seat not cracked, recalled, etc.

Latch buckled

Locking clip used and correctly placed

Figure 9–2. ▶ Correct use of a child safety seat. Source: Centers for Disease Control and Prevention (1998) Improper use of child safety seats—Kentucky, 1996. *MMWR Morbidity and Mortality Weekly Report 47*(26), 541–543.

should be restrained in a safety seat when riding in a car, and parents who are not compliant may be fined. The proper method of using a car seat is shown in Figure 9–2. The AAP recommends that infants ride in rear-facing safety seats until they weigh at least 20 lb and are 1 year old. They should never be placed in the front seat of a vehicle with a passenger-side air bag. Children older than 1 year who weigh between 20 and 40 lb should ride in a forward-facing child safety seat as long as the seat fits well (CDC, 1999b).

Other Preventive Health Measures

Infants and children of all ages should be protected from the harmful effects of the sun. The number of skin cancer cases has increased in the United States with more than 1.3 million new cases diagnosed in 2000. Anyone can get skin cancer, but individuals with certain risk factors are particularly at risk. Some risks for skin cancer are the following (CDC, 2000b):

▶ Lighter natural skin color
▶ Family history of skin cancer
▶ Personal history of skin cancer
▶ Constant exposure to the sun through work and play
▶ A history of sunburns early in life
▶ Skin that burns, freckles, get red easily, or becomes painful in the sun
▶ Blue or green eyes
▶ Blond or red hair
▶ Certain types and a large number of moles

COMMUNITY-BASED TEACHING

Safety Guidelines for Parents of Children of All Ages

- Use smoke detectors in your home. Change the batteries every year and check once a month to see that they work.
- If you have a gun in your home, make sure that the gun and ammunition are locked up separately and kept out of children's reach.
- Never drive after drinking alcohol.
- Use car safety belts at all times.
- Teach your child traffic safety. Children under 9 years of age need supervision when crossing streets.
- Teach your children how to and when to call 911.
- Learn basic life-saving skills (CPR).
- Keep a bottle of ipecac at home to treat poisoning. Call a doctor or local Poison Control Center before using it. Post the telephone number of the Poison Control Center near your telephone. Also, be sure to check the expiration date on the bottle of ipecac to make sure it is still good.

Agency for Healthcare Research and Quality. (2000). *Child health guide: Put prevention into practice*. Rockville, MD. Available at: http://www.ahcpr.gov/ppip/ppchild.htm.

COMMUNITY-BASED TEACHING

Ways to Prevent Child Abuse

- Teach your child not to let anyone touch his or her private parts.
- Tell your child to say "NO" and run away from sexual touches.
- Take any reports by your child of physical or sexual touches seriously.
- Report any abuse to your local or state child protection agency.
- If you feel angry or out of control, leave the room, take a walk, take deep breaths, or count to 100. Don't drink alcohol or take drugs. These can make your anger harder to control.
- If you are afraid you might harm your child, get help NOW. Call someone and ask for help. Talk with a friend or relative, other parents, your clergy, or your health care provider. Take time for yourself. Share child care between parents, trade babysitting with friends, or use day care. Call a hotline. The National Child Abuse Hotline number is (800) 422-4453.

Agency for Healthcare Research and Quality. (2000). *Child health guide: Put prevention into practice*. Rockville, MD. Available at: http://www.ahcpr.gov/ppip/ppchild/htm.

COMMUNITY-BASED TEACHING

Ways to Protect Children from Overexposure to the Sun

- *Seek shade* from ultraviolet (UV) rays, especially during midday.
- *Cover up* to protect exposed skin.
- *Get a hat* with a wide brim.
- *Grab shades* that block both UVA and UVB rays.
- *Rub on sunscreen*—at least SPF 15 or higher, with both UVA and UVB protection.

Centers for Disease Control and Prevention. (2000). *Facts and statistics about skin cancer.* National Center for Chronic Disease Prevention and Health Promotion, Division of Cancer Prevention and Control. Available at: http://www.cdc.gov/chooseyourcover/skin.htm.

Poor nutrition and dental hygiene contribute to dental caries. Dental caries is the single most common chronic disease of childhood, occurring five to eight times as frequently as asthma, the second most common chronic condition among children. Unless identified and addressed early, caries are irreversible (DHHS, 2000b).

Handwashing is a simple and effective disease-prevention measure (Fig. 9–3). It is important to teach children handwashing skills. *Those Mean Nasty Dirty Downright Disgusting but . . . Invisible Germs,* a children's book by Judith Rice, is a good resource for educating children and is also available in Spanish.

As with all assessment, the effectiveness lies in the strength of the questions asked. General interview and developmental surveillance questions for children of all ages and their parents can be found at http://www.brightfutures.org.

COMMUNITY-BASED TEACHING

Recommendations for Oral Health for Infants and Older Children

Infants

- If most of the child's nutrition comes from breast-feeding, or if there is too little fluoride in the drinking water, the child may need fluoride drops or tablets.
- Don't use a baby bottle as a pacifer or put a child to sleep with a baby bottle. This can cause tooth decay and ear infections.
- Keep an infant's teeth and gums clean by wiping with a moist cloth after feeding.
- After the infant has several teeth, then brush with a soft toothbrush.

Older Children

- Use dental floss to help prevent gum disease.
- Discourage smoking and smokeless tobacco.
- Sealants prevent cavities in permanent teeth.

Agency for Healthcare Research and Quality. (2000). *Child health guide: Put prevention into practice.* Rockville, MD. Available at: http://www.ahcpr.gov/ppip/ppchild.htm.

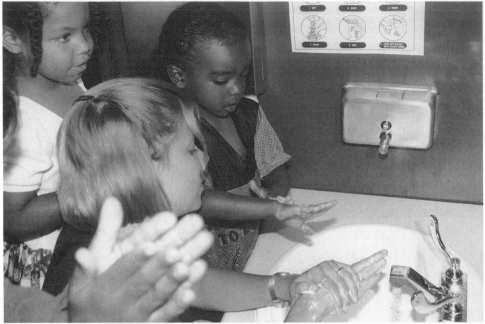

Photo by: Tom Heaney

Figure 9–3. ▶ Good handwashing skills have been associated with a decrease in colds and influenza.

 SCHOOL-AGED CHILDREN

The leading cause of death for all children between ages 5 and 14 years is motor vehicle accidents. Factors that contribute to these fatalities include drunk drivers and unrestrained children. In 1996, about 62% of all children who died in motor vehicle crashes were unrestrained (CDC, 1999b). Pedestrian deaths account for 15% of all motor vehicle-related deaths sustained by children (CDC, 1997).

Middle childhood is when the foundations of a healthy lifestyle are formed and when health promotion programs are likely to have the greatest impact (Polivka & Ryan-Wenger, 1999). A survey of elementary school-aged children examined health and lifestyle behaviors. This research found that 68% did not always

COMMUNITY-BASED NURSING CARE GUIDELINES

Guidelines for Health Promotion and Disease Prevention in Children

- Use the *Child Health Guide.*
- Identify recommended screening for the age group.
- Determine developmental tasks for the age group.
- Use general interview questions and developmental surveillance questions.
- Formulate interventions accordingly.

▶ **Box 9–6.** *Healthy People 2010* Objectives
for School-Aged Children and Adolescents ◀

Reduce the rate of child (ages 5–9 years), adolescent, and young adult deaths.
Reduce coronary heart disease deaths.
Reduce or eliminate indigenous cases of vaccine-preventable disease.
Reduce the suicide rate.
Reduce iron deficiency among young children and females of childbearing age.
Reduce the proportion of children and adolescents who are overweight or obese.
Increase the proportion of persons aged 2 years and older who consume at least
 two daily servings of fruit.
Increase the proportion of persons aged 2 years and older who consume at least
 three daily servings of vegetables.
Reduce the proportion of children and adolescents who have dental caries
 experience in their primary or permanent teeth.
Increase the proportion of adolescents who engage in moderate physical activity
 for at least 30 minutes on 5 or more of the previous 7 days.
Increase the proportion of adolescents who engage in vigorous physical activity
 that promotes cardiorespiratory fitness 3 or more days per week for 20 or
 more minutes per occasion.
Increase the proportion of children and adolescents who view television 2 hours
 or less per day.
Increase the proportion of the nation's public and private schools that provide
 access to their physical activity spaces and facilities for all persons outside of
 normal school hours (before and after the school day, on weekends, and
 during summer and other vacations).
Reduce the proportion of adolescents and young adults with *Chlamydia
 trachomatis* infections.
Reduce tobacco use by adolescents.

U.S. Department of Health and Human Services. (2000). Maternal, infant, and child health. In
Healthy people 2010. National health promotion and disease prevention objectives.
Washington, DC: U.S. Government Printing Office.

---

sleep 8 hours a night, only 50% brushed their teeth, and fewer than 50% reported
having annual dental visits. The youngest children reported always eating unhealthy snacks and never eating vegetables daily. Only 50% of the children always followed bicycle safety rules, and fewer than 30% always wore a bicycle
helmet. Only 60% of the children reported always using a seatbelt. Fewer than
50% of the students reported always swimming with someone else.

Healthy People 2010 objectives for middle childhood are given in Box 9–6.

Screening

The growth rate slows somewhat in the middle childhood years. Children's
readiness for school depends on prior experiences in the first 5 years of life.
Nurses should assess the achievement of the child and provide guidance to the
family on anticipated tasks. See the Bright Futures Web site for information on
developmental tasks.

At age 5 years, screening should include vision and hearing, blood pressure,
risk for lead exposure (with blood draw if deemed necessary), blood cholesterol,
and developmental screening. Weight and height should also be assessed.

Safety

The most important topic to cover with all families with children is safety, and the one intervention that prevents the most loss of life and injury is using appropriate restraints when riding in an automobile.

Children over 40 lb can begin to safely wear a seatbelt. At this time, air bags are not safe for children younger than 13 years and can cause fatalities. Until passenger vehicles are equipped with air bags that are safe and effective for children, those younger than 13 years should not ride in a front passenger seat that is equipped with an air bag.

Another important safety intervention is use of bike helmets. Bicycling is a popular activity in the United States. About half a million people are injured in bike mishaps each year. Of these injuries, head injury is the most common cause of death and serious disability. The use of bike helmets is effective in preventing head injury. Community programs to increase bike helmet use can reduce the incidence of head injury among bicycle riders. All people should wear a helmet when riding a bike (CDC, 1995).

Prevention of Chronic Conditions

As the child enters middle childhood, even more emphasis should be placed on secondary prevention, which allows early intervention for health conditions that may develop to chronic conditions in adulthood. The primary contributors to chronic conditions that can be addressed are weight, nutrition, and physical activity level.

Weight

Overweight and obesity are increasing among children and adolescents in the United States. The rate of overweight among children ages 6 to 17 years has more than doubled in the past 30 years, with most of the increase since the late 1970s. Eleven percent of those between 6 and 17 are seriously overweight. Elevated blood cholesterol levels and high blood pressure are associated with obesity, which is in turn associated with heart disease and stroke, two leading causes of death in adulthood. Being overweight in childhood and adolescence has been associated with increased adult morbidity (CDC, 1996). Disease prevention and health promotion activities that decrease the incidence of obesity are directed at improving nutrition and increasing physical activity levels.

Nutrition

Reviewing basic information about the recommended intake by food groups with parent and child is another important intervention in helping families improve their nutrition.

Physical Activity

Many states have eliminated physical education programs and after-school sports programs. Physical education programs are determined by state, but only one state follows the American Heart Association recommendation of daily physical education from kindergarten through 12th grade. These changes have had an impact on the daily reported activity of children. Further, children participate in more sedentary activities after school, such as watching television and playing computer games, than children did 10 years ago. *Healthy People 2010* recommends children watch less than 2 hours of television a day.

Discussing the need for daily physical activity is an important strategy for nurses in community-based settings. Encouraging children to participate in activities that provide an aerobic component such as riding bikes every day (wearing a helmet, of course), walking instead of riding in a car from place to place, and playing outside every day. Swimming, playing organized or unorganized sports, or doing physical activities as a family are other ways to increase a child's activity level.

Pointing out the benefits of exercise may also help parents encourage children to be more physically active. Helping parents understand the relationship between activity and normal weight, future health, and the threat of developing chronic disease are a few of the strategies the nurse can use to help parents understand the importance of structuring family life and the child's life to include physical activity.

 ## ADOLESCENTS

The leading cause of death for adolescents between 15 and 19 years of age is motor vehicle accidents, which cause 36% of total deaths. Other unintentional injuries such as falls, drowning, and poisoning cause 9%; homicides, 20%; suicides, 12.4%; and acquired immunodeficiency syndrome (AIDS), 0.3%. The majority (78%) of the total mortality in this age group can be attributed to preventable causes (CDC, 1999c).

The leading cause of death for persons ages 20 to 24 is motor vehicle accidents, at 30%. Other unintentional injuries, such as falls, drowning, and poisoning caused 10%; homicides, 20.4%; suicides, 14%; AIDS, 2%. Teens are far less likely to use seatbelts than any other age group (CDC, 1999c). Alcohol is involved in about 35% of adolescent fatalities and 40% of all adolescent drownings. Suicide is the third leading cause of death among those ages 15 to 24. As with the 15- to 19-year-old group, 76% of the deaths in this age group can be attributed to preventable causes. At this time, most of the new human immunodeficiency virus (HIV) infections occur each year among those between ages 13 and 21 years.

One comprehensive survey of high school students in 1999 found that 85% rode bicycles without a helmet, 17% carried a weapon, and 8% had attempted suicide in the 12 months preceding the survey. Thirty-five percent smoked cigarettes, 50% had at least one drink of alcohol, and 32% had 5 or more drinks of alcohol on at least one occasion during the 30 days preceding the survey (CDC, 1999c).

Of the 36% who had sexual intercourse during the previous 3 months, 58% used a condom during the last intercourse, with 16% of all currently sexually active students using birth control before the last sexual intercourse. As far as dietary behaviors, 10% were overweight, 24% ate 5 or more serving of fruits and vegetables during the 7 days preceding the survey, and 5% took laxatives or vomited to lose weight during the 30 days preceding the survey. Related to physical activity, 65% did vigorous physical activity and 27% did moderate physical activity for at least 20 minutes on 3 or more of the 7 days preceding the survey, and 56% were enrolled in physical education class with 29% attending physical education class daily (CDC, 1999a). These results compare to other surveys, which show that nearly half of American youths ages 12 to 21 years are not vigorously active on a regular basis (CDC, 1999a).

When results from 1999 were compared with results from 1991 and 1995, the percentage of students who felt unsafe going to school increased from 6% to 26%. Students were smoking more cigarettes in 1999, with an increase in those smoking more than 10 cigarettes per day from 1% to 11%. There was also an increase in those having sexual intercourse before 13 years of age, from 3% to 16%. The percentage of students attending physical education class increased from 6% to 16%.

Healthy People 2010 objectives for school-aged children and adolescents are shown in Box 9–6.

Screening

Recommendations for screening in early and later adolescence are found in the Bright Futures guidelines. Some other areas for screening adolescent clients include smoking, alcohol and drug use, sexual activity, and injury prevention behaviors. Teens' behaviors often place them at risk for serious injury, sexually transmitted diseases (STDs), and chronic diseases. Bright Futures provides excellent developmental surveillance questions that address these issues. It is also important to keep developmental tasks in mind when assessing health issues and planning health promotion and disease prevention activities.

Because such a large proportion of deaths in this age group are preventable, safety should be the number one priority for health promotion and injury prevention. However, because of the nature of the adolescent client, this is a formidable challenge.

Adolescence is one of the most dynamic stages of human development. It is accompanied by dramatic physical, cognitive, social, and emotional changes that present both opportunities and challenges for the adolescent, the family, and the broader community. Nurses must be sensitive to the dynamic nature of this stage as well as the increasing need for independence balanced with dependence. Further, as adolescents progress through the teen years, they become increasingly able and desiring to make their own health care decisions.

Prevention of Chronic Conditions

Smoking Cessation

Several excellent resources on the Internet address smoking cessation. Some are very colorful, specifically designed by teens for teens. One site is http://www.cdc.gov/tobacco/tipsteen.htm.

Nutrition

Teaching teens about nutrition is challenging. *Bright Futures in Practice: Nutrition* is an excellent resource for nutrition information for infancy through adolescence (Fig. 9–4). This resource is available through http://www.brightfutures.org.

Physical Activity

Adolescents and young adults benefit from physical activity. Moderate amounts of daily physical activity are recommended for people of all ages. This amount can be obtained in longer sessions of moderately intense activities, such as brisk walking for 30 minutes, or in shorter sessions of more intense activities, such as jogging or playing soccer or basketball for 15 to 20 minutes. Physical activity helps build and maintain healthy bones, muscles, and joints; controls weight; builds lean muscle; and reduces fat. Most importantly, physical activity prevents or delays the development of high blood pressure and helps reduce blood pressure in some adolescents with hypertension.

COMMUNITY-BASED TEACHING
WHAT YOU(TH) SHOULD KNOW ABOUT TOBACCO

Tobacco and Athletic Performance

- Don't get trapped. Nicotine in cigarettes, cigars, and spit tobacco is addictive.
- Nicotine narrows your blood vessels and puts added strain on your heart.
- Smoking can wreck lungs and reduce oxygen available for muscles used during sports.
- Smokers suffer shortness of breath (gasp!) almost 3 times more often than nonsmokers.
- Smokers run slower and can't run as far, affecting overall athletic performance.
- Cigars and spit tobacco are NOT safe alternatives.

Tobacco and Personal Appearance

- Yuck! Tobacco smoke can make hair and clothes stink.
- Tobacco stains teeth and causes bad breath.
- Short-term use of spit tobacco can cause cracked lips, white spots, sores, and bleeding in the mouth.
- Surgery to remove oral cancers caused by tobacco use can lead to serious changes in the face. Sean Marcee, a high school star athlete who used spit tobacco, died of oral cancer when he was 19 years old.

SO . . .
- Know the truth. Despite all the tobacco use on TV and in movies, music videos, billboards and magazines—most teens, adults, and athletes DON'T use tobacco.
- Make friends, develop athletic skills, control weight, be independent, be cool . . . play sports.
- Don't waste (burn) money on tobacco. Spend it on CDs, clothes, computer games, and movies.

Get involved: make your team, school, and home tobacco-free; teach others; join community efforts to prevent tobacco use.

Available at: http://www.cdc.gov/tobacco/educational_materials/Yuthfax1.htm.

Health Promotion

Sexual Health Promotion

The incidence of STDs has skyrocketed, and most new HIV infections occur in people between 13 and 21 years of age. As part of holistic care, nurses in community-based settings should always assess sexuality. When assessing and teaching teens in this area, an open, frank, direct, and nonjudgmental approach is best. Talking openly and frankly with young teens about the benefits and risks of being sexually active may allow teens, especially girls, to understand that being sexually active is a choice. Earlier age of first coitus is a well-established risk factor for STDs because there is greater opportunity for exposure to pathogens. Early coitus is also associated with later high-risk cognitive, affective, and behavioral choices. Self-esteem and empowerment activities contribute to delay of first intercourse (Beitz, 1998).

Other primary prevention strategies to promote sexual health include comprehensive sex education beginning in primary school. Abstinence is a highly

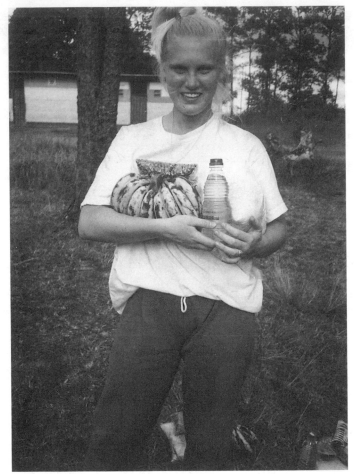

Photo by: Roberta Hunt

Figure 9–4. ▶ Suggestions for teaching adolescents about nutrition include instilling a sense of pride in identifying and choosing healthy meals and snacks.

positive choice for both sexes until they are ready to deal with the responsibility of being sexually active. However, it is not realistic as a sole strategy. The emphasis must be that sexual health promotion is for life and that contraception is useless if not practiced consistently.

Some sexuality health promotion programs use a more dramatic approach, with speakers who are HIV positive or have AIDS. These speakers tell their stories to teen groups, often with great success. Nurses can develop audiovisual aids (diagrams, pictures, and videos) to make sex education unforgettable. Nurses can explore with teens the differences between the facts of physiology and untrue but fervently held beliefs. Helping teens understand the relationship between substance abuse and STDs is another important issue to address. Peer education is a program model that is highly successful and inexpensive to implement.

Nurses can play a critical role in the improvement of sexual health counseling by using a direct and frank approach in interactions with individual teens, parents, groups, and peers. They play a pivotal role in community education by highlighting the relationship between substance abuse and unsafe sexual activity. Nurses in community-based settings can have enormous impact on sexual health promotion by acting as a positive role model for sexual health and being involved in issues related to sexual health.

Suicide Prevention

Suicide is a complex condition that can, in some cases, be prevented by early recognition and treatment of mental disorders. At least 90% of people who kill themselves have mental or substance abuse disorders (DHHS, 2000b). Thus, early identification and treatment of these disorders is paramount in the prevention of suicide. The recommendations from a national report on suicide prevention programs for adolescents and young adults are listed in Box 9–7.

Health Prevention and Disease Prevention Activities With Teens

When teaching teens about health, it is particularly important to base the teaching on what the teen already knows about the subject. Cognitively, many teens are not able to conceptualize or hypothesize. This, coupled with the fact that teens tend to be egocentric, complicates determining the best teaching modalities to reach the teen population. Successful disease prevention and health promotion activities for teens incorporate these considerations. Thus, it is most effective when teaching teens about physical activity or nutrition to talk about the immediate, particular, personal impacts in areas of importance to them.

For instance, a teen-aged girl who is overweight may respond to information on nutrition with the incentive of losing weight so she can wear the latest clothing style. A boy may respond to the suggestion to increase physical activity in his daily life if the nurse talks about the benefits of belonging to a team or being a sports hero. When taught about smoking cessation, teens respond to the idea that if they smoke, they are less desirable to kiss, or that their hands, clothes, and hair will smell, but not to the notion that smoking increases the chances of developing lung cancer. Nor do teens respond to the idea that if they are not physically fit and well nourished there is an increased chance that they will develop heart disease, diabetes, stroke, or cancer. They are developmentally unable to value such notions.

▶ Box 9–7. Recommendations for Suicide Prevention Among Adolescents ◀

- Ensure that suicide prevention programs are linked as closely as possible with professional mental health resources in the community.
- Avoid reliance on one prevention strategy.
- Incorporate promising but underused strategies into current programs where possible.
- Restrict access to lethal means.
- Gun control strategies.
- Parental education of warning signs.
- Collaboration with other prevention programs.

Source: O'Carroll, P. W., Potter, L. B., & Mercy, J. A. (1994). Programs for the prevention of suicide among adolescent and young adults. *MMWR Morbidity and Mortality Weekly Report, 43*(RR-6), 7.

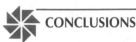
CONCLUSIONS

The primary issues involved in health promotion and disease prevention, based on *Healthy People 2010,* have been discussed from infancy through adolescence. Providing early prenatal care would eliminate many health conditions for newborn babies, save precious health care dollars and improve the quality of life for countless infants. During infancy and childhood, periodic screening allows for early identification and intervention of common and preventable conditions. Helping young children and teens value and adopt healthy lifestyle choices by improving nutrition, increasing physical activity, and following basic safety recommendations is an important contribution nurses in community-based settings can make. Advocating and participating in activities related to these issues in their own communities is another way nurses can contribute to the health of children. Lastly, being vocal and involved in public policy issues such as gun control and allocation of health care dollars for public health, as well as supporting political candidates who value public health, are all ways that nurses can improve the health of the nation's children.

What's on the Web

Bright Futures

Internet address: http://www.brightfutures.org

This Web site provides information about preventive and health promotion needs of infants, children, adolescents, families, and communities. A number of publications, including hand-outs in Spanish, can be downloaded or ordered through the site.

CDC Tobacco Information and Prevention Source
Tips4Youth Web page

Internet address: http://www.cdc.gov/tobacco/tips4youth.htm

This page compiles sites listing smoking cessation programs geared toward children and teens.

Child Health Guide: Put Prevention into Practice

Internet address: http://www.ahcpr.gov/ppip/ppchild.htm

This on-line consumer guide from the Agency for Healthcare Research and Quality explains children's preventive care. Print copies, available free of charge, can be requested by calling (800) 358-9295. The guide is also available in Spanish.

Healthfinder

Internet address: http://www.healthfinder.gov

Healthfinder is a search engine for consumer health education material, maintained by the U.S. Department of Health and Human Services.

Healthy People 2010

Internet address: http://www.health.gov/healthypeople

This document outlines the nationwide health promotion and disease prevention initiative designed to improving health for all people in the United States.

La Leche League
1400 North Meacham Road
Schaumburg, IL 60173-4048
Telephone: (847) 519-7730

Internet address: http://www.lalecheleague.org

This Web site provides information on breast-feeding, on-line discussion groups, and listings of local groups.

National Institute of Child Health and Human Development

Internet address: http://www.nichd.nih.gov

This site is an excellent resource for health education information for nurses to use with parents and families. It includes research about the health status of children.

WHY HOW WHEN to Wash Hands: A Handwashing Curriculum

Internet address: http://www.co.ramsey.mn.us/PH/hdwsh.htm

Studies have found that caregivers who teach and model good hand-washing can reduce illness by 50%. A creative and engaging curriculum to teach children why, when, and how to wash their hands can be ordered through this site. This resource, available as a video, curriculum booklet, and book, provides an easy, entertaining way to teach preschoolers the importance of handwashing. All materials are available in Spanish, Hmong, and English.

References and Bibliography

Agency for Healthcare Research and Quality. (2000). *Child health guide: Put prevention into practice.* Rockville, MD. Available at: http://www.ahcpr.gov/ppip/ppchild.htm.
American Academy of Pediatrics, Committee on Practice and Ambulatory Medicine. (1995). Recommendations for pediatric health care. *Pediatrics, 96*(2) 373–374.
Beitz, J. (1998). Sexual health promotion in adolescents and young adult: Primary prevention strategies. *Holistic Nursing Practice, 12*(2), 27–38.
Bond, L. A., & Burns, C. E. (1998). Investing in parents' development as an investment in primary prevention. *Journal of Mental Health, 7*(5), 493–503.
Centers for Disease Control and Prevention. (1995). Injury-control recommendations: Bicycle helmets. National Center for Injury Prevention and Control. *MMWR Morbidity and Mortality Weekly Report, 44*(RR-1), 1–18. Available at: http://aepo-xdv-www.epo.cdc.gov/wonder/prevguid/m0036941/m0036941.htm.
Centers for Disease Control and Prevention. (1996). Guidelines for school health programs to promote lifelong healthy eating. *MMWR Morbidity and Mortality Weekly Report, 45*(RR-9), 1–41. Available at: http://aepo-xdv-www.epo.cdc.gov/wonder/prevguid/m0042446/m0042446.htm.
Centers for Disease Control and Prevention. (1997). Childhood pedestrian deaths during Halloween—United States, 1975–1996. *MMWR Morbidity and Mortality Weekly Report, 46*(42), 987–990.
Centers for Disease Control and Prevention. (1998). Improper use of child safety seats—Kentucky, 1996. *MMWR Morbidity and Mortal Weekly Report, 47*(26), 541–543.

Centers for Disease Control and Prevention. (1999a). Adolescents and young adults fact sheet. In *Surgeon General's report on physical activity and health.* Available at: http://www.cdc.gov/nccdphp/sgr/adoles.htm.

Centers for Disease Control and Prevention. (1999b). *Child passenger safety fact sheet.* National Center for Injury Prevention and Control. Available at: http://www.cdc.gov/ncipc/factsheets/childpas.htm.

Centers for Disease Control and Prevention. (1999c). *Facts on adolescent injury.* National Center for Injury Prevention and Control. Available at: http://www.cdc.gov/ncipc/factsheets/adoles.htm.

Centers for Disease Control and Prevention. (2000a). *Early hearing detection and intervention program Web site.* National Center for Environmental Health Division of Birth Defects, Child Development, and Disability and Health. Available at: http://www.cdc.gov/nceh/cddh/ehdi.htm.

Centers for Disease Control and Prevention. (2000b). *Facts and statistics about skin cancer.* National Center for Chronic Disease Prevention and Health Promotion, Division of Cancer Prevention and Control. Available at: http://www.cdc.gov/chooseyourcover/skin.htm.

Dougherty, G., Schiffrin, A., White, D., Soderstrom, L., & Sufrategui, M. (1999). Home-based management can achieve intensification cost-effectively in type-I diabetes. *Pediatrics, 103*(1), 122–128.

Federal Interagency Forum on Child and Family Statistics. (1999). *American's children: Key national indicators of well-being.* Federal Interagency Forum on Child and Family Statistics. Washington, DC: U.S. Government Printing Office.

Green, P. M., & Adderley-Kelly, B. (1999). Partnership for health promotion in an urban community. *Nursing and Health Care Perspectives, 20*(2), 76–81.

Grunbaum, J., Kann, L., Kinchen, S., Ross, J., Gowda, V., Collins, J., & Kolbe, L. (2000). Youth risk behavior surveillance. National alternative high school youth risk behavior survey, United States, 1998. *Journal of School Health, 70*(1), 5–17.

Havas, S., Anliker, J., Damrohn, D., Langenberg, P., Ballesteros, M., & Feldman, R. (1998). Final results of the Maryland WIC 5—a day promotion program. *American Journal of Public Health, 88*(8), 1161–1167.

Hodnett, E. D. (1999). Caregiver support for women during childbirth. *Cochrane Database System Review, 2.* CD000199.

Kawabata, T., Cross, D., Nishioka, N., & Satoshi, S. (1999). Relationship between self-esteem and smoking behavior among Japanese early adolescents: Initial results from a three-year study. *Journal of School Health, 69*(7), 280–284.

Korinis, M., Korslund, M., Gavriella, B., Donohue, J., & Johnson, J. (1998). Comparison of calcium and weight loss information in teen-focused versus magazines over two 4-year periods. *Journal of Nutrition Education, 30*(3), 149–155.

Levin, D. (1997). Young people's lifestyles. *World Health, 50*(3), 21.

Lumley, J., Oliver, S., & Waters, E. (1999). Interventions for promoting smoking cessation during pregnancy. *Cochrane Database System Review.*

Mann, R., Abercrombie, P., DeJoseph, J., Norbeck, J., & Smith, R. (1999). The personal experience of pregnancy for African-American women. *Journal of Transcultural Nursing, 10*(4), 297–305.

McIntyre, L., Belzer, E., Manchester, L., Blanchard, W., Officer, S., & Simpson, A. (1996). The Dartmouth health promotion study: A failed quest for synergy in school health promotion. *Journal of School Health, 66*(4), 132–136.

Minnesota Department of Health, Division of Family Health, Minnesota Healthy Beginnings. (1999). *Promoting Minnesota healthy beginnings: Finding from focus groups with expecting moms and new parents.* Minneapolis: Minnesota Department of Health.

Monteiro, L. (1985). Florence Nightingale on public health nursing. *American Journal of Public Health, 75*(2), 181–185.

O'Carroll, P. W., Potter, L. B., & Mercy, J. A. (1994). Programs for the prevention of suicide among adolescent and young adults. *MMWR Morbidity and Mortality Weekly Report, 43*(RR-6), 1–7.

Patterson, D., & Lanier, C. (1999). Adolescent health transitions: Focus group study of teens and young adults with special health care needs. *Family Community Health, 22*(2), 43–58.

Pillitteri, A. (1999). *Maternal & child health nursing: Care of the childbearing & childrearing family* (3rd ed.). Philadelphia: Lippincott Williams & Wilkins.

Pizzi, E., & Wold, Z. (1998). Health risk and health promotion for older women: Utility of health promotion diary. *Holistic Nursing Practice, 12*(2), 62–73.

Polivka, B., & Ryan-Wenger, N. (1999). Health promotions and injury prevention behaviors of elementary school children. *Pediatric Nursing, 25*(2), 127.

Poss, J. (1999). Providing culturally competent care: Is there a role for health promoters? *Nursing Outlook, 47*(1), 30–36.

Ray, K. L., & Hodnett, E. D. (1997). Caregiver support for postpartum depression. *Cochrane Database System Review.*

Roberts-Gray, C. (1998). Heart partners: A strategy for promoting effective diffusion of school health promotion programs. *Journal of School Health, 68*(3), 106–109.

Roth, J., Hendrickson, J., Schilling, M., & Stowell, D. (1998). The risk of mothers having low weight babies: Implications of recent medical research for school health personnel. *Journal of School Health, 68*(7), 271–275.

Siarkowski, K. (1999). Children's adaptation to insulin dependent diabetes mellitus: A critical review of the literature. *Pediatric Nursing, 15*(6), 627–645.

Sullivan, L. (1998). How effective is preschool vision, hearing and developmental screening? *Pediatric Nursing, 14*(3), 181–183, 204.

Thomas, M., Benton, D., Keirle, K., & Pearsal, R. (1998). A review of the health promotion status of secondary schools in Wales and England. *Health Promotion International, 13*(2), 121–129.

U.S. Department of Health and Human Services, Public Health Service Center for Disease Control and Prevention. (1991). *Preventing lead poisoning in young children.* Available at http://aepo-xdv-www.epo.cdc.gov/wonder/prevguid/p0000029/entire.htm.

U.S. Department of Health and Human Services. (2000a). *Bright futures.* National Center for Education in Maternal Child Health. Maternal and Child Health Bureau. Arlington, VA. Available at: http://www.brightfutures.org.

U.S. Department of Health and Human Services. (2000b). Maternal, infant, and child health. In *Healthy people 2010. National health promotion and disease prevention objectives.* Washington, DC: U.S. Government Printing Office.

U.S. Department of Health and Human Services. (2000c). *Project to promote health education among children wins top prize in HHS secretary's award for health innovation.* Washington, DC: U.S. Government Printing Office.

Vickers, A., Ohlsson, A., Lacy, J. B., & Horsley, A. (1999) Massage for promoting growth and development of preterm and/or low birthweight infants. *Cochrane Database System Review, 2*, CD000390.

Weitzman, M., Fisch, S., Holmberg, R., Jackson, R., Lisbin, A., McKay, C., et al. (1996). Health needs of homeless children and families. *Pediatrics, 98*(40), 789–791.

Wright, A., Bauer, M., Naylor, A., Sutcliffe, E., & Clark, L. (1998). Increasing breastfeeding rates to reduce infant illness at the community level. *Pediatrics, 101*(5), 838–839.

Zahn, L., Cloutterbuck, J., Keshian, J., & Lombardi, L. (1998). Promoting health: Perspectives from ethnic elderly women. *Journal of Community Health Nursing, 15*(1), 31–44.

LEARNING ACTIVITIES

LEARNING ACTIVITY 9-1

▶ **Client Case Study:** Health Promotion and Disease Prevention for the Pregnant Teen

You are working as a community-based nurse making home visits to pregnant teens through the clinic where you are employed. The school nurse calls the clinic and requests that a home visit be made to Shantrell, who has shared with the school nurse that she is pregnant. She has been to your clinic for health care but has not had prenatal care. All you know is that Shantrell is 16-years-old and pregnant and is no longer going to school.

When you drive to the client's home you notice that the house is very old, with old cars and debris in the yard.

What else do you assess as you drive through the neighborhood?

You knock on the door. You notice that the paint is peeling on the outside of the house and looks like it hasn't been painted in a long time. Your client, Shantrell, comes to the door. You greet her, tell her your name, the name of the clinic you work for, and why you are visiting. During the first part of the visit, you spend some time getting to know Shantrell.

What could you use for a guide for interview questions?

You learn that Shantrell found out she was pregnant 1 month ago and is 3 months pregnant. She has not come in to the clinic because she thought that she only needed to see the doctor the month before the baby is born.

What would you want to screen for?
What topics would you want to address during the rest of the visit?
What other questions would you ask?
What will be your number one priority?
What do you hope to screen for and teach about in the next visit?

LEARNING ACTIVITY 9-2

▶ **Client Care Study:** Infant and Newborn

Shantrell has given birth to a baby girl who was 7 lb, 6 oz. She named the baby Precious. Both mom and baby did well during and after delivery. The baby is crying when you arrive for the visit. Shantrell picks up the baby, holds her close, and quietly talks to her.

What does this tell you about Shantrell's ability to comfort the newborn?
What do you do at this point?

Shantrell says she is breast-feeding Precious because "You told me that if I breast-feed my baby, I will lose my big tummy, and look slimmer faster." You ask how the feeding is going and she states, "Good. When I am at school, my mom gives her a bottle of milk."

What screening would you do at every visit?
What special risks may this infant have?
What would your priority be at this visit?

LEARNING ACTIVITY 9-3

▶ **Critical Thinking Exercise:** Self-Evalution

1. In your clinical journal, describe a situation you have encountered when screening and doing health promotion activities.

   What did you learn from this experience?
   How will you practice differently based on this experience?

2. In your clinical journal, describe a situation in which you have observed infants or children not receiving the health care that they needed.

   How could or would you like to advocate for this issue when you begin to practice as an RN?
   What could you do now?

Health Promotion and Disease Prevention for Adults

R O B E R T A   H U N T

► L E A R N I N G   O B J E C T I V E S ◄

- Identify the leading causes of death for adults.
- Discuss the major diseases and threats to health for adults.
- Summarize the primary health issues for adults.
- Identify nursing roles for each level of prevention for primary health issues for adults.
- Compose a list of nursing interventions for the primary health issues for adults.
- Determine health needs for adults for which a nurse could be an advocate.

► K E Y   T E R M S ◄

health disparity   overweight
health indicator   obese
moderate physical activity

Health Status of Adults

Eliminating Disparity in Health Care

Health Screening for Adults

Interventions for Leading Health Indicators

Conclusions

HEALTH STATUS OF ADULTS

The major causes of death in the United States (Table 10–1) generally result from a mix of behaviors that contribute to injury, violence, and other environmental factors, as well as lack of access to quality health services. For the nurse, this points to the importance of understanding and monitoring health behaviors, environmental factors, and community health systems. This chapter will assist the nurse to understand and learn to monitor health behaviors that affect health and contribute to the major causes of death and disability.

Because the average person is living longer, more attention is now focused on preserving quality of life rather than only extending length of life. Chief among the factors involving preserving quality of life is the prevention and treatment of musculosketetal conditions. Demographic trends also indicate that people will need to continue to work at older ages. Nurses will increasingly be involved in efforts to decrease the adverse social and economic consequence of high rates of activity limitation and disability of older persons.

Leading **health indicators** are seen in Box 10–1. These illuminate individual behavioral, physical, social, and environmental factors and health systems issues that affect the health of individuals. "The health indicators are intended to help everyone more easily understand the importance of health promotion and disease prevention and to encourage wide participation in improving health in the next decade" (U.S. Department of Health and Human Services [DHHS], 2000, p. 25).

ELIMINATING DISPARITY IN HEALTH CARE

The central goals of *Healthy People 2010* are to increase quality and years of healthy life and to eliminate health disparities. **Health disparities** exist by gender, race or ethnicity, education or income, disability, living in rural localities, or sexual orientation. Men have a life expectancy that is 6 years less than women's, and they have a higher rate of death for each of the 10 leading causes of death. Women have had an increasing rate of death from lung cancer in the past 20 years, whereas the men's rate has decreased.

Disparity by ethnicity is believed to be a result of complex interactions among genetic variations, environmental factors, and specific health behaviors. Heart disease death rates are more than 40% higher for African Americans than for whites. Hispanics living in the United States are almost twice as likely to die from diabetes than are non-Hispanic whites. American Indians and Alaska Na-

TABLE 10–1 • Leading Causes of Death in Adults, United States, 1997

Age (y)	Cause of Death	Number
25–44	Unintentional injuries	27,129
	Cancer	21,706
	Heart disease	16,513
45–65	Cancer	131,743
	Heart disease	101,235
	Unintentional injuries	17,521

U.S. Department of Health and Human Services. (2000). *Healthy people 2010. National health promotion and disease prevention objectives.* Washington, DC: U.S. Government Printing Office.

> ▶ **Box 10–1.** Leading Health Indicators From *Healthy People 2010* ◀
>
> | | |
> |---|---|
> | 1. Physical activity | 6. Mental health |
> | 2. Overweight and obesity | 7. Injury violence |
> | 3. Tobacco use | 8. Environmental quality |
> | 4. Substance abuse | 9. Immunization |
> | 5. Responsible sexual behavior | 10. Access to health care |

tives have twice the rate of diabetes that whites have and disproportionately high rates of death from unintentional injuries and suicide. Asians and Pacific Islanders, on average, have health indicators that suggest they are one of the healthiest population groups in the United States.

Income and education underlie many health disparities in the United States. Income and education are intrinsically related; people with the worst health status are among those with the highest poverty rates and least education. Income inequality in the United States has increased over the past 3 decades.

People with disabilities are identified as people who have activity limitation, people who need assistive devices, or people who perceive themselves as having a disability. Roughly 21% of the population reports some level of disability. Many people with disabilities lack access to health services and medical care.

Rural localities are home to 25% of Americans. Those living in rural areas are less likely to use preventive screening services, exercise regularly, or wear seatbelts, and are more likely to be uninsured.

The gay and lesbian populations have health problems unique to their population. Gay men are more likely than heterosexual men to have human immunodeficiency virus (HIV), other sexually transmitted diseases (STDs), substance abuse, depression, and suicide. Some studies show that lesbian women have higher rates of smoking, obesity, alcohol abuse, and stress than heterosexual women do.

Nurses can help reduce health disparities by (1) educating themselves regarding issues of disparity, (2) identifying vulnerable populations in their communities, and (3) advocating for vulnerable populations. Suggestions for advocacy activities for nurses include:

▶ Empowering each client and family they care for that experiences disparities in health care
▶ Discussing disparities in their communities with colleagues
▶ Writing about disparities for hospital, clinic, or professional organization newsletters
▶ Writing letters to, or calling and making an appointment to speak to, local or state politicians to describe evidence of health disparities that they encounter

Diversity is one of our nation's greatest assets, but in the case of health disparity it presents a great challenge. Regardless of age, gender, race, ethnicity, income, education, geographic location, disability, or sexual orientation, everyone deserves equal access to health care.

HEALTH SCREENING FOR ADULTS

As with clients at other ages, health screening for adults is intended for primary, secondary, or tertiary prevention. Primary prevention to prevent the initial occurrence of a disease with an adult client could be immunization screening and recommendation of an annual flu shot. Secondary prevention could be screening for hypertension at a health fair or yearly mammography for women over 50 years of age. Tertiary prevention could be initiating an exercise program for an obese client who has type 2 diabetes. Screening is always intended to identify people who are at risk for developing a health condition so that appropriate intervention can be undertaken.

The nurse should encourage the client to actively practice prevention. One way to accomplish this is to use the *Personal Health Guide: Put Prevention into Practice* available from the Agency for Healthcare Research and Quality at http://www.ahcpr.gov/ppip/ppadult.htm or by calling (800) 358-9295. This guide makes it easier for clients to keep accurate information about their health and for the nurse to guide clients in identifying and planning health promotion and disease prevention activities. The guide contains information on screening as well as on topics related to the leading health indicators. It also contains forms for record-keeping essential for health promotion and disease prevention.

General Screening

Major areas of adult health screening covered in the *Personal Health Guide* include blood pressure, cholesterol, weight, and immunizations. Maintaining a normal blood pressure protects from heart disease, stroke, and kidney problems. It is recommended that all adults have their blood pressure checked regularly. Those with high blood pressure should work with their health care provider to lower it by changing their diet, losing weight, exercising, and, if prescribed, taking medication.

Cholesterol should be checked in men ages 35 to 65 years and woman ages 45 to 65. Cholesterol can be lowered by changing diet, losing excess weight, and getting exercise. The client's knowledge about cholesterol and heart disease can be assessed by using quizzes available from the National Heart, Lung, and Blood Institute at http://www.nhlbi.nih.gov/health/public/heart/chol/chol_iq.htm and http://www.nhlbi.nih.gov/health/public/heart/other/hh_iq.htm.

Weighing too much or too little can lead to health problems. Healthy diet and regular exercise are factors that contribute to weight loss. Assessment should include the evaluation of body mass index (BMI), waist circumference, and overall medical risk.

Immunizations are cited as one of the greatest achievements of public health in the 20th century. Immunizations needed by adults are shown in Box 10–2. It is important to continue to increase the proportion of children who receive all vaccines as well as the proportion of adults who are vaccinated annually against the flu.

Oral health care is also very important for overall general health. Not only will proper oral care preserve teeth for a lifetime, but flossing every day contributes to a longer life.

Cancer Screening

Colorectal cancer is the third leading cause of death from cancer. The risk of developing colorectal cancer increases with advancing age. African Americans are more likely than whites to be diagnosed at a later stage and die from colorectal cancer. Risk factors include inflammatory bowel disease and a family or personal history of colorectal cancer or polyps. Lack of regular physical activity, low fruit

---

▶ **Box 10–2.** Recommended Immunizations for Adults ◀

- Tetanus-diphtheria: every 10 years
- Rubella: for women considering pregnancy
- Pneumoococcal (pneumonia): at about age 65
- Influenza: for people who have a chronic condition, work with high-risk populations or live with someone who works with high-risk populations, pregnant woman after the first trimester, or anyone over 50 years of age
- Hepatitis B: for people who have contact with human blood or body fluids, have unprotected sex, or share needles during intravenous drug use. Health professionals should also consider hepatitis B immunization.

Agency for Healthcare Research and Quality. (2000). *Personal health guide: Put preventon into practice.* Rockville MD. Available at: http://www.ahcpr.gov/ppip/ppadult.htm.

---

and vegetable intake, a low-fiber diet, obesity, and alcohol consumption are other contributing factors. Reducing the number of deaths from colorectal cancer chiefly depends on detecting and removing precancerous colorectal polyps, as well as detecting and treating the cancer in its early stages. People 50 years and older should been screened regularly with a fecal occult blood test yearly and sigmoidoscopy every 5 to 10 years.

Regular mammography screening for women age 50 and older has been shown to be effective in reducing deaths from breast cancer (Centers for Disease Control and Prevention [CDC], 1999). Some women may need to begin mammograms earlier, depending on their health history. All women should have an annual Pap smear at age 18 or when they become sexually active. Those who have three or more normal annual tests may be tested less frequently, at the discretion of the nurse practitioner or physician.

The CDC National Breast and Cervical Cancer Early Detection Program provides free screening exams for all women. throughout the United States. Consult the Web site at http://www.cdc.gov/cancer/nbccedp/index.htm or call (888) 842-6355 for more information or to find out where your client can get a free or low-cost mammogram and Pap test in your area.

Prostate cancer is the most commonly diagnosed form of cancer, second to skin cancer, and is second to lung cancer as a cause of cancer-related death among men. Scientific evidence is insufficient to determine if screening for prostate cancer reduces deaths or if treatment in early stages is more effective

---

COMMUNITY-BASED TEACHING

Basic Principles of Oral Health

- Visit your dentist regularly for checkups.
- Brush after meals.
- Use dental floss daily.
- Limit the amount of sweets, especially between meals.
- Do not smoke or chew tobacco products.

than no treatment in prolonging a man's life. Thus, widespread screening and testing for early detection of prostate cancer are not scientifically justified at this time. The two common methods for detecting prostate cancer are digital rectal examination and prostate-specific antigen testing.

Screening for High-Risk Groups

The following conditions may require additional screening. If the client falls into any of these categories, he or she should discuss it with a nurse practitioner or physician.

- ▶ Has diabetes, or is older than 40 and African American, or older than 60 years of age—requires additional eye exams
- ▶ Has had intercourse without condoms, has had multiple partners, or has had an STD—may require screening for STDs
- ▶ Has injected illegal drugs, had a blood transfusion between 1978 and 1985— may need an HIV or hepatitis test
- ▶ Has a family member with diabetes, is overweight, or has had diabetes during pregnancy—may need a glucose test
- ▶ Over age 65—needs a hearing test
- ▶ Now or in the past, has consumed a lot of alcohol, smoked, or chewed tobacco—may need a mouth exam
- ▶ Male and over age 50—needs a prostate exam
- ▶ Male and age 14 to 35 years, particularly if a testicle is abnormally small or not in the normal position—may need a testicular exam
- ▶ Has had a family member with skin cancer, or has had a lot of sun exposure— may need a skin exam
- ▶ Has had radiation treatments of the upper body—may need a thyroid exam
- ▶ Has been exposed to tuberculosis; has recently moved from Asia, Africa, Central or South American, or the Pacific Islands; has kidney failure, diabetes, HIV, or alcoholism; or uses illegal drugs—may need a tuberculosis (PPD) test (*Personal Health Guide: Put Prevention into Practice,* April 1998. Publication No. APPIP 98-0027. Agency for Health Care Policy and Research, Rockville, MD. Available at: http://www.ahrq.gov/ppip/ppadult.htm)

 INTERVENTIONS FOR LEADING HEALTH INDICATORS

Evidence exists that some of the leading causes of death and disability in the United States, such as heart disease, cancer, stroke, some respiratory diseases, unintentional injuries, and HIV and acquired immunodeficiency syndrome (AIDS), can often be prevented by making lifestyle changes. Staying physically active, eating right, and not smoking (or quitting if you do smoke) are the three most important strategies to better health (Fig. 10–1).

Physical Activity

Engaging in regular physical activity on most days of the week reduces the risk of developing or dying from some of the leading causes of illness and death. Box 10–3 presents an overview of the relationship between physical activity and morbidity and mortality.

More than 60% of adults in the United States do not engage in recommended

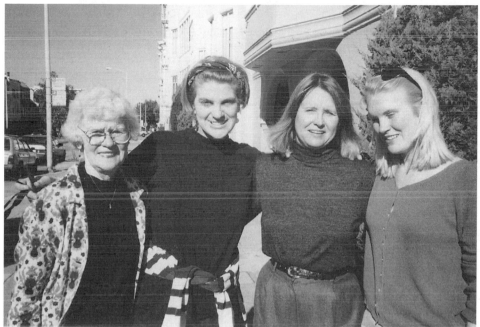

Photo by: Tim Heaney

Figure 10–1. ▶ A healthy lifestyle incorporating physical activity, good nutrition, social support, and avoidance of activities that are detrimental to health can improve quality of life for adults of all ages.

▶ **Box 10–3.** The Effects of Physical Activity on Health ◀

Regular physical activity reduces the risk of:

- Dying prematurely
- Dying prematurely from heart disease
- Developing diabetes
- Developing high blood pressure
- Developing colon cancer

Regular physical activity helps:

- Reduce blood pressure in those with hypertension
- Reduce feeling of depression and anxiety
- Control weight
- Build and maintain healthy bones, muscles and joints
- Promote psychological well-being

Health burdens that could be reduced through regular physical activity:

- 13.5 million people have coronary heart disease
- 1.5 million individuals have an myocardial infarct each year
- 8 million people have type II diabetes (adult-onset)
- Over 60 million individuals (one third of the population) are overweight

Centers for Disease Control and Prevention. (1999). *The link between physical activity and morbidity and mortality. Physical activity and health: A report of the Surgeon General.* Available at: http://www.cdc.gov/nccdphp/sgr/mm.htm.

amounts of physical activity. Physical inactivity is more common among women than men, African American and Hispanic adults than white adults, older adults than younger adults, and less affluent people than more affluent people.

"How much activity?" and "How do I start?" are two common questions clients may ask regarding physical activity. Clients who have been very sedentary or are obese may want to start by reducing sedentary time and gradually building physical activity into each day. A client may begin by gradually increasing daily activities such as taking the stairs or walking or swimming at a slow pace.

The need to avoid injury during physical activity is a high priority. Walking is an ideal activity to use to increase physical activity because it is safe and accessible to most people. For those who have been physically inactive, a starting point can be walking 10 minutes, 3 days a week, building to 30 to 45 minutes of more intense walking and gradually increasing to most if not all days. **Moderate physical activity** for 30 to 45 minutes, 3 to 5 days per week, is a reasonable initial goal. Most adults should be encouraged to set a long-term goal of 30 minutes or more of moderate-intensity physical activity on most, preferably all, days of the week. Table 10–2 shows examples of moderate amounts of physical activity achieved from both common chores and sporting activities.

With time, weight loss, and increased functional capacity, the client may want to engage in more strenuous activities. These include fitness walking, cycling, rowing, cross-country skiing, aerobic dancing, and jumping rope. If jogging is desired, the client's ability to jog must be assessed first. Competitive sports such as tennis, soccer, or volleyball provide enjoyable physical activity for some individuals, but again, care must be taken to avoid injury.

Individuals who are not physically active cite many reasons for their inactivity. Appendix H of the National Institutes of Health (NIH) *The Pratical Guide: Identification, Evaluation, and Treatment of Overweight and Obesity in Adults,* available online at http://www.nhlbi.nih.gov/guidelines/obesity/ob_home.htm, gives the nurse

---

TABLE 10–2 • Examples of Moderate Amounts of Physical Activity*

Common Chores	Sporting Activities	
Washing and waxing a car for 45–60 min	Playing volleyball for 45–60 min	Less Vigorous, More Time
Washing windows or floors for 45–60 min	Playing touch football for 45 min	
Gardening for 30–45 min	Walking 1¾ miles in 35 min (20 min/mile)	
Wheeling self in wheelchair for 30–40 min	Basketball (shooting baskets) for 30 min	↑
Pushing a stroller 1½ miles in 30 min	Bicycling 5 miles in 30 min	
Raking leaves for 30 min	Dancing fast (social) for 30 min	
Walking 2 miles in 30 min (15 min/mile)	Water aerobics for 30 min	
Shoveling snow for 15 min	Swimming laps for 20 min	↓
Stairwalking for 15 min	Basketball (playing a game) for 15–20 min	More Vigorous, Less Time
	Jumping rope for 15 min	
	Running 1½ miles in 15 min (10 min/mile)	

*A moderate amount of physical activity is roughly equivalent to physical activity that uses approximately 150 calories of energy per day, or 1,000 calories per week.
Some activities can be performed at various intensities; the suggested durations correspond to expected intensity of effort.
National Institutes of Health. (1998). *The practical guide: Identification, evaluation, and treatment of overweight and obesity in adults.* National Heart, Lung and Blood Institute Obesity Education Initiative.

some pointers for helping the client overcome obstacles to regular activity. It also includes two sample exercise programs. Social support from family and friends has been consistently and positively related to regular exercise. Nurses who work closely with clients in community-based settings have ample opportunity to encourage daily moderate physical activity for 30 minutes a day for all adults.

Overweight and Obesity

Overweight and obesity are major contributors to many preventable causes of death, with a general rule that higher body weight is associated with higher death rates. Being overweight or obese substantially raises the risk of illness from high blood pressure; high cholesterol; type 2 diabetes; heart disease and stroke; gallbladder disease; arthritis; sleep disturbances; and endometrial, breast, prostate, and colon cancers.

Women from lower income households are more likely to be overweight. Obesity is more common among African American and Hispanic women than among white women. Eighty percent more African American women than men are overweight (DHHS, 2000).

A person with a BMI between 25.0 and 29.9 is considered **overweight.** A person with a BMI of 30.0 or greater is considered **obese.** Box 10–4 shows how to calculate BMI and waist circumference. Table 10–3 contains a BMI estimation table.

Dietary therapy, physical activity, and behavioral therapy are the usual interventions for overweight and obesity. For the morbidly obese, pharmacotherapy and weight loss surgery may be considered. A combination of diet modification, increased physical activity, and behavior therapy can be effective for most obese individuals. A guide to selecting appropriate treatment is found in the NIH *Practical Guide.*

Weight loss therapy is not appropriate for some individuals, including most pregnant or lactating women, people with uncontrolled psychiatric illness, and people with serious illnesses that might be exacerbated by caloric restriction. Clients with active substance abuse or a history of anorexia nervosa or bulimia nervosa should receive care by a specialist.

It is recommended that health care providers first complete a behavioral assessment to determine a client's readiness for weight loss. One example is found in the NIH *Practical Guide.* A guide to behavior change is seen in Appendix I of the NIH publication, which can be used to help the client plan a weight loss program.

Next, a diet with a 500- to 1,000-calorie deficit should be planned. This usually means 1,000 to 1,200 calories for women and 1,200 to 1,600 calories for men. Sample diets for American, Asian, Southern, Mexican American, and lacto-ovo vegetarian clients are found in the appendices of the NIH *Practical Guide,* along with tips for weight loss including methods of food preparation and how to choose food when dining out.

The nurse and client can plan and monitor the weight loss program by using a weight and goal record. The client can keep a record of food consumption and physical activity each week by using a diet and activity tracking sheet. Samples of these resources are found in the appendices of the *Practical Guide,* along with additional resources for healthy eating and physical activity. Through health education, nurses can help reduce the proportion of adults who are obese.

Tobacco Use

Cigarette smoking, responsible for more than 430,000 deaths annually, continues to be the main preventable cause of disease and death in the United States

▶ **Box 10–4.** Calculating Body Mass Index and Waist Circumference ◀

You can calculate BMI as follows:

$$BMI = \frac{weight\ (kg)}{height\ squared\ (m^2)}$$

If pounds and inches are used:

BMI = weight (lb) × 703 height squared (inches²)

Calculation Directions and Sample.

Here is a shortcut method for calculating BMI. (Example: for a person who is 5 feet 5 inches tall weighing 180 lbs)

1. Multiply weight (in pounds) by 703 180 × 703 = 126,540
2. Multiply height (in inches) by
   height (in inches)   65 × 65 = 4225
3. Divide the answer in step 1 by the answer
   in step 2 to get the BMI.   126,540/4225=29.9

   BMI = B29.9

Waist Circumference Measurement

To measure waist circumference, locate the upper hip bone and the top of the right iliac crest. Place a measuring tape in a horizontal plane around the abdomen at the level of the iliac crest. Before reading the tape measure, ensure that the tape is snug, but does not compress the skin, and is parallel to the floor. The measurement is made at the end of a normal expiration.

High-Risk Waist Circumference

Men: F > 40 in (> 102 cm)
Women: F > 35 in (> 88 cm)

Measuring-Tape Position for Waist (Abdominal) Circumference in Adults

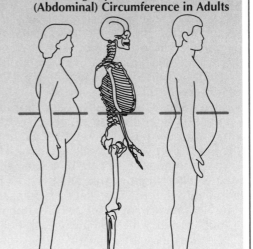

National Institutes of Health. (1998). *The practical guide: Identification, evaluation, and treatment of overweight and obesity in adults.* National Heart, Lung and Blood Institute Obesity Education Initiative.

(*Treating tobacco use and dependence,* 2000). Smoking is a major risk factor for developing heart disease, stroke, lung cancer, and chronic lung disease. The percentage of adolescents who smoke has increased in the past decade, and each day, more than 3,000 children and adolescents start using tobacco (*Treating tobacco use and dependence,* 2000). This trend is of great concern because most adult smokers tried their first cigarette before 18 years of age. Half of all adolescent smokers who continue to smoke in adulthood will die from smoking-related

TABLE 10–3 • Body Mass Index Estimation

Body Weight (pounds)

BMI	Healthy Weight						Overweight					Obese									Very Obese															
Height (inches)	19	20	21	22	23	24	25	26	27	28	29	30	31	32	33	34	35	36	37	38	39	40	41	42	43	44	45	46	47	48	49	50	51	52	53	54
58	91	96	100	105	110	115	119	124	129	134	138	143	148	153	158	162	167	172	177	181	186	191	196	201	205	210	215	220	224	229	234	239	244	248	253	258
59	94	99	104	109	114	119	124	128	133	138	143	148	153	158	163	168	173	178	183	188	193	198	203	208	212	217	222	227	232	237	242	247	252	257	262	267
60	97	102	107	112	118	123	128	133	138	143	148	153	158	163	168	174	179	184	189	194	199	204	209	215	220	225	230	235	240	245	250	255	261	266	271	276
61	100	106	111	116	122	127	132	137	143	148	153	158	164	169	174	180	185	190	195	201	206	211	217	222	227	232	238	243	248	254	259	264	269	275	280	285
62	104	109	115	120	126	131	136	142	147	153	158	164	169	175	180	186	191	196	202	207	213	218	224	229	235	240	246	251	256	262	267	273	278	284	289	295
63	107	113	118	124	130	135	141	146	152	158	163	169	175	180	186	191	197	203	208	214	220	225	231	237	242	248	254	259	265	270	278	284	289	295	301	304
64	110	116	122	128	134	140	145	151	157	163	169	174	180	186	192	197	204	209	215	221	227	232	238	244	250	256	262	267	273	279	285	291	296	302	308	314
65	114	120	126	132	138	144	150	156	162	168	174	180	186	192	198	204	210	216	222	228	234	240	246	252	258	264	270	276	282	288	294	300	306	312	318	324
66	118	124	130	136	142	148	155	161	167	173	179	186	192	198	204	210	216	223	229	235	241	247	253	260	266	272	278	284	291	297	303	309	315	322	328	334
67	121	127	134	140	146	153	159	166	172	178	185	191	198	204	211	217	223	230	236	242	249	255	261	268	274	280	287	293	299	306	312	319	325	331	338	344
68	125	131	138	144	151	158	164	171	177	184	190	197	203	210	216	223	230	236	243	249	256	262	269	276	282	289	295	302	308	315	322	328	335	341	348	354
69	128	135	142	149	155	162	169	176	182	189	196	203	209	216	223	230	236	243	250	257	263	270	277	284	291	297	304	311	318	324	331	338	345	351	358	365
70	132	139	146	153	160	167	174	181	188	195	202	209	216	222	229	236	243	250	257	264	271	278	285	292	299	306	313	320	327	334	341	348	355	362	369	376
71	136	143	150	157	165	172	179	186	193	200	208	215	222	229	236	243	250	257	265	272	279	286	293	301	308	315	322	329	338	343	351	358	365	372	379	386
72	140	147	154	162	169	177	184	191	199	206	213	221	228	235	242	250	258	265	272	279	287	294	302	309	316	324	331	338	346	353	361	368	375	383	390	397
73	144	151	159	166	174	182	189	197	204	212	219	227	235	242	250	257	265	272	280	288	295	302	310	318	325	333	340	348	355	363	371	378	386	393	401	408
74	148	155	163	171	179	186	194	202	210	218	225	233	241	249	256	264	272	280	287	295	303	311	319	326	334	342	350	358	365	373	381	389	396	404	412	420
75	152	160	168	176	184	192	200	208	216	224	232	240	248	256	264	272	279	287	295	303	311	319	327	335	343	351	359	367	375	383	391	399	407	415	423	431
76	156	164	172	180	189	197	205	213	221	230	238	246	254	263	271	279	287	295	304	312	320	328	336	344	353	361	369	377	385	394	402	410	418	426	435	443

National Institutes of Health. (1998). *The practical guide: Identification, evaluation, and treatment of overweight and obesity in adults.* National Heart, Lung and Blood Institute Obesity Education Initiative.

illness. Whites are more likely than African Americans and Hispanics to use tobacco (DHHS, 2000).

The financial costs of smoking and smoking-related disease, including lost earnings and productivity, approach $100 billion per year. It is estimated that a program to provide 75% of adult smokers with a smoking cessation intervention (nicotine replacement therapy, counseling, or a combination) would be cost effective in relation to other interventions, such as blood pressure screening and mammography. Currently, most medical schools do not require clinical training in techniques for smoking cessation (*Treating tobacco use and dependence,* 2000).

The community-based nurse should screen for tobacco use and encourage cessation with every client. Current research in the area of smoking cessation is shown in Research Box 10–1.

Substance Abuse

Many serious problems are associated with alcohol and illicit drug use. The financial costs of substance abuse are high, estimated at $276 billion per year (DHHS, 2000). Substance abuse is associated with child and spousal abuse, STDs, motor vehicle accidents, escalation of health care costs, low worker productivity, and homelessness. Alcohol abuse alone is associated with motor vehicle accidents, homicides, suicides, and drownings. Chronic alcohol use can lead to heart disease, cancer, liver disease, and pancreatitis (DHHS, 2000).

The rate of adult drinking and illicit drug use has been constant since 1980. Whites and Hispanics are more likely than African Americans to use alcohol. Whites are more likely than African Americans and Hispanics to use illicit drugs (DHHS, 2000).

Assessment and intervention with substance-related health issues is an important role for the nurse in community-based settings. The more direct, honest, and open the nurse is when addressing this issue, the more likely clients will be to view their own patterns of use of alcohol as an important aspect of health promotion.

RESEARCH IN COMMUNITY-BASED NURSING CARE

Research Box 10–1 ▶ Nursing Interventions
for Smoking Cessation

This integrative literature review of 19 studies was conducted to determine the effectiveness of nursing-delivered smoking cessation interventions. It was found that smokers who were offered advice by nursing professionals had an increased likelihood of quitting compared to smokers without such nursing interventions. This result reflected a significantly positive effect for smoking cessation interventions by nurses. The challenge to nurses is to incorporate smoking cessation interventions as part of standard practice so that the nurse discusses tobacco use with all clients, gives advice to quit, and uses behavioral counseling. Nurses interface with clients in numerous settings allowing them to play an important role in reducing cigarette smoking by adults.

Rice, V. H., & Stead, L. F. (1999). Nursing interventions for smoking cessation. *Cochrane Database System Review, 2,* CD001188.

COMMUNITY-BASED NURSING CARE GUIDELINES

Guidelines for Smoking Cessation Intervention

Ask
Ask clients if they smoke and how much. Congratulate ex-smokers. Record their smoking status.

Advise
Ask clients about the benefits of not smoking. Express concern and recommend that clients quit.

Prepare
Set a quit date. Review tips for quitting. Tell clients you will follow-up or you will think of them on quit day.

Follow up
Ask clients if they still smoke. Give ex-smokers a pat on the back. Send cards or call clients soon after their visit and/or just before quit day.

U.S. Department of Health and Human Services. (1993) *Nurses: Help your patients stop smoking*. Washington, DC: National Heart, Lung and Blood Institute.

An assessment for alcohol abuse is given in Box 10–5. Teaching the client about avoiding substance abuse issues is the next step after assessment.

Interventions targeted to groups and communities have demonstrated some efficacy in reducing substance abuse. School-based prevention programs directed toward altering perceived peer-group norms about alcohol use and helping develop skill in resisting peer pressure to drink are successful in reducing alcohol use among participants. Raising the minimum legal drinking age has reduced alcohol consumption, traffic accidents, and related fatalities among young persons under 21 years of age. Higher cost for alcohol is also associated with lower alcohol consumption and lowered adverse outcomes. In college settings, one-to-one motivational counseling has been effective in reducing alcohol-related problems. It is important that the nurse direct efforts to reduce the proportion of adults using illicit drugs and engaging in binge drinking of alcoholic beverages.

▶ Box 10–5. Quick Assessment for Alcohol Abuse ◀

A "yes" answer to any of the following questions may be a warning sign that the client has a drinking problem and should talk to a health care provider.

- Have you ever felt that you should cut down on your drinking?
- Have people annoyed you by criticizing your drinking?
- Have you ever felt bad or guilty about drinking?
- Have you ever had a drink first thing in the morning to steady your nerves or to get rid of a hangover?

Personal health guide: Put prevention into practice. (1998, April). Publication No. APPIP 98-0027. Rockville, MD: Agency for Health Care Policy and Research. Available at: http://www.ahrq.gov/ppip/ppadult.htm.

COMMUNITY-BASED TEACHING

Tips to Reduce Substance Abuse Behaviors

- Don't use illegal (street) drugs of any kind, at any time.
- Use prescription drugs only as directed by a health care provider.
- Use nonprescription drugs only as instructed on the label.
- Tell your health care provider all of the medications you are currently taking.
- If you drink alcohol, do so only in moderation—no more than one drink daily for women and two drinks daily for men.
- Do not drink alcohol before or while driving a motor vehicle.
- If you have concerns about your alcohol or drug use, talk to your health care provider.

Personal health guide: Put prevention into practice. (1998, April). Publication No. APPIP 98-0027. Rockville, MD: Agency for Health Care Policy and Research. Available at: http://www.ahrq.gov/ppip/ppadult/htm.

Responsible Sexual Behavior

Unprotected sex can result in unintended pregnancies and STDs, including HIV. About half of all new HIV infections in the United States are among individuals over 25 years of age, with the majority being infected through sexual behavior. Recently, there has been an increase in abstinence among youth and an increase in condom use among sexually active adults. Condoms, used correctly and consistently, can prevent STDs, including HIV.

COMMUNITY-BASED NURSING CARE GUIDELINES

Guidelines for Alcohol and Substance Use Intervention

Ask
Ask clients if they use alcohol or other drugs, how much, and the frequency. Ask about binge drinking (more than 3 drinks per occasion or 7 drinks per week). Congratulate recovering alcoholics and drug users.
Ask clients the assessment questions in Box 10–5. Also ask about any adverse consequences they have experienced from their drinking.

Advise
Ask what benefits the clients would enjoy if they reduced alcohol or drug intake.

Prepare
Set a date to quit drinking, attend Alcoholics Anonymous, or get counseling for concerns related to the client's substance use.

Follow-up
Follow-up by asking about progress. Be straightforward, matter of fact, and nonjudgemental. Praise and encourage any small steps taken. Continue to validate any effort.

Health teaching is the most important disease prevention activity the nurse can use to address health issues related to sexual behavior. Again, sexuality must always be assessed, with teaching and interventions based on the client's knowledge base, concerns, and cultural sensitivities. As discussed in Chapter 9, young teens should be encouraged to delay age of first intercourse. Teaching about the effectiveness of various contraceptive methods, and always providing condoms, are interventions that have been shown again and again to be essential to sexual health promotion.

Mental Health

Twenty percent of the population is affected by mental illness during a given year, with depression the most common disorder. Mental health is not just the absence of illness but a "state of successful mental functioning, resulting in productivity, fulfilling relationships and ability to adapt to change and cope with adversity" (DHHS, 2000, p. 37).

Depression is a common condition that is often not recognized by health care providers. The warning signs of depression are outlined in Box 10–6. Depression affects daily functioning and in some cases incapacitates the individual. Major depression is the leading cause of all disabilities and the cause of more than two thirds of suicides each year. Financial costs from lost work time are high. Unfortunately, there is still widespread misunderstanding about mental illness and associated stigmatization, which often prevents individuals with depression from getting professional help.

Adults and older adults have the highest rates of depression, with major depression affecting twice as many women as men. Depression is also high among those with chronic conditions; 12% of patients hospitalized with heart disease or hip fracture are diagnosed with depression (DHHS, 2000).

Depression is a treatable condition—medications and psychological treatment are effective in 80% of people suffering from depression. But to receive treatment, people with depression have to be identified and encouraged to seek help. An important role of the nurse in community-based care is to identify those experiencing depression and convince them to seek assistance early.

At least 90% of people who commit suicide have or are experiencing mental illness, a substance abuse disorder, or a combination; therefore, it is essential that health care professionals be diligent about screening and intervention when

---

▶ **Box 10–6.** Warning Signs of Depression ◀

- Feeling sad, hopeless, or guilty most of the time
- Loss of interest and pleasure in daily activities
- Sleep problems (either too much or too little)
- Fatigue, low energy, or feeling "slowed down"
- Problems making decisions or thinking clearly
- Crying a lot
- Changes in appetite or weight (up or down)
- Thoughts of suicide or death

Personal health guide: Put prevention into practice. (1998, April). Publication No. APPIP 98-0027. Rockville, MD: Agency for Health Care Policy and Research. Available at: http://www.ahrq.gov/ppip/ppadult.htm.

mental illness is suspected. Again, nurses should not be afraid to ask questions regarding mental health concerns and to refer accordingly. It is very important that the proportion of adults with recognized depression who receive treatment continues to rise.

Injuries and Violence

Motor vehicle accidents are the most common cause of serious injury among adults. The current yearly cost of injury and violence is estimated at more than $224 billion, which is an increase of 42% over the previous decade. Nearly 40% of all traffic fatalities in 1997 were related to alcohol use, with drivers between 21 and 24 years having the highest intoxication rate (CDC, 1999).

Certain types of injuries appear to affect some groups more frequently. American Indians and Alaska Natives have disproportionately high death rates from motor vehicle accidents, residential fires, and drowning. There are higher rates of death from unintentional injury among African Americans. In every age group, drowning rates are almost 2 to 4 times greater for males than females. Homicide is especially high among African American and Hispanic youths. Nurses must be involved in efforts to reduce death caused by motor vehicle accidents and by homicide.

Injuries are among the leading causes of death for women in the United States. Many injuries to women result from violent acts; others are caused by unintentional events such as falls, motor vehicle accidents, burns, drowning, and poisonings. Some injuries affect women more frequently than men, with hip fractures and domestic violence being the most common.

Intentional injury, or physical assault, is a leading cause of injury to women. Research indicates that as many as 30% of women treated in emergency departments have injuries or symptoms related to physical abuse. A poll in 1993 found that 14% of women reported that a husband or boyfriend had been violent with them (CDC, 1999).

COMMUNITY-BASED TEACHING

Recommendations for Preventing Injuries

- Always wear a seatbelt while in the car.
- Never drive after drinking alcohol.
- Always wear a safety helmet while riding a motorcycle or bicycle.
- Use smoke detectors in your home; check to make sure they work every month, and change the batteries every year.
- Keep the temperature of hot water less than 120°F, particularly if there are children or older adults living in your home.
- If you choose to keep a gun in your home, make sure that the gun and the ammunition are locked up separately and out of the reach of children.
- Prevent falls by older adults by repairing slippery or uneven walking surfaces, improving poor lighting, and installing secure railings on all stairways.
- Be alert for hazards in your workplace and follow all safety rules.

Personal health guide: Put prevention into practice. (1998, April). Publication No. APPIP 98-0027. Rockville, MD: Agency for Health Care Policy and Research. Available at: http://www.ahrq.gov/ppip/ppadult.htm.

Environmental Quality

An estimated 25% of preventable illnesses worldwide can be attributed to poor environmental quality. Poor air quality, including both ozone (outside air) and tobacco smoke (inside air), is one of the prime contributors. In the United States, air pollution alone is estimated to contribute to 50,000 premature deaths annually. Incidence of asthma has been on the rise for the past few decades among adults and children.

It is important that the proportion of individuals exposed to poor air quality is reduced as well as reducing the proportion of nonsmokers exposed to second-hand smoke. Teaching clients about the importance of maintaining smoke-free indoor air and the hazards of second-hand smoke is one intervention. Second, the nurse can teach clients the threat that poor outdoor air quality poses for health and the importance of supporting political candidates and legislation that protects air quality.

Immunizations

Immunizations are cited as one of the greatest achievements of public health in the 20th century. It is important to continue to increase the proportion of chil-

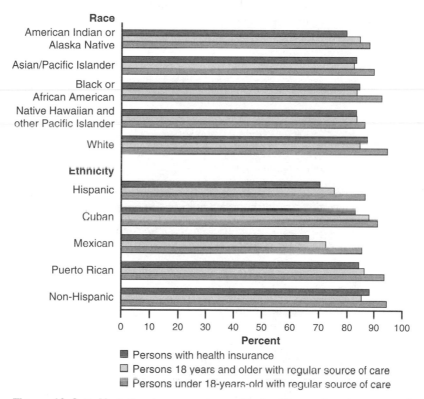

Figure 10–2. ▶ Variation in access to quality health services by race and ethnicity, United States, 1997. Source: U.S. Department of Health and Human Services. (2000). *Healthy people 2010. National health promotion disease prevention objectives.* Washington, DC: U.S. Government Printing Office.

dren who receive all vaccines as well as the proportion of adults who are vaccinated annually against the flu.

Access to Health Care

According to *Healthy People 2010,* access to quality care is important to eliminate health disparities and increase the quality and years of healthy life for all Americans. One way to improve access is to improve continuum of care. Until the 1980s, there was a gradual decline in the proportion of people without health insurance. Since the late 1980s, this proportion has remained the same, at 15%. The variation in access to health care by race and ethnicity is seen in Figure 10–2.

 ## CONCLUSIONS

Current critical issues of health and health care have changed dramatically in the past 100 years. Today, most diseases and deaths result from preventable causes. The nurse plays an essential role in early identification of and intervention in these conditions. Nurses can be successful in this charge by screening, particularly in high-risk groups. By identifying conditions early in their course, they can provide interventions that will substantially minimize the effects of these conditions. By following the health indicators identified by *Healthy People 2010,* nurses can help adults live longer and healthier lives.

What's on the Web

Personal Health Guide: Put Prevention into Practice

Internet address: http://www.ahrq.gov/ppip/ppadult.htm

This on-line consumer guide from the Agency for Healthcare Research and Quality explains preventive care for adults. Print copies, available free of charge, can be requested by calling (800) 358-9295. The guide is also available in Spanish.

RESOURCES FOR CANCER SCREENING
National Cancer Institute

Internet address: http://www.nci.nih.gov

National Cancer Institute Cervical Cancer Information

Internet address: http://cancernet.nci.nih.gov

National Cervical Cancer Coalition

Internet address: http://www.nccc-online.org

American Cancer Society

Internet address: http://www.cancer.org

Center for Cervical Health

Internet address: http://www.cervicalhealth.com

COOKBOOKS

Heart-Healthy Home Cooking African American Style

Internet address:
http://rover.nhlbi.nih.gov/health/public/heart/other/chdblack/cooking.htm

Delicious Heart-Healthy Latino Recipes (bilingual cookbook)

Internet address: http://rover.nhlbi.nih.gov/health/public/heart/other/sp_recip.htm

Print copies can be ordered for a small fee by phone at (301) 592-8573 or on the Web at http://www.nhlbi.nih.gov/health/infoctr/ic-ordr.htm.

Obesity Education Initiative

Internet address: http://www.nhlbi.nih.gov/about/oei/index.htm

An excellent Web site with abundant information for provider, patient, and public education related to obesity, produced by the National Heart, Lung, and Blood Institute.

RESOURCES FOR SMOKING CESSATION

Nursing Center for Tobacco Intervention

Internet address: http://www.con.ohio-state.edu/tobacco

Designed to increase nurse provider participation in the delivery of tobacco cessation interventions with all tobacco users, this site has excellent information as well as links to other sites with outstanding teaching materials for health education.

TIPS: Tobacco Information and Prevention Source

Internet address: http://www.cdc.gov/tobacco

National Center for Chronic Disease Prevention and Health Promotion
Chronic Disease Prevention: Risk Behaviors-Tobacco Use

Internet address: http://www.cdc.gov/nccdphp/tobacco.htm

Virtual Office of the Surgeon General

Reducing Tobacco Use Report

Internet address: http://www.surgeongeneral.gov/library/tobacco_use

American Lung Institute
Tobacco Control

Internet address: http://www.lungusa.org/tobacco

References and Bibliography

Agency for Healthcare Research and Quality. (1998). *Personal health guide: Put prevention into practice.* Rockville, MD. Available at: http://www.ahcpr.gov/ppip/ppadult.htm.

Banks-Wallace, J. (1998). Emancipator potential of storytelling in a group. *Image: Journal of Nursing Scholarship, 30*(1), 17–25.

Berg, A., Dencker, K., & Skarsatter, I. (1999). *Evidence-based nursing in the treatment of people with depression.* Swedish Council on Technology Assessment in Health Care (SBU), Swedish Nurses Association (SSF), Report No. 3, p. 62.

Centers for Disease Control and Prevention. (1999). *Violence and injury.* Office of Women's Health. Available on-line at: http:/www.cdc.gov.od/owh/whvio.htm.

Centers for Disease Control and Prevention. (2000). *The National Breast and Cervical Cancer Early Detection Program. Cancer prevention and control.* Available on-line at: http:/www.cdc.gov/cancer.

Choudhry, U. K. (1998). Health promotion among immigrant women from India living in Canada. *Image: Journal of Nursing Scholarship, 30*(3), 269–274.

Dille, J. (1999). Worksite influenza immunization: Successful program. *AAOHN Journal, 47*(7), 293–299.

Gibson, P. G., Coughlan, J. ,Wilson, A. J., Abrahmson, M., Bauman, A., Hensley, M. J., & Walters, E. H. (1999). Self-management education and regular practitioner review for adults with asthma. *Cochrane Database System Review, 2,* CD001117.

Gibson, P. G., Coughlan, J., Wilson, A. J., Hensley, M. J., Abrahmson, M., Bauman, A., & Walters, E. H. (1999). Limited (information only) patient education programs for adults with asthma. *Cochrane Database System Review, 2,* CD001005.

Hannigan, B. (1999). Mental health nursing in the community: A United Kingdom perspective. *Home Health Care Management, 11*(4). 60–66.

Lancaster, T., & Stead, L. F. (1999). Self-help interventions for smoking cessation. *Cochrane Database System Review, 2,* CD001118.

Morin, K. (1998). Promoting gynecologic health in young and middle-age women. *Holistic Nursing Practice, 12*(2) 17–27.

National Institutes of Health. (1998). *The practical guide: Identification, evaluation, and treatment of overweight and obesity in adults.* National Heart, Lung and Blood Institute Obesity Education Initiative. Bethesda, MD: U.S. Department of Health & Human Services.

Rice, V. H., & Stead, L. F. (1999). Nursing interventions for smoking cessation. *Cochrane Database System Review, 2,* CD001188.

Treating tobacco use and dependence. Fact sheet, June 2000. U.S. Public Health Service. http://www.surgeongeneral.gov/tobacco/smokfact.htm.

U.S. Department of Health and Human Services. (1993). *Nurses: Help your patients stop smoking.* National Institutes of Health, National Heart, Lung, and Blood Institute. Available on-line at: http://www.nhlbi.nih.gov/health/prof/lung/other/nurssmok.txt.

U.S. Department of Health and Human Services. (2000). *Healthy people 2010. National health promotion and disease prevention objectives.* Washington, DC: U.S. Government Printing Office.

Walder, C., & Nies, M. (1998). Health promoting lifestyles: Health women and women with breast cancer. *Nurse Educator, 23*(3), 6–7.

Wells, B., & Horm, J. (1998). Targeting the underserved for breast and cervical cancer screening: The utility of ecological analysis using the National Health Interview Survey. *American Journal of Public Health, 88*(10), 1484–1486.

Williams, R., Lethbridge, D., & Chamber, W. (1997). Development of a health promotion in inventory for poor rural women. *Family and Community Health, 20*(2), 13–24.

L E A R N I N G   A C T I V I T I E S

LEARNING ACTIVITY 10-1

▶ **Client Care Study:** Health Promotion and Disease Prevention for the Healthy Adult

You are working as a home care nurse caring for a Richard, a 45-year-old client who has advanced chronic obstructive pulmonary disease (COPD) and is on oxygen constantly. Richard, a former smoker, has had several upper respiratory infections this winter, with one resulting in hospitalization for a week. Richard lives with his 25-year-old daughter and her husband, who are both teachers and heavy smokers.

  Which health indicators contribute to Richard's health status?
  What could you as the nurse for this family do to promote Richard's health?
  What steps will you take to address this issue?

LEARNING ACTIVITY 10-2

▶ Health Promotion and Disease Prevention for Adults

During a weekend visit to your parents' home, you are visiting with a friend of your parents, who asks you about what you are studying in your nursing classes. You explain that you are studying about disease prevention and health promotion. The friend, who is 45-years-old, says, "I am not sick. What would someone my age need to do to prevent disease?"

  What would be your response to his question?

LEARNING ACTIVITY 10-3

▶ **Critical Thinking Exercise:** Self-Evaluation

  1. In your clinical journal, describe a situation you have encountered when screening and doing health promotion and disease prevention teaching and planning with an adult client.

    What did you learn from this experience?
    How will you practice differently based on this experience?

  2. In your clinical journal, describe a situation in which you have observed an adult client who was not receiving the health promotion or disease prevention care that he or she needed.

    How could or would you advocate for these issues when you begin to practice as an RN?
    What could you do now?

Health Promotion and Disease Prevention for Elderly Adults

R O B E R T A   H U N T

▶ LEARNING OBJECTIVES ◀

- Identify the major causes of death for the elderly.
- Discuss the major diseases and threats to health of elderly adults.
- Summarize the major health issues for older adults.
- Identify nursing roles for each level of prevention for major health issues for elderly adults.
- Compose a list of nursing interventions for the major health issues for older adults.
- Determine health needs of the elderly for which a nurse could be an advocate.

▶ KEY TERMS ◀

life expectancy at birth
life expectancy at 65 or 85
medication safety

personal definition of health
polypharmacy

Health Status of Elderly Adults

Health Screening in Elderly Adults

Interventions for Leading Health Indicators

Conclusions

HEALTH STATUS OF ELDERLY ADULTS

Life expectancy at birth, as well as life expectancy at age 65 and 85, has increased over time as death rates for many causes of death have declined. **Life expectancy at birth** is the number of years that a person born in that year can expect to live. **Life expectancy at 65 or 85** is the number of years that a person who is 65 or 85 years old can expect to live. The leading causes of death for elderly adults are listed in Table 11–1. The largest decrease in mortality has been in death rates for heart disease and stroke; death rates for pneumonia and influenza have increased in the past 2 decades (National Center for Health Statistics [NCHS], 1999).

The elderly population in the United States is growing in number. Life expectancies at ages 65 and 85 have increased over the past 50 years. People who live to age 65 can expect to live, on average, nearly 18 more years. Since 1900, the percentage of people over 65 years and older has tripled. This growth is expected to continue for some time, eventually accounting for over 20% of all Americans by 2030. In addition, the elderly population will continue to be more and more diverse (NCHS, 1999).

This growing segment of the population has health care needs that are different from those of other segments of the population. Of people older than 70 years, 80% have one or more chronic conditions (Fig. 11–1). Visual impairments affect 13% of people at age 70 and 31% at age 85, and hearing impairments affect 26% at age 70 and 50% at age 85 (NCHS, 1999).

Living arrangements of persons over 65 years of age reveal that as people age, they are more likely to live alone. Further, they are more likely to have difficulty performing one or more physical activities, activities of daily living (ADL), or instrumental activities of daily living (IADL). Figure 11–2 shows the percentage of people older than 70 who are unable to perform certain daily activities. All of these factors have implications for the ability of the elderly to perform self-care and live independently while managing a chronic illness, and the amount of nursing care this population may need as they age (NCHS, 1999). Research Box 11–1 examines self-perceptions of health in the elderly.

HEALTH SCREENING IN ELDERLY ADULTS

As with clients at other ages, health screening for the elderly is intended for primary, secondary, or tertiary prevention. Primary prevention (to prevent the initial occurrence of a disease) with an elderly client could be immunization screening and recommendations of an annual flu shot. A second example of primary prevention could be a safety assessment of the home to identify potential areas

TABLE 11–1 • Leading Causes of Death in Adults 65 Years and Older, United States, 1997

Cause of Death	Number
Heart disease	606,913
Cancer	382,913
Stroke	140,366

U.S. Department of Health and Human Services. (2000). *Healthy people 2010. National health promotion and disease prevention objectives.* Washington, DC: U.S. Government Printing Office.

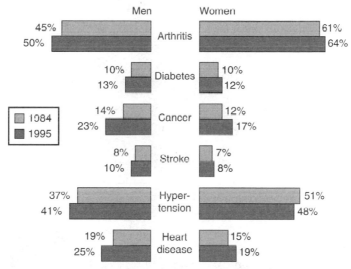

Figure 11–1. ▶ Percentage of people 70 years of age and older who reported having selected chronic conditions, by sex, United States, 1984 and 1995. These data refer to the civilian noninstitutionalized population. 1984 percentages are age-adjusted to the 1995 population. Source: Supplement on aging and Second supplement on aging. In National Center for Health Statistics. (2000). *Chartbook 2000. Federal interagency forum on aging-related statistics. Older Americans 2000: Key indicators of well-being.* http://www.agingstats.gov/chartbook2000/healthstatus.html.

where a fall could occur. Examples of secondary prevention would be hypertension screening or a nurse teaching breast self-examination to a group or an individual. Tertiary prevention could be initiating an exercise program for an elderly client who has heart disease. Screening is always performed so that people at risk for certain conditions can be identified, with interventions as appropriate.

One way to encourage the elderly client to put prevention into practice is to use the *Staying Healthy at 50+* guide developed by the Agency for Healthcare Research and Quality (AHRQ). This guide is available on line at http://www. ahcpr.gov/ppip/50plus/index.htm or can be ordered free by calling (800) 358-9295. It includes recommendations about lifestyle choices that prevent certain chronic diseases, primary prevention screening, and immunizations.

General Screening

All screening discussed for adults also applies to elderly adults. This section discusses screening that is of particular importance to elderly adults.

High blood pressure is more common for people older than 45, especially African Americans. Therefore, the elderly should have their blood pressure checked periodically. How often will be determined by their nurse practitioner or physician. Cholesterol levels start to increase in middle-aged men and women just before menopause, and in anyone who has just gained weight; cholesterol should be measured in people meeting these descriptions. Type 2 diabetes is more common in people older than 45, with one in five individuals over 65 developing diabetes. Screening for diabetes is recommended for people with a fam-

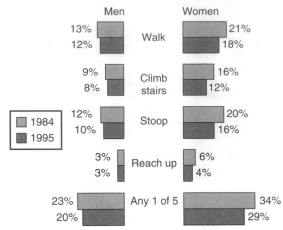

Figure 11–2. ▶ Percentage of people age 70 and older who are unable to perform certain physical functions, by sex, 1984 and 1995. The nine physical functioning activities are: walking a quarter mile; walking up 10 steps without resting; standing or being on your feet for about 2 hours; sitting for about 2 hours; stooping, crouching or kneeling; reaching up over your head; reaching out as if to shake someone's hand; using your fingers to grasp or handle; lifting or carrying something as heavy as 10 lbs. A person is considered disabled if he or she is unable to perform an activity alone and without aids. Rates for 1984 are age-adjusted to the 1995 population. These data refer to the civilian noninstitutionalized population. Based on interviews conducted between October 1994 and March 1996 with noninstitutionalized persons. Caregivers provide help or supervision with at least one ADL or IADL. Source: Supplement on aging and second supplement on aging. In National Center for Health Statistics. (2000). *Chartbook 2000. Federal interagency forum on -aging related statistics. Older Americans 2000: Key indicators of well-being.* Available at: http://www.agingstats.gov/chartbook2000/healthstatus.html.

ily member with diabetes, who are overweight, or who had diabetes during pregnancy. Elderly individuals should also be screened for osteoporosis risk, depression, alcohol abuse, and violence.

The adult immunization schedule applies to elderly adults as well. However, the current recommendation is that everyone older than 50 years receive an annual flu shot. Elderly people should be screened for tuberculosis (TB) if they have been in close contact with someone with TB; have recently moved from Asia, Africa, Central or South America, or the Pacific Islands; have kidney failure, diabetes, alcoholism, or are positive for human immunodeficiency virus (HIV); or have injected or now inject illegal drugs.

Cancer Screening

Most breast cancer occurs in women older than 50, so mammography is recommended yearly. Women should have a Pap test every 3 years except in the presence of genital warts, multiple sex partners, or abnormal Pap tests, in which cases testing should be done annually. Women older than 65 with a history of normal Pap smears or with a hysterectomy may stop having Pap tests after consulting with a nurse practitioner or physician.

Colon cancer is more common in the elderly than in younger adults. Starting at age 50, fecal occult blood testing should be done every year and sigmoidoscopy every 5 to 10 years.

RESEARCH IN COMMUNITY-BASED NURSING CARE

Research Box 11–1 ▶ Personal Definitions of Health Among Elderly People: A Link to Effective Health Promotion

Older persons tend to listen to advice about health that agrees with their **personal definition of health.** Because personal definitions of health are an important link to effective health promotion, this study explored how the elderly define health. The sample consisted of 67 individuals all over 65 years of age and able to participate in eight focus groups. These participants were urban dwellers with middle to low income levels, and mobile enough to travel to the study site. They were all African American or white and English-speaking individuals who needed help with at least one ADL in the past 12 months or had received at least one community-based service. Participants' focus group statements pertaining to health definitions were used as the data for this study. These statements were grouped into five general categories seen below.

Frequency of Categories of Health Definition Statements by Race and Gender

| Category | African American | | White | | |
	Female	Male	Female	Male	Total
Activity definitions	10	10	3	8	30
Attitude definitions	8	14	1	0	23
Basic functions definitions	0	4	2	4	10
Absence of medical attention definitions	4	1	1	1	7
Medical definition	1	2	0	2	7

Frequency of Activity Definitions of Health Statement by Race and Gender

| Category | African American | | White | | |
	Female	Male	Female	Male	Total
Getting up and out	5	7	2	3	17
Exercise	4	3	0	4	11
Volunteering	1	0	1	0	2
Independence	0	0	0	1	1

With one exception, the African American participants defined health in terms of attitudes. There was little evidence of significant overall gender differences in statements. This study shows that health is a relative term, and that the meaning changes for people as they age. There is a clear distinction between white and African American participants' perceptions of health. This research applies to nursing interventions in that health promotion programs are more effective if they relate to the targeted individual's personal definition of health.

Kaufman, J. (1996). Personal definitions of health among elderly people: A link to effective health promotion. *Gerontological Health Promotion, 19*(2), 58 69.

Prostate cancer is most common in men older than 50 years, African Americans, and men with a family history of prostate cancer. Screening includes rectal examination and prostate-specific antigen blood testing. However, research has not demonstrated that these tests save lives.

Additional Screening

Environmental screening with a home safety check is an essential component of health promotion and disease prevention for the elderly client. As discussed in Chapter 5, other screening for elderly clients involves hearing and vision, assessment of functional status, and cognition. With all clients it is important to screen for all leading health indicators. Refer to Box 10–1 for a list of the leading health indicators from *Healthy People 2010*. Interventions to address these are covered in the next section.

INTERVENTIONS FOR LEADING HEALTH INDICATORS

Once screening has been done, conditions that put the client at risk are addressed. Many factors have contributed to the decline in mortality from heart disease and stroke. Some of these include changes in health behaviors, decrease in smoking, improvements in nutrition, increases in the overall educational level of the older population, and innovations in medical technology (NCHS, 1999).

Because the average person is living longer, more attention is now focused on preserving quality of life than on extending length of life. Most elderly people have one or more chronic conditions, and as a result of increased longevity, they will be living longer with these conditions. Nurses will increasingly be involved in efforts to decrease the adverse social and economic consequences of a high rate of activity limitation and disability of older persons. Thus, health promotion and disease prevention interventions for this segment of the population are important (Fig. 11–3).

This shift in focus requires dispelling myths commonly held about the elderly, including seeing the elderly as sick and sedentary, sexless, senile, and spent down. Nurses can facilitate successful aging by considering the elderly client holistically and can maximize functioning by addressing physical and psychological well-being as well as competence in adaptation (Fig. 11–4).

Physical Activity

Older adults, both male and female, can obtain significant health benefits with a moderate amount of daily physical activity. Additional health benefits can be gained through greater amounts of physical activity. Care should always be taken to avoid injury (Centers for Disease Control and Prevention [CDC], 1999b).

Previously sedentary older adults who begin physical activity programs should start with short intervals of moderate physical activity, from 5 to 10 minutes, and gradually build up to the desired amount. Benefits of physical activity include cardiorespiratory endurance and muscle strengthening. Stronger muscles reduce the risk of falling and improve the ability to perform routine tasks of daily life (CDC, 1999b). Other benefits of physical activity include:

▶ Helps maintain the ability to live independently and reduces the risk of falling and fracturing bones
▶ Reduces the risk of dying from coronary heart disease and of developing high blood pressure, colon cancer, and diabetes
▶ Can help reduce blood pressure in some people with hypertension

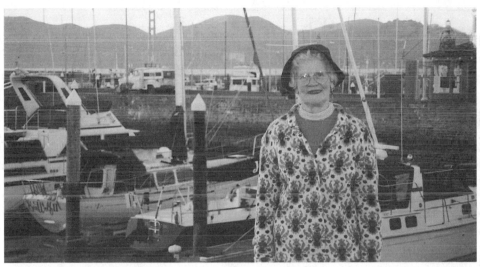

Figure 11-3. ► Using health promotion and disease prevention strategies can create a longer and healthier life.

► Helps people with chronic, disabling conditions improve their stamina and muscle strength
► Reduces symptoms of anxiety and depression and fosters improvements in mood and feelings of well-being
► Helps maintain healthy bones, muscles, and joints
► Helps control joint swelling and pain associated with arthritis (CDC, 1999b)

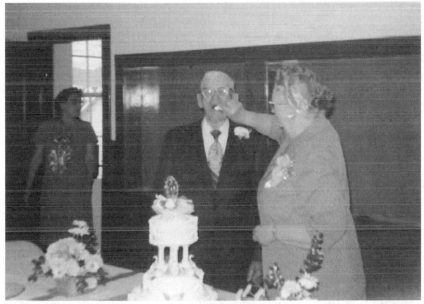

Figure 11-4. ► A satisfying marital relationship contributes to longevity.

▶ **Box 11–1.** What Communities Can Do to
Promote Physical Activity in Elderly Adults ◀

- Provide community-based physical activity programs that offer aerobic, strengthening and flexibility components specifically designed for older adults.
- Encourage mall and other indoor or protected locations to provide safe places for walking in any weather.
- Ensure that facilities for physical activity accommodate and encourage participation by older adults.
- Provide transportation for older adults to parks or facilities that provide physical activity programs.
- Encourage health care providers to talk routinely to their older adult clients about incorporating physical activity into their lives.
- Plan community activities that include opportunities or older adults to be physically active.

Centers for Disease Control and Prevention. (1999). National Center for Chronic Disease Prevention and Health Promotion. *Physical activity and health: A report of the Surgeon General.* Available at: http://www.cdc.gov/nccdphp/sgr/olderad.htm.

Ways that communities can promote physical activity for elderly adults are listed in Box 11–1.

Overweight and Obesity

Because no consensus exists regarding optimal weight for older persons, it is difficult to make recommendations regarding weight loss with the elderly. It is currently believed that lean body weight throughout life is optimal, but stability in weight after age 50 is recommended.

Tobacco Use

Smoking among adults has declined. However, because smoking remains the health indicator that is known to most negatively affect health, it is important to address the question of smoking with elderly clients and encourage them to quit. Box 11–2 can be used for health assessment and teaching older clients about the advantages of quitting at any age.

Substance Abuse

Not everyone who drinks regularly has a drinking problem. The questions in Box 10–5 can be used to help an elderly client recognize a drinking problem.

Older problem drinkers have a very good chance for recovery because once they decide to seek help, they usually stay with treatment programs. Resources include Alcoholics Anonymous (AA); local chapters can be found in the phone book. The National Institute on Alcohol Abuse and Alcoholism (NIAAA) at (301) 443-3860 is another resource.

Responsible Sexual Behavior

Understanding normal changes in sexual response is the first step to sexual health promotion. With aging, women may notice changes in the shape and

▶ Box 11–2. Check Your Smoking I.Q. ◀

If you or someone you know is an older smoker, you may think that there is no point in quitting now. Think again. By quitting smoking now, you will feel more in control and have fewer coughs and colds. On the other hand, with every cigarette you smoke, you increase your chances of having a heart attack, a stroke, or cancer. Need to think about this more? Take this older smokers' I.Q. quiz. Just answer "true" or "false" to each statement below.

True or False

1. ○ True ○ False If you have smoked for most of your life, it's not worth stopping now.
2. ○ True ○ False Older smokers who try to quit are more likely to stay off cigarettes.
3. ○ True ○ False Smokers get tired and short of breath more easily than nonsmokers the same age.
4. ○ True ○ False Smoking is a major risk factor for heart attack and stroke among adults 60 years of age and older.
5. ○ True ○ False Quitting smoking can help those who have already had a heart attack.
6. ○ True ○ False Most older smokers don't want to stop smoking.
7. ○ True ○ False An older smoker is more likely to smoke more cigarettes than a younger smoker.
8. ○ True ○ False Someone who has smoked for 30 to 40 years probably won't be able to quit smoking.
9. ○ True ○ False Very few older adults smoke cigarettes.
10. ○ True ○ False Lifelong smokers are more likely to die of diseases like emphysema and bronchitis than nonsmokers.

Answers

1. **False.** Nonsense! You have every reason to quit now and quit for good—even if you've been smoking for years. Stopping smoking will help you live longer and feel better. You will reduce your risk of heart attack, stroke, and cancer; improve blood flow and lung function; and help stop diseases like emphysema and bronchitis from getting worse.
2. **True.** Once they quit, older smokers are far more likely than younger smokers to stay away from cigarettes. Older smokers know more about both the short- and long-term health benefits of quitting.
3. **True.** Smokers, especially those over 50 years old, are much more likely to get tired, feel short of breath, and cough more often. These symptoms can signal the start of bronchitis or emphysema, both of which are suffered more often by older smokers. Stopping smoking will help reduce these symptoms.
4. **True.** Smoking is a major risk factor for four of the five leading causes of death including heart disease, stroke, cancer, and lung diseases like emphysema and bronchitis. For adults 60 and over, smoking is a major risk factor for six of the top 14 causes of death. Older male smokers are nearly twice as likely to die from stroke as older men who do not smoke. The odds are nearly as high for older female smokers. Cigarette smokers of any age have a 70 percent greater heart disease death rate than do nonsmokers.

(continued)

> ► **Box 11–2.** Check Your Smoking I.Q. (*Continued*) ◄

5. **True.** The good news is that stopping smoking does help people who have suffered a heart attack. In fact, their chances of having another attack are smaller. In some cases, ex-smokers can cut their risk of another heart attack by half or more.

6. **False.** Most smokers would prefer to quit. In fact, in a recent study, 65% of older smokers said that they would like to stop. What keeps them from quitting? They are afraid of being irritable, nervous, and tense. Others are concerned about cravings for cigarettes. Most don't want to gain weight. Many think it's too late to quit—that quitting after so many years of smoking will not help. But this is not true.

7. **True.** Older smokers usually smoke more cigarettes than younger people. Plus, older smokers are more likely to smoke high-nicotine brands.

8. **False.** You may be surprised to learn that older smokers are actually more likely to succeed at quitting smoking. This is more true if they're already experiencing long-term smoking-related symptoms like shortness of breath, coughing, or chest pain. Older smokers who stop want to avoid further health problems, take control of their life, get rid of the smell of cigarettes, and save money.

9. **False.** One of five adults aged 50 or older smokes cigarettes. This is more than 11 million smokers, a fourth of the country's 43 million smokers! About 25% of the general U.S. population still smokes.

10. **True.** Smoking greatly increases the risk of dying from diseases like emphysema and bronchitis. In fact, over 80% of all deaths from these two diseases are directly due to smoking. The risk of dying from lung cancer is also a lot higher for smokers than nonsmokers: 22 times higher for males, 12 times higher for females.

National Heart, Lung, and Blood Institute.
Available at: http://www.nhlbi.nih.gov/health/public/lung/other/smoking.html.

flexibility of the vagina and a decrease in vaginal lubrication. This can be addressed by using a vaginal lubricant. Men may find that it takes longer to get an erection or that the erection may not be as firm or large as in earlier years. As men get older, impotence increases, with some chronic conditions contributing to this change (eg, heart disease, hypertension, and diabetes). For many men, impotence can be managed and reversed.

Having safe sex is imperative for people at all ages. In some areas of the country, the incidence of HIV among the elderly is on the rise. It is always essential that the nurse discuss the importance of safe sex, particularly regarding having sex with a new partner or multiple partners.

Mental Health

Many issues related to mental health emerge as individuals age. The losses associated with aging, including loss of health, friends, and spouses, all contribute to the development of depression among the elderly. Depression rates among older Americans who experience a physical health problem are 12% for persons hospitalized for problems such as hip fracture or heart disease. Depression rates for older persons in nursing homes range from 15% to 25%. Prevalence of dementia, such as Alzheimer's disease and other severe losses of mental abilities, is estimated at 12% at age 65 and over 25% at age 85. The rate of completed suicide is highest among elderly men, who account for about 80% of suicides among persons age 65 and older. Elderly men have a suicide rate six times the national average (DHHS, 2000).

Common signs of depression are listed in Box 10–6. Once depression is identified, it can be treated successfully. Support groups, other talk therapy, antidepressant drugs, and electroconvulsive therapy are some forms of treatment that may be used for clients with depression.

Preparing for major changes in life, keeping and maintaining friendships, developing interests or hobbies, and keeping the mind and body active may help prevent depression. Being physically fit, eating a balanced diet, and following the nurse practitioner's or physician's recommendations regarding medication can also minimize depression. Other suggestions for the client facing depression include:

▶ Accept the fact that help is needed.
▶ Consult a health care provider who has special training in mental health issues of the elderly.
▶ Do not be afraid of getting help because of the cost.

If the depressed older person will not seek help, friends or relatives can help by explaining how treatment may help the person feel better. Sometimes the family can arrange for the health care provider to call the family member or make a home visit to start the process. Community mental health centers offer treatment and often have resources. Additional resources on depression can be found in Appendix 11–1.

Safety and Injury Prevention

Injuries are a leading cause of morbidity and mortality among the elderly. The primary causes of injury among this age group are motor vehicle accidents, falls, and mishaps related to polypharmacology.

Motor vehicle-related death rates for the elderly are the highest of any age group. Per miles driven, drivers older than 75 years have higher rates of vehicle-related death than all other age groups except teenagers. Measures that could benefit older people as well as other age groups are increased use of public transportation and restricted driving privileges when circumstances warrant. For example, in some states, the length of the license term for older drivers has been reduced to 2 years rather than 4. In some states, physicians are required to report to the state's licensing agency cases of certain medical conditions that could affect a person's ability to drive.

Falls are recognized as a leading cause of injury and death among the elderly. In the United States, one of every three people 65 years and older falls each year. Half of those older than 75 who fracture a hip as a result of a fall die within 1 year of the incident (Rawsky, 1998). By 2020, the cost of fall injuries is expected to reach $32 billion (CDC, 2000b). The elderly are at increased risk for injury from falls because of the high incidence of osteoporosis in this age group. Prevention of fractures is related to increasing bone density and preventing falls.

Polypharmacy, or the prescription of more than one medication, resulting in a complex medication regimen, is becoming more common. Elderly clients typically take more medications than other age groups. **Medication safety** is increasingly being recognized as an area with potential for injury. Taking medication the wrong way or with other medications that cause harmful interactions can make the client worse rather than better. *Prescription Medicines and You* is an

COMMUNITY-BASED TEACHING

Tips for Prevention of Fractures in the Elderly

Osteoporosis can be prevented by:
- Doing weight-bearing exercises, such as walking, stair climbing, jogging, yoga, and lifting weights
- Getting 1,000 to 1,300 mg of calcium per day
- Not smoking
- Taking hormone replacement therapy (HRT) if you are a woman

For adults 65-years-old or older, 60% of all falls happen at home, 30% in public places, and 10% in health care institutions.

The risk of falling can be reduced by:
- Maintaining a regular exercise program
- Taking steps to make living areas safer
    Remove tripping hazards
    Use nonskid mats in the bathtub
    Have handrails on both side of all stairs
- Reviewing all medication with the nurse practitioner or physician to reduce side effects and interactions
- Having a vision check every year

Adapted from Centers for Disease Control and Prevention. (2000). *Falls and hip fractures among older adults.* National Center for Injury Prevention and Control. Available on-line at: http://www.cdc.gov/ncipc/factsheets/falls.htm.

excellent guide designed to help avoid medication errors and get the most from the medication. See What's on the Web for information on how to obtain a copy.

Environmental Quality

Because the elderly are more vulnerable to alterations in environmental conditions, poor air quality has a greater impact on this age group. The proportion of elderly individuals exposed to poor air quality, both second-hand smoke and other air pollution, must be reduced. With the elderly population increasing, maintaining air quality is even more essential to maintaining and improving the health of the nation.

Immunizations

The most important intervention to improve health of the elderly related to immunizations is to increase the number of elderly people vaccinated against influenza every year. Nurses play an important role in organizing, staffing, and evaluating immunization clinics. As nurses, we have some work to do in this area, particularly with diverse populations.

Access to Health Care

Access to care is important to increase the quality and years of health life for all Americans. Elderly individuals may perceive that they do not have access because they have unfounded concerns about cost for services. They also may have limited mobility, as a result of either a chronic condition or lack of transportation. Perhaps the elderly person has limited ability to speak English or is distrustful of health care providers. These are all issues of access that may affect the client's health. The nurse must always assess the client's perception of access and intervene accordingly.

 CONCLUSIONS

Life expectancy at birth, as well as at 65 and 85 years of age, has increased over the past decades. The elderly are growing in number and have special health needs. Because elderly people are living longer with more chronic conditions, attention is now focused on preserving quality of life. Nurses can use the leading health indicators to illuminate individual behaviors and physical, social, and environmental factors that require intervention to prevent disease and promote health in the older segment of the population.

What's on the Web

Health, United States, 1999 With Health and Aging Chartbook

Internet address: http://www.cdc.gov/nchs/products/pubs/pubd/hus/2010/2010.htm

This 1999 resource from the CDC National Department of Health Statistics includes a special report on the aging population in the United States.

Older Americans 2000: Key Indicators of Well-Being

Internet address: http://www.agingstats.gov/chartbook2000/default.htm

This report of the Federal Interagency Forum on Aging-Related Statitics provides information on indicators that address the lives of the older population, including access to health care, home care, vaccinations, social activity, and dietary quality.

Prescription Medicines and You

Internet address: http://www.ahrq.gov/consumer/ncpiebro.htm

This consumer guide from the National Council on Patient Information and Education and the AHRQ can be used as a teaching tool to facilitate medication safety. Print copies, available in six languages, can be ordered for a small fee at http://www.talkaboutrx.org or by calling (800) 358-9295.

Put Prevention Into Practice: Staying Healthy at 50+

Internet address: http://www.ahrq.gov/ppip/50plus/index.html.

This on-line consumer guide from the AHRQ explains preventive care for older adults. Print copies, available free of charge, can be requested by calling (800) 358-9295. The guide is also available in Spanish.

AgePage: Depression, a Serious but Treatable Illness

Internet address: http://www.nih.gov/nia/health/agepages/depresti.htm

This document from the National Institute on Aging addresses depression as it relates to older people and provides a list of resources.

Alzheimer's Association

Internet address: http://www.alz.org

Provides consumer and professional information, including a section dedicated to family caregivers and friends of people with Alzheimer's disease. Contains links to local chapters and other support groups and resources. Includes information in Spanish.

National Council on the Aging

Internet address: http://www.ncoa.org

This site provides information geared toward elderly people on topics including finances, housing, long-term care, rural aging, employment, health care, Social Security, senior centers, and end-of-life care.

Resource Directory for Older People

Internet address: http://www.aoa.gov/aoa/resource.html

This site features a list of organizations compiled by the Administration on Aging and the National Institute on Aging.

POTENTIAL PARTNERS FOR HEALTH PROMOTION ACTIVITIES FOR THE ELDERLY

American Association of Retired Persons

Internet address: http://www.aarp.org

American Council on Science and Health

Internet address: http://www.acsh.org

American Federation of Home Health Agencies

Internet address: http://www.his.com/~afhha/usa.html

American Health Foundation

Internet address: http://www.ahf.org

American Society on Aging

Internet address: http://www.asaging.org

National Association for Home Care

Internet address: http://www.nahc.org

National Health Policy Forum

Internet address: http://www.nhpf.org

National Wellness Institute

Internet address: http://www.nationalwellness.org

People's Medical Society

Internet address: http://www.peoplesmed.org

References and Bibliography

Appling, S. (1997). Wellness promotion and the elderly. *Medical Surgical Nursing, 6*(1), 45–47.

Chatten, D. (1998). Walks on the wild side. *Nursing Times, 94*(14), 38–39.

Centers for Disease Control and Prevention. (1999a). *Motor vehicle-related deaths among older Americans fact sheet.* National Center for Injury Prevention and Control. Available on-line at http://www.cdc.gov/ncipc/factsheets/older.htm.

Centers for Disease Control and Prevention. (1999b). *Surgeon General's report on physical activity and health.* National Center for Chronic Disease Prevention and Health Promotion. Available on-line at: http://www.cdc.gov/nccdphp/sgr/olderad.htm.

Centers for Disease Control and Prevention. (2000a). *Falls and hip fractures among older adults.* National Center for Injury Prevention and Control. Available on-line at: http://www.cdc.gov/ncipc/factsheets/falls.htm.

Centers for Disease Control and Prevention. (2000b). *The costs of fall injuries among older adults.* National Center for Injury Prevention and Control. Available on-line at: http://www.cdc.gov/ncipc/factsheets/fallcost.htm.

Fowler, S. (1997). Health promotion in chronically ill older adults. *Journal of Neuroscience Nursing, 29*(1), 39–44.

Gillespie, L. D., Gillespie, W. J., Cumming, R., Lamb, S. E., & Rowe, B. H. (2000). Interventions for preventing falls in the elderly. *Cochrane Database System Review, 2,* CD000340.

Haber, D., Looney, C., Babola, K., Hinmand, M., & Utsey, C. (2000). Impact of a healthy promotion course on inactive, overweight or physically limited older adults. *Family and Community Health, 22*(4), 48.

Kaufman, J. (1996). Personal definitions of health among elderly people: A link to effective health promotion. *Family and Community Health, 19*(2), 58–69.

Kessenich, C. (1998). Tai chi as a method of fall prevention in the elderly. *Orthopaedic Nursing, 17*(4), 2–30.

Maddox, M. (1999). Older women and the meaning of health. *Journal of Geronotological Nursing, 25*(12), 26–33.

Mouton, C., & Espino, D. (1999). Health screening in older women. *American Family Physician, 59*(7), 1035–1041.

Murashima, S., Hatono, Y., Whyte, N., & Asahara, K. (1999). Public health nursing in Japan: New opportunities for health promotion. *Public Health Nursing, 16*(2), 133–139.

National Center for Health Statistics. (1999). *Health, United States, 1999 with health and aging chartbook.* Hyattsville, MD: Author.

Poss, J. (1999). Providing culturally competent care: Is there a role for health promoters? *Nursing Outlook, 47*(1), 30–36.

Prescription medicines and you. (1999). AHCPR Publication No. 96-0056. Agency for Health Care Policy and Research, National Council on Patient Information and Education, Rockville, MD and Washington, DC. Available on-line at: http://www.ahrq.gov/consumer/ncpiebo.htm.

Rawsky, E. (1998). Review of the literature on falls among the elderly. *Image: Journal of Nursing Scholarship, 30*(1), 47–51.

Sharkey, P., & Bey, J. (1998). Designing an incentive based health promotion program. *AAOHN Journal, 46*(3), 133–144.

Staying healthy at 50+. (2000). Agency for Healthcare Research and Quality, Rockville, MD. AHRQ Publication No. 00-0002. Available on-line at: http://www.ahrq.gov/ppip/50plus/index.html.

Turkoski, B. (1997). Negative behavior in elderly home care patients. *Home Healthcare Nurse, 15*(7), 474–484.

U.S. Department of Health and Human Services. (1995a). *AgePage: Aging and alcohol abuse.* National Institute on Aging. Available on-line at: http://www.nih.gov/nia/health/agepages/alcohol.htm.

U.S. Department of Health and Human Services. (1995b). *AgePage: Depression, a serious but treatable illness.* National Institute on Aging. Available on-line at: http://www.nih.gov/nia/health/agepages/depresti.htm.

U.S. Department of Health and Human Services. (2000). *Healthy people 2010. National health promotion disease prevention objectives.* Washington, DC: U.S. Government Printing Office.

Wallace, J., Buccaneer, D., Grottos, L., Alveoli, S., Tell, L., Lcrois, A., & Wagner, E. (1998). Implementation and effectiveness of a community-based health promotion program for older adults. *Journal of Gerontology, 53*(4), 301–307.

Williams, S., Drew, J., Wright, B., Seidman, R., McGann, M., & Boulan, T. (1998). Health promotion workshops for seniors: Predictors of attendance and behavioral outcomes. *Journal of Health Education, 29*(3), 166–175.

LEARNING ACTIVITIES

LEARNING ACTIVITY 11-1

▶ **Client Care Study:** Health Promotion and Disease Prevention for the Elderly Adult

You are working in a community clinic that serves many senior citizens from the surrounding area. Last year, you noted that in November through March the clinic visits were for colds, influenza, sore throats, bronchitis, and pneumonia, in order of frequency. As you are reviewing the clinic records, you learn that 80% of the clinic visits resulting in hospitalization resulted from bronchitis, pneumonia, and influenza.

What clinic activities related to health promotion and disease prevention would you plan for the late fall?

LEARNING ACTIVITY 11-2

▶ **Critical Thinking Exercise:** Self-Evaluation

1. In your clinical journal, describe a situation you have encountered when screening and doing health promotion and disease prevention teaching and planning with an elderly adult.

   What did you learn from this experience?
   How will you practice differently based on this experience?

2. In your clinical journal, describe a situation in which you have observed an elderly client who was not receiving the health promotion or disease prevention care that was needed.

   How could you advocate for these issues when you begin to practice as an RN?
   What could you do now?

Resources for Depression and the Elderly

The National Institute of Mental Health's (NIMH) special DEPRESSION Awareness, Recognition, and Treatment Program offers several publications, including "If You're Over 65 and Feeling Depressed: Treatment Brings New Hope." Contact the Information Resources and Inquiries Branch, NIMH, Room 7C-02, MSC 8030, Bethesda, MD 20892-8030; (800) 421-4211. Visit the website at http://www.nimh.nih.gov.

The National Depressive and Manic Depressive Association (National DMDA) has over 200 chapters in the United States and Canada offering support to people with depression and their families. They sponsor education and research programs and distribute brochures, videotapes, and audio programs. Write to the National DMDA, 730 N. Franklin Street, Suite 501, Chicago, IL 60610-3526; call (800) 826-3632. Visit their Web site at http://www.ndmda.org.

The National Alliance for the Mentally Ill (NAMI) has a Medical Information Series that provides patients and families with information on several mental illnesses and their treatments, including the publication "Understanding Major Depression: What You Need to Know About This Medical Illness." NAMI state affiliates provide emotional support and can help find local services. Write or call NAMI at 200 North Glebe Road, Suite 1015, Arlington, VA 22203-3754; (800) 950-NAMI (6264). The Web site is http://www.nami.org.

The National Mental Health Association (NMHA) publishes information on a variety of mental health issues and has special information on depression and its treatment. NMHA also provides referrals and support. Write or call the NMHA Information Center, 1021 Prince Street, Alexandria, VA 22314-2971; (800) 969-6642. Visit the Web site at http://www.nmha.org.

The American Association for Geriatric Psychiatry (AAGP) is a national professional organization of specialists in geriatric psychiatry. It provides teaching materials and brochures about selected mental health disorders, including depression. Write to Publications, AAGP, 7910 Woodmont Avenue, Suite 1350, Bethesda, MD 20814-3004. Visit the Web site at http://www.aagpgpa.org.

The American Psychological Association (APA), the professional and scientific organization for the practice of psychology, has several brochures and fact sheets for consumers and health professionals, including a pamphlet "What You Should Know About Women and Depression." Write or call APA Public Affairs, 750 First Street, NE, Washington, DC 20002-4242; (800) 374-3120. The Web site is http://www.apa.org.

The National Institute on Aging (NIA) distributes Age Pages and other materials on a wide range of topics related to health and aging. For a list of free publications, write to the NIA Information Center, P. O. Box 8057, Gaithersburg, MD 20898-8057; or call (800) 222-2225, or (800) 222-4225 (TTY). Visit the Web site at http://www.nih.gov/nia.

The Alzheimer's Disease Education and Referral (ADEAR) Center is a clearinghouse supported by the NIA with information on Alzheimer's disease and related disorders. For information about depression for Alzheimer's patients and caregivers, contact the ADEAR Center at P. O. Box 8250, Silver Spring, MD 20907-8250; (800)438-4380. Visit the ADEAR Center's Web site at http://www.alzheimers.org.

U.S. Department of Health and Human Services. (1995). *AgePage: Depression: A Serious but Treatable Illness. National Institute on Aging.* Available on-line at: http://www.nih.gov/nia/health/agepages/depresti.htm.

Settings for Practice

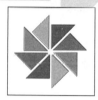 The settings and roles of the nurse have changed over time. In the late 1800s, a nurse was a woman in a black dress and a long black cape with a black satchel, visiting homes to care for the sick. A health care shifted toward care of the ill in the hospital, the nurse was a woman with a severely starched white uniform, white stockings, and a starched white cap, bending over the bed of a sick person.

Today, male and female nurses work in a wide variety of settings, taking on many roles. These settings are discussed in Chapter 12. The nurse working in the community is no longer recognizable by sex, uniform, or setting, for nurses are now involved in all levels of health care delivery. Nurses practice in corporations, neighborhood schools, day surgery centers, churches, long-term care facilities, and a variety of ambulatory clinics. Their clients may be well children or they may be older people, abused women, homeless families, prisoners, or drug addicts.

Increasingly, the home is becoming the focus for many nurses practicing in the current health care system. Agencies providing home care, the significance of home care, and the transfer of acute care nursing to home care nursing skills are discussed in Chapter 13. Barriers to successful home care and skills and competencies are included. The first visit is described, along with safety issues and lay caretaker involvement. The chapter ends with a discussion of hospice care in the home.

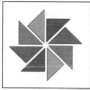

Practice Settings and Specialties

ROBERTA HUNT

►LEARNING OBJECTIVES◄

- Describe health care opportunities involving care for older adults.
- Identify issues involved in decisions related to residential care of an older adult.
- Create a list of health care settings in your community in which you could work as a nurse.
- Compare and contrast the roles of the nurse in a school setting and an industrial setting.

►KEY TERMS◄

adult foster care homes
advanced practice nurse
ambulatory care centers
assisted living facilities
boarding care homes
case manager
clinical nurse specialist
day surgery centers
detoxification facilities
employee assistance programs
employee wellness programs
extended care facilities
gerontology nursing
home health care
homeless shelter
hospice care
nurse midwife

nurse practitioner
nursing centers
occupational health nurse
outpatient services
parish nurse
practice settings
rehabilitation centers
residential centers
retirement communities
school nurse
skilled nursing facilities
sliding fee scale
specialized care centers
subacute rehabilitation centers
transitional housing
wellness promotion
work site health promotion

Gerontology Nursing

Practice Settings and Practice Opportunities

Nursing Specialties

Conclusions

The settings for health care delivery have undergone rapid and dramatic changes in the past decade. This is due, in part, to escalating health care costs. It is also attributable to the self-care movement. Reduced infant mortality, control of communicable diseases, and the aging of "baby boomers" have increased the number of people living to older age. Life span has also increased for those with specific chronic diseases such as cystic fibrosis, sickle cell anemia, diabetes, and acquired immunodeficiency syndrome (AIDS) and for those who have been paralyzed by stroke or trauma.

These recent changes have made it possible for nurses to choose fields or specialization from an infinite number of choices. Unlike the past, fewer than 60% of nurses currently work in hospital inpatient and outpatient departments, with more than 17% working in community or public health settings. Employment of registered nurses is expected to grow faster than the average for all occupations through 2008, with many new jobs being created. Although there will always be a need for traditional hospital nurses, a large number of new nurses will be employed in home health, long-term, and ambulatory care. Technologic advances in client care, which allow a greater number of health problems to be treated, will drive this growth. Further, as discussed in Chapter 11, the number of older people, who typically have more health care needs than other segments of the population, is increasing (Bureau of Labor Statistics, 2000).

This chapter discusses the different settings for practice a nurse may encounter. Schools of nursing are widening the experiences for clinical training of their students. However, no one school can cover all these settings within its curriculum. People entering nursing today must seek out ways of venturing into new and different settings by reading about, observing, and volunteering in some of the settings.

 GERONTOLOGY NURSING

Older adults, particularly those older than 65 years, are the most rapidly growing segment of our population. According to the National Center for Health Statistics (1999), by the year 2030, 20% of the population will be older than 65. This sector of the population has unique needs and problems that must be met. Because it is a growing field in which nurses are employed, gerontologic specialization is a focus of this chapter.

Research on aging during the past 30 years has provided new information that has contributed greatly to a better understanding of the physical and psychological changes that accompany aging. Nursing has played a major role in assisting the aging. **Gerontology nursing** has become a growing specialty in the past decade. All nurses who work with older people must have an understanding of the theoretical concepts of aging and the physical, emotional, and psychosocial changes occurring in later years.

Goals for the Aging Population

Healthy People 2010 (U.S. Department of Health and Human Services [DHHS], 2000) outlines a national strategy for improving the health of United States citizens during the 2000–2010 decade. This strategy focuses on the prevention of major chronic illnesses, injuries, and infectious diseases. The primary goals of *Healthy People 2010*, to increase quality and years of healthy life and eliminate health disparities, benefit the elderly population.

  Healthy People 2010 seeks to help the elderly population achieve a longer and healthier life by assisting individuals to gain the knowledge, motivation, and opportunities to make informed decisions about their health. Secondarily, *Healthy People 2010* encourages state and local leaders to develop community- and state-wide efforts that promote healthy behaviors, healthy environments, and increased access to high-quality health care. High-quality health care includes services recognized as essential, an increase in home food services, participation in the organization of health promotion programs, oral health, and various health examinations, such as breast screening, Pap smears, and hearing and vision screening. Thousands of organizations focus on care and services for the older person. Those with a health promotion and disease prevention focal point were discussed in Chapter 11. As one individual relates, these services assist in the development of independence.

> Several years ago I fractured my hip and had to have it nailed back together. Because of my age (77) the doctor and the physical therapist wanted to put me in a nursing home. When I insisted on a referral to a rehabilitation center, the social service department helped me find the best one in the area. Today, I can walk again, not as well as I used to, but I am walking and living at home. If I hadn't insisted on the rehab center I'd be immobile in a nursing home today.

Care in the Home

Home health care, the most common means of providing nursing care in the home through home visits, will be covered in Chapter 13. However, other programs exist to extend the period of time that seniors are able to remain in their homes. Most seniors prefer to stay in their own homes and communities rather than enter long-term care or assisted living facilities. One program, the Living at Home/Block Nurse Program, developed in Minnesota almost 20 years ago, is a community-based service that depends on professional and volunteer services of neighborhood residents to provide information, social and support services, skilled nursing care, and other assistance to the elderly to promote self-sufficiency. This concept depends on the grassroots community interest and active commitment of service groups, churches, businesses, schools, colleges, and universities. Evaluation of this program demonstrates that $3 is saved for every $1 spent keeping the elderly at home and out of long-term care facilities, which are primarily funded by Medicare. This model has been duplicated throughout the United States with great success. The program provides skilled nursing, case management, and supervision of home health aides and homemakers, often with nursing students as the care providers. The Web page for further information is http://www.elderberry.org.

Care Outside the Home

Adult Day Care Centers

The adult day care center offers social, recreational, and therapeutic activities to seniors who are in need of supervision during the day. Nurses are frequently part of the professional staff and are responsible for health assessments and designing and managing therapeutic regimens and medications. Often, physical care (eg, bathing) takes place at the day care center. These vital organizations offer more personal attention and have a quieter atmosphere than most senior centers. In addition, they provide care for the dependent individual who cannot manage alone but is not in need of nursing home placement. Adult day care is not reimbursable through Medicare.

Adult Foster Care Homes

Adult foster care homes (AFCs), also known as board and care homes or family care homes, are safe, small (usually fewer than six clients per home) residential sites that provide housing and protective oversight. Many AFCs provide care to frail elderly adults and those with dementia. Nationwide, these facilities maybe referred to by many names, including residential, adult, foster, family, boarding, or assisted living. There is a lack of federal guidelines to standardize this type of care.

Residential Opportunities

Some older adults, particularly those with chronic conditions, maybe very isolated living at home. Living arrangements for these individuals in a **residential center** may be a better option. Successful placement, however, requires research, client and family involvement, planning, and a focus on the client's maintaining control of his or her own life. There are multiple levels of residential living from which to choose, including:

Retirement communities: Designed for the functionally and socially independent, these provide a community living style for individuals who choose to live with other seniors. Accommodations include homes or apartments with supportive services provided by the retirement community.

Assisted living facilities: Geared toward the individual who has need for some assistance in daily activities (medications, meals, dressing, bathing) but who is able to function fairly independently, these facilities generally house residents in bedrooms located in a homelike environment.

Extended care facilities and **skilled nursing facilities:** More institutional in their design, with ongoing medical and nursing services and supervision, extended care facilities (known in some areas as nursing homes) provide care for individuals who need ongoing daily care, generally for the rest of their lives. Skilled nursing facilities provide nursing, medical, and therapy services for elderly people requiring ongoing medical or rehabilitative services but not hospitalization. Most individuals stay for a few weeks in a skilled facility and are then discharged home or transferred into an extended care facility because they can no longer manage at home after an acute illness or injury.

Subacute rehabilitative centers: Focused on the rehabilitation of individuals who have suffered an illness or accident, rehabilitative centers provide longer-term rehabilitative services such as nursing and medical care and physical, occupational, and speech therapy. Residence in this category is for a limited time. Individuals are discharged when they have reached their rehabilitative goals or when they are no longer making progress.

Boarding care homes: Providing personal custodial care for residents who are not able to live independently, boarding homes do not have nursing or medical supervision or care. Residents generally stay indefinitely.

Extended care facility residents were queried in a study about factors that influence the quality of care they receive. They responded that the most important aspect was their ability to retain control of their lives. To provide effective care, the nurse must be familiar with the resident's health problems and needs. Aging is a normal, irreversible process. Many of the problems of aging can be prevented by considering that the older adult's physical, emotional, social, and spiritual needs are complex and interrelated. These factors are important to any older adult living in any kind of residential setting.

Senior Citizen Health Clinics
Clinics designed to provide health care for seniors are found in senior high rises, neighborhood senior centers, and other locations where high concentrations of seniors live. These clinics provide blood pressure screening, medication review, hospital discharge follow-up, basic nursing screening and assessment, and disease prevention and health promotion interventions. Some clinics offer home visits.

In this setting, the clinic nurse may identify older adults who are in need of companionship or friendship. In some community-based senior citizen clinics, volunteers provide friendship on a one-to-one basis. These types of programs

---

COMMUNITY-BASED NURSING CARE GUIDELINES

Nursing Home Residents: Important Factors for Quality of Care

- Positive staff attitudes and relationships with residents
- Adequate wages and other rewards for staff
- Wide variety of activities
- Fresh, tasty food that is varied to reflect ethnic differences and individual needs
- Explicit, workable channels for problem resolution (accompanied by love and understanding)
- Safe environment
- Maximum possible independence for residents
- Strong, enforced regulations
- Resident participation in policy making and quality control both in their own facilities and at state and federal levels
- Active, concerned, informed administrator
- Community involvement

A consumer perspective on quality care: The residents' point of view, published by the National Citizens' Coalition for Nursing Home Reform. In P. B. Doress, D. L. Siegal, & the Midlife and Older Women Book Project. (1987). *Ourselves, growing older.* New York: Simon and Schuster.

demonstrate success by providing older adults with the opportunity to have support and friendship, which has been shown to reduce depression and the number of clinic visits.

Decisions Regarding Residential Care

When faced with the possibility of residential living, families are generally ill prepared to make decisions. Extended care facility placement is the only alternative some know. However, many alternatives exist for older adults who need new or temporary living arrangements. A skilled nursing facility may provide temporary care during recovery from a broken hip. A residential community may have an assisted living section where residents may recover from surgery and then return to their own apartments. These are only two of a variety of cost-effective alternatives.

When a client is considering leaving his or her home to live in another environment, certain questions can be asked to assist in determining what level and type of residential facility are most appropriate. Community-based nurses focus on continuity of care for their clients by collaborating with the client, family, and other health care providers to plan care at various levels.

What services are available in the community/facility? The ideal situation is to keep the older person in his or her own home or in a nearby facility that will allow friends and relatives to visit, in surroundings similar to the present living situation. Moving out of state will not be helpful for a person who enjoys close relationships with family and friends near his or her present location. Someone who lives in the country will probably not enjoy a residence in the city.

The nurse first looks at available services that could help the older person remain in his or her present living situation. Home health care, homemaker assistance, personal care, Meals On Wheels or an on-site dining room, emergency alert systems in the rooms, shopping and chore services, assisted living environments, and respite care are some of the services that may be available to assist the client. If the person already lives in a retirement community, can services be provided within the community?

What is the client's housing situation now? When adults reach a certain age, they may choose to simplify their lives by moving. They may be lonely, unwilling or unable to maintain a house, or simply feel more comfortable having people available to help them if needed. They may feel unsafe in their neighborhood because of crime. There are many options in settings, including subsidized housing, a retirement community, assisted living communities, high-rise apartments, and senior communities.

COMMUNITY-BASED NURSING CARE GUIDELINES

Questions to Ask When Considering Residential Care

- What services are available in the community/facility?
- What is the client's housing situation now?
- What are the client's nutritional needs? How is exercise obtained?
- Is there need for social interaction and companionship?
- What are the client's safety needs?
- What can the client afford?
- What financial assistance can the family provide?

What are the client's nutritional needs? How is exercise obtained? As people grow older, their nutritional needs change. Many require special diets; reduction in salt, fat, and carbohydrates; or an increase in protein, fiber, and bulk. Problems with vision, dentures, or feelings of isolation may cause an individual to eat little or not at all. Will residential care provide better nutrition for the client? Or will a program such as Meals On Wheels suffice?

Exercise is important at any age. Physical activity improves the quality of life. Daily walks, swimming, water aerobics, gardening, and biking increase physical well-being and provide social and emotional gratification. Some of these activities may be performed in and around the home. However, to be able to exercise, some older adults may need safety, companions, and facilities provided only by residential care.

Is there need for social interaction and companionship? Are people able to cope with loss? Loss of loved ones, friends, family, spouse, or siblings becomes a common theme as people age. Along with this loss also comes the loss of material possessions, such as a house, because it is no longer affordable or is physically impossible to maintain. The older adult is at risk for depression and suicide. *Healthy People 2010* (DHHS, 2000) cited that depression rates for older persons in nursing homes range from 15% to 25%. Depression and suicide resulting from bereavement can be prevented through appropriate nursing intervention. Living in a residential community may alleviate depression and create an opportunity for new social interactions. Companionship and relationships add meaning to life. Residential living may provide both.

What are the client's safety needs? As they age, people become more vulnerable to falls and injury. Reduced sensory perception, circulatory changes resulting in unsteadiness or dizziness, slower reaction time, and confusion often occur, all of which put the older adult at high risk for accidents. Can the client safely remain at home? Can the house be made safe so that the client may remain in the home?

When evaluating a residential living setting, the safety of the client must be considered and is often the determining factor in deciding what level will be chosen. If the client is unsafe, falls often, or is confused and forgetful, he or she cannot live safely alone.

What can the client afford? People are living many years past retirement. The fear of not having adequate financial resources can result in skimping on meals, not buying necessary medication, or not undergoing routine health examinations. When residential placement is considered, financial resources must be reviewed thoroughly.

The client's ability to pay will affect health care choices. Medicare will pay a skilled nursing facility for rehabilitative care but will not pay for a stay in an extended care facility. Medicaid will pay for extended care if the client qualifies. If money is an issue, financial assistance programs and services may be available in the community. Points that have to be considered include the level of residential care, whether the facility is nonprofit or publicly subsidized, and if a **sliding fee scale** is used.

What financial assistance can the family provide? It is important to consider early on the amount of financial assistance the family can or will provide. Depleting the family's resources to place the client in a residential setting may be counterproductive. It is important to determine how involved family members are, what their financial resources are, and what is realistic for everyone involved. Respite care provided by a community organization may be a viable alternative for some.

With the family and client, the nurse reviews the issues related to these questions. Sometimes the nurse and a social worker may collaborate and solve problems with the client. The client's physician may be contacted concerning the client's condition and what type of residence may be necessary.

PRACTICE SETTINGS AND PRACTICE OPPORTUNITIES

With the increased emphasis on self-care, disease prevention, and health promotion, health care delivery is needed in settings other than traditional hospitals. Further, health care has had to extend to where the population is (eg, to people who live in remote rural areas of the country).

As the need for local health care facilities that provide comprehensive services increases, the way the services are made available to consumers is changing. The growing number of nontraditional health care facilities reflects this trend. A glance at our social systems reveals that almost every established institution provides some type of health care. Industrial plants, businesses, schools, prisons, churches, and civic groups provide varying degrees of care, usually with a focus on prevention. Although state laws govern the tasks nurses may perform, it is usually the work setting or the agency that determines day-to-day activities.

The number and type of **practice settings** for community-based nursing exceeds our capacity to count or examine in this book. However, an overview of a number of settings will be given. Further, it is difficult to place health care settings in precise categories; many of them overlap. For instance, a clinic may be located in a hospital, or some long-term care facilities may be specialized facilities. The categories in this section are arbitrary and were chosen for ease in identifying some of the settings and types of care that community-based nurses may provide.

Acute Care: Hospitals

Hospitals remain the major site where nurses practice. Technically, acute care nursing is community-based nursing because acute care nurses do take care of individuals and families in a specific community. They also perform much of the initial teaching of clients and caregivers for procedures to be done in the home. Most hospital nurses are staff nurses who provide bedside care and carry out the medical regimen prescribed by physicians. They may also supervise licensed practical nurses and aides. Hospital nurses usually are assigned to one specialty area.

Nursing Centers

Among the newer forms of community-based nursing are **nursing centers.** They may be located at various sites within a community. Managed by nurses, they deliver primary health care to specific populations. Physician backup is available, and consultation is used as needed. The National League for Nursing gives the following definition of a community nursing center (Murphy, 1995, p. 3):

▶ A nurse occupies the chief management position.
▶ Accountability and responsibility for client care and professional practice remain with the nursing staff.
▶ Nurses are the primary providers seen by clients visiting the center.

COMMUNITY-BASED NURSING CARE GUIDELINES

Sampling of Variety of Nursing
Functions in Health Care Settings

Hospital: Acute Care
Serves as administrator or manager
Assesses and monitors client's
  health status
Provides direct care
Coordinates care of others
Teaches client and family
Provides support for family members
Makes referrals

Home Care
Assesses client, family, and culture
Assesses home and community
  environment
Develops relationship based on
  mutual trust
Contacts physician regarding
  client's condition
Plans, implements, and evaluates
  plan of care
Provides direct care
Coordinates care given by others
Teaches client and family
Provides support for family members
Makes referrals

Clinic (Ambulatory) Care
Makes health assessments
Assists primary care provider (may
  be primary care provider)
Provides direct care
Coordinates care given by others
Teaches client and family
Plans, implements, and evaluates
  the plan of care
Provides health promotion and
  disease prevention
Serves as a client advocate

Long-Term Care
Serves as administrator
Coordinates care given by others
Provides direct care
Teaches client and families
Plans, implements, and evaluates
  the plan of care
Makes referrals

Nursing Home
Serves as administrator
Coordinates care of others
Assesses client's condition
Develops treatment plans
Provides direct care
Maintains contact with the client's
  physician

Residential Centers
Provides direct care
Provides health assessments
Provides health promotion and
  prevention
Provides counseling and support
Makes referrals
Collaborates with other health team
  members
Coordinates services

Schools and Industry
Conducts health screening
Completes health assessments
Provides first aid or initial
  emergency care
Provides health education
Provides health promotion and
  disease prevention
Provides counseling and support
Makes referrals

A nursing center is not only a setting for care, it is also a concept. A nursing center shapes broader services offered to the community. "It must allow for an actual site for care but also support nurse-managed services to clients in their home, community, hospital, nursing home, or a site across the healthcare continuum" (Murphy, 1995, p. 3). Nursing centers bring nursing care directly to communities to help maximize the health of diverse populations. One of the two broad goals for *Healthy People 2010* is to eliminate health disparities. As a setting for community-based nursing, nursing centers are the perfect design to meet this charge.

Most academic nursing centers focus on community health, outreach, and **wellness promotion,** and many operate out of schools of nursing with faculty and students providing the services. They often provide services to the underserved, uninsured, or disadvantaged populations including women and children, the homeless, and minorities (LaMone, McDaniel, & Sullivan, 1998). However, there are nursing centers that serve insured populations as well. Many nursing centers exist in the midwestern United States.

Research on nursing centers is limited, but studies document changes in client and family knowledge, attitudes, behavior, and health status; client satisfaction; cost effectiveness; and quality of care (Frenn, Lundeen, Martin, Riesch, & Wilson, 1996). Several factors impede research on nursing centers, primarily lack of resources, time, staff, and money. Other factors affecting integration of research into nursing centers include community mistrust, the need for participatory recruitment strategies, and the need for multiple data collection methods (Zachariah & Lundeen, 1997).

Parish Nursing

Parish nursing is "a health promotion and disease prevention role based on the care of the whole person which encompasses seven functions" (Solari-Twadell & McDermott, 1999, p. 3). These functions are integrator of faith and health, health educator, health counselor, referral agent, trainer of volunteers, developer of support groups, and health advocate. Parish nursing has been in existence in the Midwest for some time. Before that, nurses sent by religious organizations practiced in many rural mountainous areas of the Southeast.

Parish nurses may offer screening, health education, resource and referral services, support groups, and holistic care to parishioners. Often, parish nurses reach out to vulnerable populations: older adults, single parents and their children, and grieving individuals. Many churches have nurses on their staff, whereas others use volunteers.

Clinics and Ambulatory Care Centers

Clients who do not require inpatient care (in an acute setting) can receive treatment, care, and education on an outpatient basis. **Outpatient services,** also called **ambulatory care centers,** are rapidly expanding and are now provided by hospitals, health maintenance organizations (HMOs), private and public hospitals, physicians' offices, community agencies, and public health departments (city, state, and federal). Services cover a broad range and include medical care, surgery, diagnostic tests, administration of medications (including intravenous therapy), physical therapy, kidney dialysis, counseling, birthing classes, aerobics classes, well-child care, and health education. Ambulatory care centers are located around the community for ease of access. They may be found in hospitals, low-income neighborhoods, and shopping malls. They may be provided contingent to a physician's practice and a managed care facility. Some settings, such as urgent care centers, offer walk-in, emergency care during extended hours when physicians' offices may be closed.

Some ambulatory clinics offer services to select groups. For instance, community-based nurses practice in migrant camps (Fig. 12–1), Native American reservations, correctional facilities, and remote rural settings such as coal min-

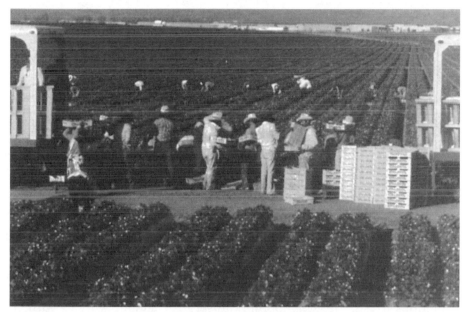

Figure 12–1. ▶ Experienced health care workers need to find ways to reach un-
deserved people, such as these migrant workers. Migrant workers are defined by their
common occupation and lifestyle, but they may cross various ethnic or racial lines

ing towns. Nurses can be an impetus for improved health and quality of life for
such client populations.

In some clinics, nurses have the primary role in conducting assessment and
caring for clients who need health maintenance or health promotion. In some locations, nurse practitioners have established their own independent ambulatory services.

Clinic nurses take on a variety of roles, depending on the medical specialty
of the physician in charge and the type of clients served. For example, a nurse
working in an HMO wound care clinic may care only for clients with private insurance. Community clinics may have a more heterogeneous population, with
some clients with and some without insurance. The clients' ability for self-care
may vary between the two clinics depending on the individual client, family and
social support, and other resources. Further, continuity of care may vary depending on what the insurance coverage will pay for as well as the family and
community support that is available for the client.

Physicians' Offices
Physicians in private and group practices, in primary care or specialties, employ
nurses. These nurses prepare clients, perform some assessments and routine
laboratory work, assist with examinations, administer injections and medications, change wound dressings, assist with minor surgery, and maintain records.

Day Surgery Centers
Advanced technologies have influenced changes in the care of the client and in
the environment where care is provided. Minimally invasive procedures (eg, lap-
aroscopy, use of flexible endoscopes and lasers, and microwave therapies) now

allow surgical procedures to be done in an ambulatory setting. Nurses working in **day surgery centers** have a range of duties: case management and direct patient care, admission and assessment, preoperative and postoperative monitoring, and discharge planning and teaching.

Community Clinics

Some communities offer special challenges to health care professionals:

▶ Transient populations with frequent moves from one geographic area to another
▶ Family violence and child abuse, a major factor in our society today
▶ Infection with human immunodeficiency virus (HIV) at epidemic proportions in urban, suburban, and rural areas
▶ Rural communities without a resident physician, with acute or emergency services long distances away
▶ Growing number of uninsured and homeless individuals and families
▶ Limited access and availability because of insufficient funding for health care services

These populations provide a challenge for experienced health care professionals to find ways to secure health care for the underserved. Innovative nursing solutions to help develop appropriate services include working with community partners to develop programs and services. Nurses can also volunteer to staff a free clinic; participate in outreach, such as launching campaigns on health education; and speak to neighborhood gatherings, community forums, or church groups.

Specialized Care Centers

Specialized care centers provide health care for a specific population or group. Some of these are walk-in clinics; others provide residential care. Specialized care differs depending on the population served. For instance, a walk-in clinic may serve only teens or homeless teens. Poor nutrition, poor hygiene, adolescent pregnancy, alcohol and drug abuse, and family violence may be prevalent in some urban and rural communities.

Specialized clinics for individuals with cancer or HIV and AIDS are available in most cities. Clients come from their homes for diagnosis, treatment, and care, including chemotherapy. These clinics are generally associated with a hospital or an HMO. Nurses provide direct client care, treatment, monitoring, and assistance with planning of interventions; they also attempt to minimize discomfort, manage pain, and maximize quality of life. The members of the multidisciplinary team collaborate closely. Nurses focus their time on care and support for the clients and significant others.

Day centers for older adults were discussed at the beginning of this chapter. Day care centers provide services for infants, children, or disabled adults. Care may be for children of working mothers after school before parents return from work. Some day care centers provide care for children with minor illnesses when the parents must work. Other centers provide day care for children with chronic illnesses who cannot attend public school or, because of physical, mental, or developmental disabilities, cannot find employment. Nurses usually serve on the staff, or a nurse may manage the day care center.

Mental health centers may be connected to a hospital or may be independent agencies. They may be part of a network of other coordinated social and health care services. Treatment provided may be short-term or long-term care or crisis intervention. The nurse may be involved in assessment, counseling, or administration of medications. Knowledge of the community for further referral is necessary. Nurses may be involved in 24-hour hotline services. Clients may vary from mentally healthy people in a situational crisis to those with acute or chronic schizophrenia or Alzheimer's disease.

Maternal/well-child health care programs may be conducted at a specialized center. Prenatal and postnatal care may be provided (Fig. 12–2) in which assessment and education are the focus. Postnatal follow-ups are sometimes made by telephone or with home visits. The nurse may advise on exercise, nutrition, and family planning. These services are discussed in more detail in Chapter 9.

Nutrition centers may provide health counseling for mothers and children, older adults, and homeless or addicted clients. Government-sponsored WIC (women, infants, and children) programs help fortify the dietary intake of infants, children, and pregnant women. For every $1 spent on WIC, $1 is saved. Meals On Wheels and food pantries may be part of the program for older adults, homebound individuals, or clients and families living in poverty. Programs for adolescents with eating disorders, nutrition counseling for people with diabetes, and programs for the overweight client illustrate the variety of nutrition programs that can be offered in specialized clinics.

Long-Term Care Facilities

These facilities have recently proliferated for two reasons: (1) early discharge from the acute care setting often requires care that cannot be provided by family caretakers in the home, and (2) the number of older adults who have no one

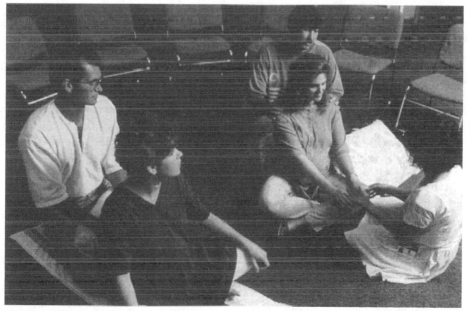

Figure 12–2. ▶ Expectant parents learn techniques to promote relaxation and comfort during birth. Classes in breast-feeding, infant care, and child care are also provided in many maternity centers.

to care for them in the home and who no longer can provide for their own activities of daily living has increased.

Long-term care may be provided for days or years. Most of these facilities focus on maintaining client function and independence, and improving quality of life. The facility may be associated with a hospital or an independent organization. Long-term care settings and centers for specialized care may overlap. For instance, a person with mental illness will seek specialized care, but it may be necessary to receive the care in a long-term setting.

There are several aspects to the role of the nurse in long-term care facilities. One important role is that of case manager. Often, the nurse working in long-term care delegates to and supervises licensed practical/vocational nurses and nursing assistants. A second role is that of care provider, because the registered nurse assesses and determines the appropriate plan of care for the residents.

Residential Programs and Facilities

Residential facilities provide a unique setting for community-based nursing because the nurse has a captive audience. Here the nurse can take advantage of the close proximity of the residents to do health teaching, health promotion, and disease prevention. By building trust through good relationships with the residents, nurses expand their roles to become counselors and advocates, providing direct support.

Residential programs may be chemical dependency treatment facilities, group homes for the mentally ill or retarded, halfway houses for recovery from addiction, detoxification units for safe withdrawal from alcohol or drugs, shelters for battered women, or hospices for the terminally ill. Nursing functions and roles vary with the kind of residential program or facility; they may include direct caregiver, case management, health education, discharge planning, counselor, and advocate.

Rehabilitation Centers

A free-standing or hospital-associated **rehabilitation center** for drug dependency treatment or for physical or emotional rehabilitation is another setting for care. The goal of this type of facility is to help clients reach optimal health so they can become part of the productive community again. Rehabilitation centers often have a philosophy of improving quality of life and facilitating independent self-care to the client's full ability. An interdisciplinary health care team collaborates to plan and implement care. The role of the nurse includes direct care, teaching, and counseling.

Detoxification Facilities

Clients are admitted to **detoxification facilities** for the express purpose of detoxifying their bodies from chemicals. Nurses are responsible for health assessment, identification of immediate physical needs, and referral to community organizations at the time of discharge. Medication administration and ongoing monitoring of the client's physical well-being from the day of admission are critical to ensure the client's safety.

Treatment Facilities for Addictions

Here again, the goal of the nurse is to return the client to optimal health. Clients in treatment facilities for addictions usually do not require close monitoring for physiologic changes after the first 48 to 72 hours of the detoxification period.

The goal of treatment is for clients to begin their own recovery process to allow them to return to the community as better functioning and productive members of society. Recovery is a lifelong commitment that clients must make to address their addiction. The nurse is responsible for health assessment, planning, and management of identified problems. Direct care is provided through medication administration and management of acute problems. A multidisciplinary approach is used, and the focus for discharge planning is the successful reentry of the client into society.

EXAMPLE OF A CLIENT SITUATION

▶ Role of the Nurse in a Residential Treatment Center for Teenagers

Marva is a nurse at a residential chemical dependency treatment program for male and female adolescents. Criteria for admission require that clients be between 11 and 17 years old and diagnosed as chemically dependent or have chronic substance abuse with legal consequences. The average length of the prescribed program is 30 to 45 days.

Marva has a small office close to the dormitory-style rooms where the clients stay. Her responsibilities include medication supervision, overseeing self-administration of medications, taking a health history and doing an assessment on each new admission, health education, disease prevention, health promotion, intervention in acute situations, collaboration during discharge planning, and teaching. She enjoys working with adolescents who have varied emotional and physical problems.

It is important that the teens trust Marva and develop a relationship with her that is different from the relationships established with the program's counselors. Establishing trust is always a challenge, but particularly so with teens with addiction problems. Another challenge in this particular facility is that the population is coed. Sex education is imperative, as is problem-solving the many "attachments" the clients develop among each other. Marva states with a smile, "I just did not learn how to handle problems like this at nursing school. Some days, I really need to use every ounce of imagination I can muster." Marva has both independence and challenge in her practice.

Shelters for Battered Women

Domestic violence crosses all social, economic, racial, and ethnic boundaries. Shelters have been built around the country to house battered women and their children. They provide a safe place where the women will have an advocate and easy access to counseling. The nurse functions primarily as advocate and collaborator and provides health assessment, referrals, and education for the women and their children. Individual and group meetings with residents are part of the nurse's regular routine. The nurse who works with battered women must have good communication skills and must be aware of the resources available to meet the needs of these women and children.

Homeless Shelters and Transitional Housing

The percentage of people who are homeless has been increasing since 1970. The fastest growing segment is women and children, making up more than 50% of the homeless population in many cities in the United States (Children's Defense Fund, 1994). Most of these families are single-parent, female-headed families with up to three children who are primarily preschoolers (Helvie & Kuntsmann,

1999). The homeless population has three to six times higher prevalence rates of physical illnesses than the general population and is twice as likely to suffer from mental illness. Further, the homeless have greater difficulty gaining access to health care than poor families with homes (Rog, Holupke, & Brito, 1996). In addition, individuals without homes are exposed to nature's elements and to society's violence, placing them at increased risk for illness or injury (Fig. 12–3). They also may be addicted to drugs and alcohol, have poor nutrition and poor hygiene, and live in overcrowded facilities.

In treating illnesses and injuries in the homeless population, the nurse practicing in a **homeless shelter** or **transitional housing** may offer a variety of services such as immunizations, referral for further diagnosis of sexually transmitted diseases, teaching for pregnant women, and instructions regarding health maintenance. Assessing and completing immunization status of children who are homeless is an important primary prevention intervention. Screenings for skin conditions, evidence of early signs of chronic conditions such as diabetes, and hypertension are secondary prevention interventions. Another example is screening for normal development in children by using the Denver Developmental Screening Tool II to identify developmental delays. Assisting the client to follow-up with existing health issues and getting access to care, such as obtaining medication for mental health conditions like depression, is tertiary prevention. Nurses play an important role in the care of homeless individuals and families.

Camps

Camp programs for children and adults employ nurses in private, church, YWCA, YMCA, and Girl Scout and Boy Scout programs. They may be employed as camp nurses for camps for children with chronic illness, such as asthma,

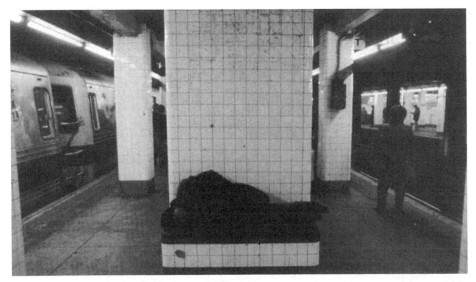

Figure 12–3. ▶ A homeless dweller takes refuge in a subway station in the city. Many times, police, social workers, and community-based health care workers comb such areas to bring homeless people in on cold nights. They are given food, shelter, clean clothing, and a health assessment.

seizure disorders, and AIDS. Direct patient care for acute situations, first aid, and health education are the primary roles. Camp nursing offers an opportunity to apply a variety of skills in a unique setting.

Schools

In 1902, Lillian Wald placed a nurse, Lina Rogers, in a school setting in New York City as an experiment. The experiment, to determine if placing nurses in schools could reduce the spread of contagious diseases, proved to be successful. Today, schools of all kinds comprise a major sector of practice for community-based nursing: day care, preschool, elementary, secondary, college, and university. Children seen by **school nurses** reflect the changing society of the nation, with different racial and ethnic backgrounds, varying socioeconomic backgrounds, and complex disabilities. Often school nurses are the major source of health assessment, health education, and emergency care for the nation's children (Taylor, Lillis, & LeMone, 1997).

The school nurse focuses on the healthy, growing individual or specializes in educational settings for the mentally or physically disabled, a role that includes health education, collaboration, and client advocacy. A school health program may include identification of communicable, chronic, or disabling diseases; immunizations; safety; and health education. State laws determine if the school can provide emergency treatment for injuries, maintenance of health records, immunizations, referral for health and social services, physical assessments, and teaching (Fig. 12–4). One school nurse relates her position as follows:

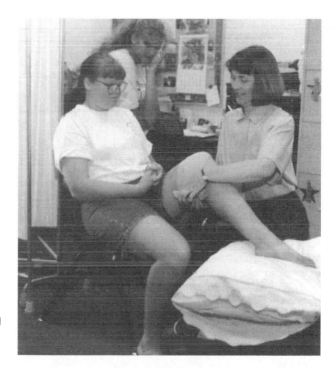

Figure 12–4. ► A school nurse assesses and treats an injured child. This is essential to a comprehensive school health program.

> ▶   I am responsible for about 1,200 high school students. Our office is open daily and we serve 50 to 60 students each day with such complaints as headaches, sore throats, fever, etc. The biggest change over the past few years has been the number of high-school-age single mothers we serve. I have developed a program of education for these young women. This includes safe sex, birth control options, child care, and child health. This takes up an enormous amount of my time. Time we could not predict was in our future as school nurses. . . . I would say I am nurse, mother, confidante, babysitter, first-aid giver, record keeper, and friend as a school nurse.

Many school nurses have become "drop-in" counselors. Often the school nurse is the one to whom a child or adolescent goes with personal questions and problems. These nurses use an established network of referrals for students' personal needs. A school nurse may refer to speech and hearing services, individual and family counseling, gay and lesbian support and youth groups, the department of social services, crisis drop-in centers, drug and alcohol programs, foster care, drop-in health clinics, and parents-in-training groups.

School nursing requires competence in the teaching, physical caregiving, and communication roles. Required educational preparation varies from registered nurse to a nurse practitioner with a graduate degree.

Most families in a community are already associated with the schools. Expansion of school-based clinics into comprehensive neighborhood health and social service centers provides another opportunity for offering nursing care to people where they live.

Industry

Business and industry provide another setting for nurses to care for people in a particular community. Occupational health nursing began in 1895 when Ida M. Steward was hired by the Vermont Marble Company to visit mothers and infants, care for the ill at home, and curb communicable diseases.

Businesses began to recognize that having healthy employees was an important factor in good management. Currently, the toll of workplace injuries and illness remains significant. Every 5 seconds a worker is injured and every 10 seconds a worker is temporarily or permanently disabled in the United States. Every year, 137 people die from work-related diseases (DHHS, 2000). Employers acknowledge that the health and well-being of employees are vital to morale and enhance the productivity of the company. Consequently, most companies provide health insurance, and many have developed programs to enhance health through the promotion of healthy lifestyles. This has spawned new language and a new focus for health care with programs such as **work site health promotion, employee wellness programs,** and **employee assistance programs,** all of which focus on the health of employees. Healthy snacks and meals, exercise programs and facilities, and educational classes are all used by companies to promote health.

The **occupational health nurse** works in a business or industry setting and fulfills a variety of roles, including health educator, advocate, collaborator, and coordinator. The focus is on keeping employees healthy, preventing illness and accidents, providing assistance to the employee who is returning to work after an illness or injury, and ensuring a safe business or industrial environment. Depending on the setting, any or all of the roles of teacher, manager, communicator, and caregiver are inherent in the occupational setting. The level of educational preparation varies.

Nurses can market their expertise to employers. They can provide programs aimed at job-related safety, weight reduction, and addiction-free lifestyles, and promote nutrition, exercise, smoking cessation, and family planning. Box 12–1 shows the priorities of the National Occupational Research Agenda (NORA) found in *Healthy People 2010.*

Hospice

Hospice care is a special service available to terminally ill individuals and their families. Care may be provided in the home, hospital, or residential hospice setting. Hospice care is more thoroughly discussed in Chapter 13.

Home Visiting

The home has been the core setting of practice for the nurse working in community-based care since the middle of the 19th century. Occupational health nursing and maternal and child care nursing originated in the home setting. In the past few decades, various studies have demonstrated how home visits improve outcomes for high-risk pregnancies and at-risk infants (Cowley & Billings, 1999). As discussed in Chapter 9, one of the goals of *Healthy People 2010* is to re

---

▶ **Box 12–1.** National Occupational Research
Agenda (NORA) Priority Research Areas ◀

Disease and Injury

Allergic and irritant dermatitis
Asthma and chronic obstructive pulmonary disease
Fertility and pregnancy abnormalities
Hearing loss
Infectious diseases
Low back disorders
Musculoskeletal disorders of the upper extremities
Traumatic injuries

Work Environment and Workforce

Emerging technologies
Indoor environment
Mixed exposures
Organization of work
Special populations at risk

Research Tools and Approaches

Cancer research methods
Control technology and personal protective equipment
Exposure assessment methods
Health services research
Intervention effectiveness research
Risk assessment methods
Social and economic consequences of workplace illness and injury
Surveillance research methods

duce the rate of low-birth-weight infants. Pregnant teenagers receiving home visits from nurses deliver heavier babies than teenagers who are not visited by a nurse. Women who smoked before pregnancy who receive home visits are less likely to smoke during pregnancy than women without home visits, which decreases the risk of having a low-birth-weight infant. Postpartum home visits are associated with a decrease in recorded child physical abuse and neglect in the first 2 years of life, especially in unmarried teen mothers of low socioeconomic status (Olds, Henderson, Chamberlin, & Tatelbaum, 1986).

Home visits with school children can facilitate case finding as well as provide more intense assessment and intervention for children with chronic conditions. Home visiting allows the nurse to establish a trusting relationship with the family and the child so that additional interventions may follow. It enhances continuity of care for all populations with all conditions. Home visiting is proven to be an effective means to enhance health outcomes, yet it is used relatively infrequently in the United States, compared with many other countries.

Home Care

Home health care is a growing area. Home health care nurses provide care mainly through home visits. Nursing agencies can contract directly with clients or with Medicare or private insurance plans to provide a selected number of visits to a particular client. Chapter 13 expands the discussion of home health care nursing.

 ## NURSING SPECIALTIES

Although all nurses need to be communicators, teachers, managers, and care providers, nurses may specialize in certain areas. Many of these specialties were discussed in the previous section on practice settings and practice opportunities. A nurse's title may reflect his or her setting, such as school nurse or occupational health nurse. Other titles may define the role the nurse plays in a setting, such as private duty nurse.

A **case manager** coordinates an individual's care and manages services supplied by various health professionals. The case manager ensures that continuity of care is provided between the acute care setting and the home, among community referrals, and among the team of practitioners. Case management is discussed in Chapter 7.

Advanced practice nurses include nurse practitioners and clinical nurse specialists. Epidemiologic studies consistently find that nurse practitioners provide client outcomes that are as good as or better than physicians' outcomes. (Brown & Grimes, 1993; Dawson & Benson, 1997; OTA, 1988; Safriet, 1992). The **nurse practitioner** is a registered nurse with advanced preparation, graduation from a nurse practitioner program, and successful completion of the licensing exam.

Nurse practitioners first began to appear in the United States and Canada in the late 1960s. Nurse practitioners may be generalists or may specialize in the care of particular types of clients. These include neonatal, pediatric, adult, geriatric, and family nurse practitioners and nurse midwives. They work in clinics, hospitals, and long-term care facilities, for public and private agencies, and in almost any setting providing health care.

Not only do nurse practitioners provide quality health care, but they also provide care at a fraction of the cost of physician care. It is estimated that nurse practitioner visits are 39% lower in cost than the average cost for comparable physician visit. The cost to society associated with not using nurse practitioners to their fullest potential is $6 billion to $9 billion a year, according to economist Nichols (1992).

A **clinical nurse specialist** (CNS) can practice in acute care or community settings. Positions generally focus on the particular expertise of the CNS (eg, diabetes CNS or oncology CNS). The specialist may develop and oversee a specialty program, act as a resource and consultant for other staff, and establish educational programs for the general public. Nurses have different degrees of autonomy and responsibility depending on the setting. Educational and professional role requirements differ as well. Most states require the nurse to have a master's degree to be a CNS. National certification by professional associations may be available.

A **nurse midwife** provides independent care for women during normal pregnancy, labor, and delivery. The nurse midwife practices in connection with a health care agency in which medical services are available if the client develops complications. In the United States, a nurse midwife is required by law to have a baccalaureate degree in nursing and a graduate degree from an accredited nurse midwife program, and to have passed the certification examination from the American College of Nurse Midwives.

 ## CONCLUSIONS

Rapid and dramatic changes have occurred in health care delivery in the community. Today opportunities exist for men and women to assume many roles in different settings in the community with a variety of clients. Because of the increasing elderly population, many nurses are entering the field of gerontology nursing, but many other opportunities exist for the practicing nurse. Such practice settings include, but are not limited to, the home, nursing centers, a variety of clinics and ambulatory care centers, specialized care centers, long-term care facilities, residential programs, schools, industry, and hospice care. The nurse may specialize in primary care, as a case manager, CNS, or nurse practitioner. Despite the variety in nursing practice, the principles of community-based care apply to all nursing roles in all settings. A creative, experienced nurse can find a variety of ways to use his or her expertise.

What's on the Web

Your Guide to Choosing a Nursing Home

Internet address: http://www.medicare.gov/publications/nhguide.pdf

This guide details a step-by-step process to help consumers make the best possible choice in a long-term care facility. A free copy can also be ordered by calling (800) 638-6833.

Allnurses.com

Internet address: http://allnurses.com

To find an exhaustive array of information on different specialties roles in nursing, consult allnurses.com and click on the Nursing Specialties category. This site provides access to resources for over 50 nursing specialties including but not limited to many community-based nursing roles such as school, ambulatory care, parish, correctional health, telephone triage, intravenous therapy, and advanced practice/nursing practitioner.

American Academy of Ambulatory Care Nursing
East Holly Avenue, Box 56
Pitman, NJ 08071
Telephone: (856) 256-2350
Toll-free: (800) AMB-NURS

Internet address: http://aaacn.inurse.com

This organization advances and influences the art and science of ambulatory care nursing practice and health care delivery systems to improve the health of individuals and communities.

American Academy of Nurse Practitioners (AANP)
Capital Station
P. O. Box 12846
Austin, TX 78711
Telephone: (512) 442-4262

Internet address: http://www.aanp.org

This organization promotes high standards of health care as delivered by nursing practitioners and acts as a forum to enhance the identity and continuity of nurse practitioners.

American Association of Occupational Health Nurses (AAOHN)
2920 Brandywine Road
Atlanta, GA 30341
Telephone: (770) 455-7757

Internet address: http://aaohn.org

This site provides information about occupational health nursing and the professional organization. AAOHN's mission is to advance the profession of occupational and environmental health nursing as the authority on health, safety, productivity, and disability management for worker populations.

American Holistic Nurses Association (AHNA)
P. O. Box 2130
Flagstaff, AZ 86003-2130
Telephone: (800) 278-2462

Internet address: http://www.ahna.org

The mission of AHNA is to unite nurses in healing. AHNA serves as a bridge between the traditional medical paradigm and universal complementary and alternative health practices. AHNA supports the concepts of holism: a state of harmony between body, mind and emotions, and spirit within an ever-changing environment.

American School Health Association (ASHA)
P. O. Box 708
Kent, OH 44240
Telephone: (330) 678-1601

Internet address: http://www.ashaweb.org

ASHA unites many professionals working in schools who are committed to safeguarding the health of school-aged children. The goals of the organization are to advocate for children and youth, represent all school health professionals, and promote professional education, public education, research, and service to children and youth. The Web site offers information about publications and conferences related to school health.

American Society for Parenteral and Enteral Nutrition (ASPEN)
8630 Fenton Street, Suite 412
Silver Spring, MD 20910
Telephone: (310) 587-6315

Internet address: http://www.clinnutr.org

This medical society is dedicated to promoting optimal nutrition and awareness of advanced clinical procedures of nutritional support.

Visiting Nurse Associations of American (VNAA)
11 Beacon Street, Suite 910
Boston, MA 02108
Telephone: (617) 523-4042

Internet address: http://www.vnaa.org

This Web site has information about visiting nurse agencies, conferences, and professional information, as well as caregiver information and home care resources.

References and Bibliography

Brown, S., & Grimes, D. S. (1993). *Nurse practitioners and certified midwives: A meta-analysis of studies on nurses in primary care roles.* Washington, DC: American Nurses Publishing.

Bureau of Labor Statistics. (2000). *Occupational outlook handbook, registered nurses.* http://stats.bls.gov/oco/ocos083.htm.

Chalmers, K., Bramadat, I., & Andrusyszyn, M. (1998). The changing environment of community health practice and education: Perceptions of staff nurses, administrators, and educators. *Journal of Nursing Education, 37*(3), 109–117.

Children's Defense Fund. (1994). *The state of America's children.* Yearbook (1994:37–44). Washington, DC: Author.

Congress of the United States, Office of Technology Assessment. (1986, December). *Nurse practitioners, physicians assistants and certified nurse-midwives.* HCS 37.

Cowley, S., & Billings, J. (1999). Identifying approaches to meet assessed needs in health visiting. *Journal of Clinical Nursing, 8*(5), 527–534.

Dawson, A., & Benson, S. (1997). Clinical nurse consultant: Defining the role. *Clinical Nurse Specialist, 11*(6), 250–254.

Doress, P. B., Siegal, D. L., & the Midlife and Older Women Book Project. (1987). *Ourselves, growing older.* New York: Simon and Schuster.

Edwards, J., Kaplan, A., Barnett, J., & Logan, C. (1998). Nurse-managed primary care in a rural community: Outcome of five years of practice. *Nursing and Healthcare Perspectives, 19*(1), 20–32.

Frenn, M., Lundeen S. P., Martin, K. S., Riesch, S. K., & Wilson, S. A. (1996). Symposium on nursing centers. Past, present and future. *Journal of Nursing Education, 35*(2), 54–62.

Gulzar, L. (1999). Access to health care. *Image: Journal of Nursing Scholarship, 31*(1), 13–19.

Hanks, C., & Smith, J. (1999). Implementing nurse home visitation programs. *Public Health Nursing, 16*(4), 235–245.

Helvie, C., & Kuntsmann, W. (1999). *Homelessness in the United States, Europe and Russia.* Westport, CT: Greenwood Publisher.

LaMone, P., McDaniel, R., & Sullivan, T. (1998). Partnership for health care: An academic nursing center in a rural community college. *Nursing and Health Care Perspective, 19*(2), 80–85.

LeMon, B. (2000). The role of the nurse practitioner. *Nursing Standard, 14*(21), 49–51.

Martin, P., & Hutchinson, S. (1999). Nurse practitioners and the problem of discounting. *Journal of Advanced Nursing, 29*(1), 9–17.

Meiner, S. (2000). Nursing documentation—Legal focus across practice settings. Thousand Oaks, CA: Sage Press.

Merrill, J., Turner, L., McLaughlin, J., & Milner, G. (1999). Following in Wald's footsteps: Bringing health to the people. *Journal of the New York State Nurses Association, 30*(1), 5–8.

Miller, B. (1999). Safe as houses. *Nursing Times, 95*(41), 32–33.

Mundinger, M. (1993). Advance practice nursing—Good medicine for physicians? *New England Journal of Medicine, 330*(3), 211–214.

Murphy, B. (1995). Nursing centers: The time is now. NLN Publication #41-2629 (ix–xxiv, 1–279). New York: National League for Nursing.

National Center for Health Statistics. (1999). *Health, United States, 1999 with health and aging chartbook*. Hyattsville, MD: Author.

Nichols, L. M. (1992). Estimating costs of under using advanced practice nurses. *Nursing Economics, 10*, 343–351.

Office of Technology Assessment. (1989). *The use of preventive services by the elderly: Preventive health services under medicare. Paper 2*. Washington, DC: Congress of the United States.

Olds, D. L., Henderson, C. R., & Kitzman, H. (1995). Does prenatal and infancy home visitation have enduring effects on qualities of parental care giving and health at 25–50 months of life? *Pediatrics, 93*, 89–98.

Olds, D. L., Henderson, C. R., Chamberlin R., & Tatelbaum, R. (1986). Preventing child abuse and neglect: A randomized trial of home visitation. *Pediatrics, 78*, 65–78.

Olds, D. L., Henderson, C. R., Tatelbaum, R., & Chamberlin R. (1986). Improving the delivery of prenatal care and outcomes of pregnancy: A randomized trial of home visitations. *Pediatrics, 77*, 16–28.

Olds, D. L., Henderson, C. R., Tatelbaum, R., & Chamberlin R. (1988). Improving the life course development of socially disadvantaged mothers: A randomized trial of home visitations. *American Journal of Public Health, 78*(11), 1436–1445.

Rog, D. J., Holupke, C. S., & Brito, M. C. (1996). The impact of housing on health: Examining supportive housing for individuals with mental illness. *Current Issues in Public Health, 2*, 153–160.

Safriet, B. (1992). Health care dollars and regulatory sense: The role of advanced practice nursing. *Yale Journal of Regulation, 9*(2), 417–487.

Salkever, D. (1992). Episode-based efficiency comparisons for physicians and nurse practitioners. *Medical Care, 20*, 143–153.

Simoni, P., & McKinney, J. (1998). Evaluation of service learning in a school of nursing: Primary care in a community setting. *Journal of Nursing Education, 37*(3), 122–128.

Solari-Twadell, P. (1999). The emerging practice of parish nursing. In Solari-Twadell, P., & McDermott, M. A. (Eds.). Parish nursing: Promoting whole person health within faith communities (pp. 3–24). Thousand Oaks: Sage Publishing.

Spradley, B. W., & Allender, J. A. (1996). *Community health nursing: Concepts and practice* (4th ed.). Philadelphia: Lippincott-Raven.

Strehlow, A., & Amos-Hones, T. (1999). The homeless as a vulnerable population. *Nursing Clinics of North America, 34*(2), 261–273.

Taylor, C., Lillis, C., & LeMone, P. (1997). *Fundamentals of nursing: The art and science of nursing care* (3rd ed.). Philadelphia: Lippincott-Raven.

U.S. Department of Health and Human Services. (2000). *Healthy people 2010. National health promotion and disease prevention objectives*. (DHHS Publication No. 91-50212). Washington, DC: U.S. Government Printing Office.

Weitzman, M., Fisch, S., Holmberg, R., Jackson, R., Lisbin, A., McKay, C., et al. (1996). Health needs of homeless children and families. *Pediatrics, 98*(40), 789–791.

Woodring, B. (2000). Home visits: Should they remain significant components of today's pediatric healthcare continuum? *Journal of Child and Family Nursing, 3*(3), 232–233.

Zachariah, R., & Lundeen, S. (1997). Research and practice in an academic community nursing center. *Image: Journal of Nursing Scholarship, 29*(3), 255–260.

LEARNING ACTIVITIES

LEARNING ACTIVITY 12-1

▶ **Client Care Study:** Gerontology Nursing

Jose Martinez is an 85-year-old man who lives in a rural area of Texas. He was discharged 2 days ago from a hospital in Austin after breaking his hip herding his sheep into the corral behind his house. His wife died last year and he has lived alone since. He has eight children; all of them live in and around the small rural town where Jose has lived after immigrating from Mexico 20 years ago.

Since fracturing his hip, Mr. Martinez has not been able to care for himself and is upset about his inability to tend to his sheep and be independent. His family has gathered to meet with the home health care nurse about plans for Mr. Martinez.

1. Discuss assessment questions related to culture that the nurse should ask when establishing a relationship with this family.
2. Identify five important questions the home health care nurse should ask during the client conference.
3. Determine what options exist for Mr. Martinez.
4. State ways the nurse can address Mr. Martinez's desire to be independent.
5. Discuss how the nurse will decide what is affordable for the client and family.
6. Determine Mr. Martinez's primary health care needs.
7. Given all the options, summarize the ideal place for Mr. Martinez to live.

LEARNING ACTIVITY 12-2

▶ **Critical Thinking Exercise:** Self-Evaluation and Reflection

1. In your clinical journal, identify a practice setting that you would like to know more about. Identify three ways you can learn more about this setting and the roles that nurses have in this setting. Implement this plan.
2. Discuss the strategies you used to explore this setting and the roles of the nurse.
3. What did you learn from this experience?
4. How will you use this information?

Home Health Care Nursing

ROBERTA HUNT

►LEARNING OBJECTIVES ◄

- Identify the purpose and goals of home care nursing.
- Discuss types of home care agencies.
- Outline the advantages and disadvantages of home care.
- Discuss barriers to successful home care nursing.
- Define the nursing skills and competencies needed in home care.
- Describe the home visit and its main components.
- Outline the role of the nurse in hospice care.

►KEY TERMS ◄

financial assessment
home care agency
home care equipment
   vendors
home infusion therapy

hospital-based home care agency
lay caregiving
official home care agency
proprietary home care agency
respite care

Historical Perspective

Significance of Home Health Care

Agencies That Provide Home Care

Acute Care Nursing Versus Home Care Nursing

Barriers to Successful Home Care

Nursing Skills and Competencies in Home Health Care

Support of the Lay Caregiver

Hospice Care

The Future of Home Care and Hospice Care

Conclusions

Home health care is the provision of health services to individuals and families in their places of residence for the purpose of promoting, maintaining, or restoring health. It is one of the most rapidly growing service industries in the United States. Nurses who work in this type of setting follow the nursing process in their provision of health care. They must be competent in their knowledge base of nursing care and in their skills of communication, teaching, management, and physical caregiving. This chapter begins with a brief introduction to the history of home health care. Home care agencies, the purposes and goals of home health care, the advantages and disadvantages of home care, and barriers to successful home care are discussed. A large part of the chapter deals with nursing skills and competencies in this setting, including a summary of the first visit. Safety issues and lay caretaker involvement are included. The nurse's participation in hospice care concludes the chapter.

 HISTORICAL PERSPECTIVE

Although the current form of home care nursing is a relatively new phenomenon, the first home care agencies were established in the 1880s. It was almost 100 years later that changes in federal reimbursement for health care brought about vast growth in home health care.

Modern home care evolved from the Visiting Nurse Association (VNA), which originated at the beginning of the 20th century in New York City. The mission of home care has changed from that of the VNA in the early part of this century, when nurses were caring for mostly indigent tuberculosis clients in the tenements. Physicians were involved in home care before World War II. The war produced a shortage of physicians, however, so the use of nurses for home care services expanded. In the 1940s, hospital-based home care agencies were established. A pivotal change in home care came from the 1965 Medicare and Medicaid legislation that allowed payment for home care services for qualified recipients. With this legislation, home care became more narrowly defined as a medical model alternative to extended hospitalizations. The impact of this legislation is seen in the monumental growth in the home care industry. In 1963, there were 1,100 home health agencies; today, there are more than 20,000.

Changes in government regulations implementing the diagnosis-related groups (DRGs) occurred for cost containment during the late 1970s and early 1980s. Most hospitals and health maintenance organizations (HMOs) began to recognize the importance of home care as a vital aspect of the health care system. Throughout the United States, insurance companies and HMOs have adopted home care as part of their standard health insurance package because the cost efficiency of care at home versus institutional care has been documented. With the trend toward shorter hospital stays, continuing care needs, and available reimbursement for home health care, the home care boom was born. Further, the increasing number of noninstitutionalized individuals older than 65 years, living long times with multiple chronic condition, has intensified the need for more home health care services. The acceleration in development of sophisticated technology that allows people to be kept alive and relatively comfortable in their own homes has also added to the need for nursing care in the home, as has consumer demand for improved end-of-life care at home.

 ## SIGNIFICANCE OF HOME HEALTH CARE

The major role of home care is to educate, reinforce, and encourage clients, families, and caregivers about ongoing care needs. The goal of home health care nursing is to provide services to individuals and families and to promote, maintain, and restore health. In most cases, this is achieved through short-term, intermittent direct nursing care made in home visits. Home care nurses provide direct services or supervise those services to assist with activities of daily living (ADL); teach clients, families, and caregivers how to provide self-care; and use communication skills to enhance continuity of care.

Governmental, private, and hospital-based programs employ home health care nurses. As most hospitals open their own home health care agencies, the fastest growing sector of home health care is the hospital-based sector. Home health care nurses are from all levels of educational preparation, but more than half are associate degree or diploma nurses. Home health care includes not only skilled nursing care but also the services of physical, occupational, and speech therapists; social workers; and home health aides.

The National Association for Home Care (NAHC) is the largest home care trade organization in the country. Its mission is to improve the quality of home care services. NAHC represents the interests of clients who need home care and caregivers who provide such services. Through a variety of activities and publications, NAHC attempts to be a unified voice for the home care and hospice community.

More than half the clients served in home care are older than 65 years. Recently hospitalized clients make up a large proportion of home care clients, with 16% of all Medicare hospitalized clients using home care within 30 days of discharge. Diseases of the circulatory system account for almost 30% of those receiving home care services with Medicare reimbursement (NAHC, 2000). There is also an increasing number of clients requiring high-technology medical interventions (intravenous therapy, mechanical ventilation, parenteral nutrition, etc).

 ## AGENCIES THAT PROVIDE HOME CARE

Home health care has evolved into a major industry with three key components: **home care agencies, home care equipment vendors,** and **home infusion therapy** companies. A change in the types of agencies that provide home care resulted from the federal legislation enacted in 1965 and 1983. Agency types today include **official, hospital-based,** and **proprietary.** These categories are described in Table 13–1.

There are a variety of home care agencies. Private duty agencies that primarily provide shift relief at health care institutions and for private clients are generally described as home care agencies. Most of the care is paid by private pay or private insurance, time is scheduled in hourly blocks, and services are largely provided by paraprofessionals (aides and homemakers) and nurses. Home care is also a generic term used for the entire industry and can include all types of agencies. In this text, the term *home care* is used to include all at-home nursing ser-

TABLE 13–1 • Description of Agencies Providing Home Care and Their Funding Sources

Type of Agency	Description	Examples
Official agency	Mandated to offer a particular group of services, and is supported by tax dollars	City and county health departments (Madera County Health Department, Madera, CA; the Health Services Agency of Fresno County)
Hospital-based agency	Has no mandates, can offer services of its own choosing, receives no tax support, and is an operating unit or department of a hospital	St. Agnes Medical Center, Fresno, CA operates St. Agnes Home Health, Private Care Home Services, and San Joaquin Healthcare, Inc. (each provides a different set of home care services)
Proprietary agency	A free-standing, for-profit home care agency, services are provided based on third-party reimbursement schedules or by self-payment	National chains/franchised agencies (Nurses Calling, Kimberly Care), locally/regionally operated agencies (Best Care Home Health Care, in California, and Interim Healthcare of Fresno, CA)

Any agency can provide home health care services. However, third-party payment (Medicare, Medicaid, or private insurance companies) depends on the mix of services available that is offered by a variety of licensed staff or contracted specialists.
Spradley, B. W., & Allender, J. A. (1996). *Community health nursing: Concepts and practice* (p. 487). Philadelphia: Lippincott-Raven.

vices. Official home care agencies are certified by the federal government to provide services for clients with Medicare and Medicaid insurance. The services have to be skilled and provide visits (30 minutes to 2 hours). Services include nursing; physical, occupational, and speech therapy; medical social work; and home health aide. Most insurance companies now pay for home health care services, but few will pay for shift nursing. Few, if any, insurance carriers will pay for paraprofessional care without skilled care services. The growing managed care movement is following the Medicare guidelines for the development of home health care services, although the number of allowed visits may be fewer and may vary among insurance companies or managed care organizations.

Today, most hospitals own or contract with home care agencies to create a continuum of care or an alternative to hospitalization. HMOs frequently choose home care services over hospitalization for clients because of its cost effectiveness. Medicare is the largest single payer of home care services (Table 13–2). Only clients who are homebound and under the care of a physician are eligible for home care services under Medicare (Box 13–1). Many insurance companies follow the same criteria. For the most part, home care has become medical care in the home; clients are given care and treatment under the specific orders of a physician. The nursing focus, consequently, has changed from a broad public health model to a focus on specific needs that have to be addressed in a limited amount of time.

TABLE 13–2 • Sources of Payment for Home Care, 1997

Source of Payment	Percent
Medicare	39.5
Medicaid	14.7
State and local government	7.0
Private insurance	11.4
Out-of-pocket	22.3
Other	12.2

Reprinted with permission. Copyright 2000. National Association for Home Care.

ACUTE CARE NURSING VERSUS HOME CARE NURSING

Because of the shift in setting for care to the home, there has been an increase in the number of nurses seeking employment outside the acute care setting. As a result, many nurses with acute care experience are now branching out into community-based care, especially home care. There are critical differences between providing client care in the acute care and home care setting.

One obvious difference in the two settings is the environment. In the home setting, the nurse is a guest in the client's home, unlike the hospital or clinic setting, where the nurse is in control of the environment. The need for the nurse to be flexible and adaptable is essential in the home setting as the nurse visits many different clients living in a variety of home situations (Cullen, 1998).

Another difference between the two settings is the type and amount of family involvement. In the acute care setting, the staff makes decisions regarding the client's care; in the home, the client and family are encouraged to make the decisions regarding care. Client and family involvement requires the nurse to use different skills in decision-making. Goals aim for long-term rather than short-term outcomes. Making decisions and setting priorities are shared activities.

A third difference is the nurse–client relationship. Often the home health care nurse cares for the same client and family over a long period of time. This allows for the development of a therapeutic relationship built on trust and caring that is much closer than in other settings.

Because home care requires assessing not only the client but also the family and environment, assessment, critical thinking, and organizational skills must be well developed. Further, because the nurse is only in the home for short

---

▶ **Box 13–1.** Medicare Home Care Coverage Criteria ◀

To be eligible for Medicare reimbursement for home health care services, clients must meet the following criteria:

1. Homebound
2. Require a skilled intervention
3. Have a plan of care signed by a physician
4. Receive care that is part-time and intermittent
5. Receive care that is reasonable and necessary

Weiss, R., & Milone-Nuzzo, P. (1999). A tool to assess homebound status. *Home Healthcare Nurse, 17*(8), 486–487.

periods of time, good communication, management, and documentation skills are essential (Cullen, 1998). Vital skills for a home care nurse are showcased in this text.

EXAMPLE OF A CLIENT SITUATION

▶ **Significance of Home Care**

Rafael is a home care nurse who visits 91-year-old Norma Wilkinson three times a week. Ms. Wilkinson has several medical problems, the major ones being high blood pressure, a heart condition, and arthritis. Rafael takes Ms. Wilkinson's blood pressure, weighs her, and sometimes draws blood. He checks on Ms. Wilkinson's general well-being. Ms. Wilkinson never married and has no relatives nearby, but Ruth, a woman from her church, looks in on her now and then and takes her shopping. Ruth has a key to the apartment. Ms. Wilkinson does not always take her medications as prescribed because some of her friends tell her she is taking too many pills.

As usual, Rafael telephones before his Friday morning visit. There is no answer, but he decides to make the visit anyway. When he knocks on the door, there is no response and the door is locked. Should he leave? He knows Ms. Wilkinson has had some dizzy spells lately and has fallen several times in the apartment. Rafael decides to call Ruth to bring the key and check the apartment with him. They search the apartment, but Ms. Wilkinson is not there, and her bed has not been slept in. They realize Ms. Wilkinson did not take her pills the previous 2 days. They begin a search of the building and discover Ms. Wilkinson in a remote part of the basement where no one ever goes. She had fallen and is confused. If the home health nurse had not made his regular visit, Ms. Wilkinson might have been in the basement for several more days before anyone discovered she was missing.

Advantages and Disadvantages of Home Health Care

There are a number of advantages to providing care in the home as opposed to the acute care setting. The primary advantage is the lower cost. The cost of inpatient care compared with home care for selected conditions is seen in Table 13–3. For clients, the advantage is the less-threatening, familiar comfort of home, which enhances care and the quality of life. Home care allows for easier access to loved ones and their support, and clients are taught self-care and encouraged to be independent, which maximizes their quality of life. Being at home also removes the family burden of traveling to and from the hospital. Being cared for at home contributes to the restoration of family control for the care being provided. These advantages are supported by the philosophy of community-based care, which focuses on enhancing self-care in the context of the family and the community.

Home care also has disadvantages. The presence of the nurse or other professional is an intrusion on the family's privacy. This may affect family decision-making and interaction among family members. The stress caused by multiple unfamiliar professionals coming into the home can also affect members of the family. In some instances, conflict may result if the nurse is not sensitive to the family's wishes and boundaries. Out-of-pocket expenses may accumulate as the result of home care not reimbursed by the third-party payer. These expenses may cause stress for the family. Financial pressure is often a precursor to the family's assuming total responsibility for their loved one's care. In a

TABLE 13–3 • Cost of Inpatient Care Compared with Home Care, Selected Conditions

Condition	Hospital Costs per Patient, per Month	Home Care Costs per Patient, per Month	Savings per Patient, per Month
Low birth weight	$26,190	$330	$25,860
Ventilator-dependent adults	$21,570	$7,050	$15,520
Oxygen-dependent children	$12,090	$5,250	$6,840
Chemotherapy for children with cancer	$68,870	$55,950	$13,920
Congestive heart failure among the elderly	$1,758	$1,605	$153
Intravenous antibiotic therapy for cellulitis, osteomyelitis, others	$12,510	$4,650	$7,860

Reprinted with permission. Copyright 2000. National Association of Home Care.

study of 18 technology-dependent children, 72% of the parents indicated that financial problems were the most serious issues confronting them once the child was at home (Leonard, Brust, & Nelson, 1993). Caring for a loved one at home may also have a negative impact on siblings and may result in aggressive behavior.

The advantages of home care far outweigh the disadvantages. Disadvantages are more of an issue if the family member is ill for a long period of time. In home care, although the client and family experience a loss of privacy and interruption of the normal family decision-making process, they still can enjoy a life together that is not possible if the client is hospitalized.

 BARRIERS TO SUCCESSFUL HOME CARE

Some of the disadvantages to home health care are also barriers to successful home care. For instance, family members express concerns about privacy, interruption of the family routine, loss of control, personality conflicts with the home care staff, and concerns about the competency of the nurses (Charkins-Drazin & Drazin, 1992). Families express their difficulty with statements like, "It changed our lives totally." Typically, loss of privacy interrupts the family structure, function, and communication patterns.

Families may understand the importance of regularity in the client's routine. Nurses can respect this concern by arriving on time for appointments and performing procedures consistent with the family's desire as long as they are within the parameters of safe care. Families tend to resent nurses who are too pushy or who try to control everything. They want the nurse to listen to them and respect the knowledge they have accumulated from being involved in care on a 24-hours-a-day, 7-days-a-week basis (Charkins-Drazin & Drazin, 1992).

 NURSING SKILLS AND COMPETENCIES IN HOME HEALTH CARE

The basic concepts of professionalism apply to nursing care in the home as they do in every setting. Promptness is imperative to good work habits. Nursing competency is critical. Families want procedures done carefully and in a manner similar to what was performed or taught in the hospital. Common needs of the home care client and family are psychosocial and learning needs, information about community resources, physical care, and management. Thus, as in other settings, communication, teaching, managing, and hands-on caregiving are important competencies and skills.

Communication

A comfortable relationship between the nurse and the client is essential to successful home care. First and foremost, the successful nurse communicates effectively with the client and family. If the nurse can build a trusting relationship, all aspects of the care will be more effective.

The nurse must be able to deal with a myriad of psychosocial issues characteristic of the home care client. The nurse wears many hats when providing care in the home including, but certainly not limited to, social worker, friend, spiritual comforter, psychologist, financial counselor, and translator of medical information (Stulginsky, 1993). As one home care nurse says:

> I was not prepared for the numerous psychosocial demands of the job. I thought I was pretty good at dealing with the psychosocial needs of clients I cared for in the hospital, but it was nothing like caring for someone in the home with the family present.

The psychosocial needs of the home care client primarily revolve around the client's adjustment to the illness, the anxiety it produces, and possible social isolation as a result. Nursing interventions that address the psychosocial needs of the client are primarily focused on building a trusting, therapeutic relationship. It is also helpful to elicit the client's and family's thoughts and feelings about this situation, which has taken control away from them (Fisch, 1993).

Teaching

Teaching is a major role for the home care nurse (Fig. 13–1). Chapter 6 addresses teaching in detail. Teaching includes explaining care and treatment at a comprehensible level. The nurse remains open minded by listening and showing respect for the client and family's knowledge. Clients and families soon become experts and are generally accurate in their observations.

The nurse can follow the teaching principles outlined in Chapter 6 when assessing the client's learning needs, remembering that the learner may be the client, family member, or caregiver. The learner's readiness to learn, need to learn, and past experiences are assessed. Learning needs are then placed in the affective, psychomotor, or cognitive domain. Finally, the learning need is validated and the teaching plan is mutually developed with the learner. After instruction, the teaching and learning are evaluated for their effectiveness. Several common areas of learning needs are the disease process, treatments, and medication.

Disease Process

Most clients and families need assistance understanding the client's diagnosis and any related disease processes. Teaching about the disease process is similar to teaching about medications or treatments and varies depending on the client's specific condition and the complexity of the diagnosis.

The client who requires only two or three home visits after routine surgery

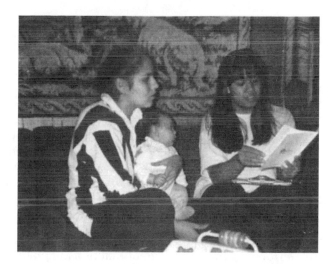

Figure 13–1. ▶ Teaching plays a major role in home care. Here a young woman is taught infant care by the community-based nurse involved in home care.

would require less information than the client with multiple chronic diseases. The most effective way to teach complex information is to divide it into small, understandable parts and instruct the client over time. When a client's condition merits many home visits with care and treatment over an extended length of time, the nurse can use that time to teach and reinforce learning without having to give all of the information in the first visit.

Treatments

Frequently, home care nurses are required to do treatments for clients and then assist the client or family to learn to complete the treatment. Treatment complexity varies. In some instances, the nurse may teach a dressing change by demonstration. In other cases, the family may have to learn to administer treatments with high-technology equipment. For example, a client may have brittle diabetes with a complicating large leg ulcer. The nurse changes the dressing, monitors the diabetes, and determines learning and teaching needs of the client and family. If the client and family are capable, the nurse teaches them to change the dressing and monitor the diabetes. It is not unusual for a client with complex technical equipment to be home with either full-time or intermittent (visits of 30–90 minutes) nursing care. Family members often provide daily intravenous line changes and irrigation, infusions of intravenous fluids, medications, or hyperalimentation through peripheral or central venous lines. They may also insert a Foley catheter or nasogastric tube and do tracheotomy care, including suctioning. Each year, more complex treatments and related equipment are available through home care. This trend requires home care nurses to provide teaching and rely on the client and family to perform procedures with a high degree of competence, identifying complicating issues and notifying the home care agency or physician appropriately.

Medication

Low adherence to prescribed medication treatment is very common, with typical adherence rates about 50% (Haynes et al., 1999). Consequently, the client and family often require assistance with medication. A thorough assessment of their ability to set up medications is the essential first step to this important intervention. This is initiated with a complete review of the medications the client is taking as compared with the most recent orders from the physician(s). The need for assistance with medications will vary from client to client according to diagnosis, age, and competency in self-care.

For example, clients recently diagnosed with diabetes may have complex learning needs for medication administration. Clients may need to learn about using a sliding scale for their insulin dosage based on a daily blood sugar level, drawing up the medication correctly, and injecting themselves. Some clients have a large number of medications with complicated doses that they must take several times a day. The more medications prescribed, the more likely the client is to not follow prescribed regimen. Comprehensive teaching enhances compliance with the home care client.

Management

As a manager of home care services, the nurse must apply leadership knowledge by performing the management functions of planning, organizing, coordinating, delegating, and evaluating care for a group of clients. The nurse must coordinate, through case management, an interdisciplinary team of multiple practitioners, the client, family, physician, and various community providers (such as Meals On Wheels and equipment vendors). The nurse's role as case manager depends on the scope of services provided by the agency and the specific providers outside the agency who are involved in the care of the client. Continuity of care is a major function accomplished by effective communication among all members of the interdisciplinary team. Management also includes delegation and evaluation of care provided by paraprofessional caregivers such as home health aides or homemakers and the family, as well as other professionals to ensure comprehensive quality care.

Physical Caregiving

Although one of the primary functions of the home care nurse is physical caregiving, the nurse is required to be flexible in this role. This means allowing the family to participate in caregiving whenever possible. Before doing a procedure, the nurse must explain to the client and the family what is being done and why, adjusting the instruction to their particular developmental stage and cognitive abilities (Fig. 13–2). It is essential for the nurse to know his or her own strengths and weaknesses and to master new skills before attempting them. Confidence is not instilled in the client if the nurse is inept and unable to provide care proficiently.

The nurse should keep the work area neat and clean by carefully disposing of laundry, trash, and equipment. People who receive nursing care in the home are at risk of acquiring infections, just as they are in the acute care setting (Centers for Disease Control and Prevention [CDC], 2000). Thorough handwashing on entering the home, after procedures, and before leaving the home is an essential aspect of good care.

The Home Visit

The skill and competency central to home health care is the home visit. However, all nurses working in the community should be prepared to make home visits. Even nurses in schools or in occupational health care are required some-

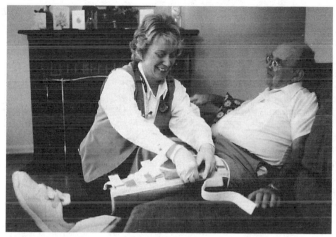

Figure 13–2. ▶ Home health nurses combine effective communication skills with their knowledge base of physical caregiving as they provide care for their clients.

times to make home visits. A home visit will often reveal information not obtained in other ways.

The main components of the home visit follow the nursing process. Observation of verbal and nonverbal patterns of family interaction help the nurse make assessments. Nursing diagnoses (or problem statements) help the nurse make joint plans with the family and establish expected outcomes. Following through with these plans helps cement a therapeutic relationship.

Preparation

Preparation for the initial visit involves reviewing the referral information to get basic information about the new client. Referrals come from a variety of sources, including hospitals, clinics, health care providers, physicians, nurses, individuals, and families. Home care referrals most often request intermittent or episodic care.

The client is contacted by telephone to inform him or her of the referral and to make an appointment for the first visit. The nurse identifies himself or herself, gives the name of the agency, and describes the purpose of the visit. A basic overview about the cost of services, eligibility, and alternative sources of support should also be discussed before the first visit. When applicable, the nurse must alert the client that he or she will need an insurance card or other evidence of coverage from a third-party payer, Medicare, or Medicaid on the first visit.

Unlike the acute care setting where a quick trip to the supply cart or utility room satisfies most equipment needs, in home health care the nurse must carry supplies. Before the first visit, the nurse should ask about supplies and determine what is needed. All home health care nurses use a bag to carry essential supplies to every home visit. This may consist of supplies and equipment the nurse uses daily for all clients, along with additional supplies. Each day the nurse should review the needs of the clients visited that day and add specific items. Essential supplies and equipment often suggested for a home visit are listed Box 13–2.

Beginning the Visit

After introductions, the visit usually begins with casual, social conversation to put the client and family at ease. A friendly, warm manner helps when the nurse be-

---

▶ **Box 13–2.** Essential Supplies and Equipment for a Home Visit ◀

- Handwashing equipment: disinfectant foam for hands, soap in container, paper towels, old newspapers (to set bag on in the home)
- Assessment equipment: thermometer, sphygmomanometer, stethoscope, tape measure, penlight, urine and blood testing equipment
- Treatment supplies: dressings, sterile and clean gloves, tape, alcohol swabs, scissors, lubricant jelly, forceps, syringes
- Occupational health and safety supplies: eye shields, mask, apron, gloves, plastic bag to double bag, sharps containers, disinfectant spray and clean-up supplies for spills, disposable scrubs, airway/mask
- Printed materials: map, agency forms, business cards
- Laboratory supplies: specimen containers, tubes, and equipment for venipuncture, culture, or urine specimen

---

gins to ask the client questions about himself or herself and the health care needs. It is important to begin building a trusting relationship from the first greeting.

During the initial interview, the nurse outlines a contract stating the purpose of the visit. The nurse uses a variety of communication tools to help the client and family understand the need for nursing care in the home.

Assessment

Assessment on a home visit differs from that in the acute care setting. The nurse incorporates the elements of community-based care into the assessment process in the home (Fig. 13–3). First and foremost, the nurse considers the issue of self-care by determining what the client's perceptions of his or her condition are and what the client identifies as personal problems and strengths. The client's ability to perform self-care or the family's acceptance of responsibility for care is explored. All assessments are made in the context of the family and community resources and support. Culture must also be considered. Continuity of care among various physicians and other professionals caring for the client is evaluated. A

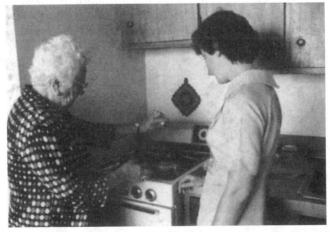

Figure 13–3. ▶ Home visits enable the nurse to assess whether the client can safely manage important self-care tasks, such as cooking.

preventive focus, keeping in mind the principles of continuity of care, is used. The nurse assesses the client and family's knowledge of the client's condition, care, and treatment. Learning needs are assessed.

PHYSICAL ASSESSMENT

Specifics of the physical assessment vary according to the client's needs. In most cases, the initial physical assessment will determine if the client is appropriate for home care services, what type of services are indicated, for how long these services will likely be needed, and who will pay for the care.

On the initial visit—and regularly throughout the care—the nurse takes vital signs and conducts a full physical assessment of the client, including a review of all systems and a focused assessment of the client's presenting condition. During this assessment the nurse collects information about the client's physical condition, functional status, ability to leave the home unassisted, ability to do self-care, and ability to perform ADL independently. Blood or urine specimens are often collected and sent to the laboratory. A sample home care laboratory request is shown in Box 13–3.

FAMILY ASSESSMENT

Because community-based care is provided in the context of the client's family and community, assessment of the family is an essential ingredient to the success of home care. Family structure, stage of illness, developmental stage, and family functions may be assessed. The nurse must also determine if the client is isolated physically or socially from other members of the family and if the family is a close-knit, nurturing, and supportive family or kinship network.

FINANCIAL ASSESSMENT

Information about the costs of home care services, insurance payment, and other financial concerns of the client and family should be discussed on the first visit.

► **Box 13–3.** Home Care Laboratory Request ◄

Laboratory: _____ Telephone: _____

Client's Name: _____ Medical Record #: _____

Client's Address: _____ Phone: _____

DOB: _____ Age: _____ Sex: _____ Diagnosis: _____

Insurance: Medicare _____ Medicaid: _____

Private Insurance: _____

Test Ordered: _____

Special Instructions: _____

Specimen Obtained By: _____ Date: _____ Time: _____

Physician(s): _____

Laboratory: Please notify Home Care Agency and Physician(s) above of the results.

© *Cheryl Skinner, RN, MPH*

Financial assessment and options to reduce the cost of care, while continuing the provision of safe, quality care, should be explored. Some clients are insured 100% for home care services as long as the services are provided within the parameters of coverage. Others may have little or no insurance coverage. Clients and families may have little knowledge about their home care coverage and may be unaware that the number of visits may be limited or that they have a lifetime maximum as stipulated in the particular health insurance policy. All of these issues must be explored.

Determination of Needs and Planning Care

After assessment, the nurse, client, and family discuss the nursing needs and develop a plan of care. They also determine who will be responsible for particular aspects of the care until the next nursing visit. The family support person may be responsible, or other professional health care or home care providers may be needed. An example of a home care interdisciplinary care plan is given in Box 13–4. Expected outcomes are developed and plans are made for a follow-up visit. Now and in the future, home health agencies have to demonstrate the client's progress toward achievement of desired outcomes (Forker, Gallagher, & Lewis, 1999).

Implementation

Physical care, teaching, counseling, and referrals are completed according to the plan of care. Because home care replaces hospitalization in meeting acute

---

► **Box 13–4.** Home Care Interdisciplinary Care Plan ◄

Client Name:_____DOB:_____Case Manager:_____

Date	Client Issue	Intervention	Facilitator	Accomplished			Comments
				Yes	No	Partially	

_____   _____   Disciplines on Case:
Date Reviewed/Initials   Date Reviewed/Initials   ☐ RN   ☐ WNA
                                                   ☐ PT   ☐ NMK
_____   _____   ☐ OT   ☐ Volunteer
Date Reviewed/Initials   Date Reviewed/Initials   ☐ ST   ☐ Chaplain
                                                   ☐ MSW   ☐ Bereavement
_____   _____   other _____
Date Reviewed/Initials   Date Reviewed/Initials

medical needs, home care focuses on physical care of the client. Short visits of 30 minutes to 2 hours focus on hands-on care of the client, incorporating a large variety of nursing skills. These include giving injections, performing venipunctures for laboratory work, doing dressing changes, giving medications, teaching the client and family how to do the care on an ongoing basis, and being the eyes and ears for the physician in observing the client's progress toward recovery. While the nurse is performing skilled nursing care, he or she is also teaching, assessing, counseling, and advising the client and family.

Termination of the Visit

The nurse reviews the purpose of the visit, outlines what was learned in the assessment phase, and reviews what was mutually agreed on for the plan of care. The time and purpose of the next visit are discussed and agreed on. The nurse may end the visit with a small amount of casual conversation. Especially if the client lives alone, conversation will be anticipated.

Follow-Up Visits and Evaluation

A thorough initial assessment allows for comprehensive planning for productive follow-up visits. A list of factors to consider when determining the need and frequency of future visits is seen in Box 13–5. Each visit should have specific goals with plans implemented to meet those goals. Subsequent visits allow the nurse to build a trusting relationship with the client, which may lead to identification of additional nursing needs. In community-based nursing, the overall goal of every home visit is to maximize health functioning and self-care.

The nurse, the client and family or caregivers evaluate the visit and the care plan. Physical care, teaching, counseling, and referrals are discussed and suggestions are made for ways to improve the care provided. The client may be asked to complete an evaluation survey (Box 13–6).

Documentation

Generally documentation for home visits follows fairly specific regulations. To ensure that the agency will qualify for payment for the visit, the client's needs and the nursing care given are documented. This includes the client's homebound status and the need for skilled professional nursing care with Medicare,

---

▶ **Box 13–5.** Factors to Consider When Determining Need and Frequency of Follow-Up Visits ◀

- Client's current health status
- Home environment
- Level of self-care abilities
- Ability of family caregivers
- Level of nursing care needed
- Prognosis
- Teaching needs
- Mental status
- Level of adherence to treatment regimen

Adapted from Smeltzer, S. C., & Bare, B. G. (2000). *Brunner and Suddarth's textbook of medical-surgical nursing* (9th ed., p. 19). Philadelphia: Lippincott Williams & Wilkins.

► **Box 13–6.** Client Satisfaction Survey ◄

To evaluate our services and continue our excellent standards of care, we need to hear from you. Please take a few minutes to complete this form and return it to us in the enclosed stamped envelope. Thank you!

1. Home health care services were provided in a timely manner when I needed them:

   _____ Very good   _____ Satisfactory   _____ Unsatisfactory

2. Home was the best setting for the care given to me for my comfort and recovery:

   _____ Very good   _____ Satisfactory   _____ Unsatisfactory

3. The number and frequency of visits provided were adequate to meet my needs:

   _____ Very good   _____ Satisfactory   _____ Unsatisfactory

4. The care I needed to improve my condition was received from home health care:

   _____ Very good   _____ Satisfactory   _____ Unsatisfactory

5. I am now able to care for myself with the procedures and instructions provided by the staff:

   _____ Very good   _____ Satisfactory   _____ Unsatisfactory

6. The home health care staff was courteous and respectful:

   _____ Very good   _____ Satisfactory   _____ Unsatisfactory

7. The names of community service agencies were given to me as needed and their services explained:

   _____ Very good   _____ Satisfactory   _____ Unsatisfactory

8. I felt my wishes about care were supported by the staff of the home health care agency:

   _____ Very good   _____ Satisfactory   _____ Unsatisfactory

9. I would use home health care services again:

   _____ Yes   _____ No

10. Home health care provided me with the following services:

    _____ Home health care   _____ Hospice   _____ Private duty

11. Comments (Please write on a separate sheet if more space is needed):

    _____
    _____
    _____
    _____
    _____
    _____
    _____
    _____

© *Cheryl Skinner, RN, MPH*

Medicaid, and most other third-party payers. If documentation is not done correctly, the agency may not be reimbursed for the visit.

At the beginning of this chapter, the Medicare coverage criteria that must be met for home care services to be reimbursed were discussed (Box 13–1). It is absolutely imperative that all of these criteria are met and documented. The nurse is responsible for documenting that the client is homebound. The primary dimensions of homebound status are that absences from the home are infrequent and for the purpose of receiving medical treatment and that leaving home requires considerable and taxing effort. Homebound status must be documented in objective and measurable terms and include the following information:

► How often a client leaves home
► For how long
► For what reason
► The effort and assisstive devices required (Stoker, 1999)

Documentation should always be focused on the client's illness, centering around the following:

► Statement of the problem(s)
► The skilled care provided to deal with the problem(s)
► Outcomes expected and achieved from the care provided (*Documentation tips,* 1999)

The plan of care must also be documented. Not only is a complete documentation of the care plan important for reimbursement and legal issues, but it is also critical to the evaluation of competent nursing practice used in quality assurance.

Confidentiality

Confidentiality is essential to quality care in community-based settings. Sometimes nurses may care for someone they know or a friend or relative of someone they know outside of their professional role. Just as in the hospital setting, nurses must never discuss individual situations or the health status of clients and families with anyone except other professional staff within professional discussions.

Safety Issues for the Nurse

The nurse should know the destination for the visit and have a route mapped out to get there. Asking directions can prove dangerous. When entering the client's neighborhood, the nurse begins an environmental assessment by doing a brief windshield survey (see Chapter 5). The purpose of the survey is to collect information about the community where the client lives and to determine if the neighborhood is safe. Occasionally the nurse may not feel safe entering a client's home. In some areas, the nurse may need to be accompanied by a policeman or security officer. No nurse should ever disregard personal safety in an effort to visit a client.

 ## SUPPORT OF THE LAY CAREGIVER

Because so many clients are discharged early with conditions more serious or less stable than in the past, the home care environment has become the site of major caretaking activities. The use of families, relatives, or support systems as

COMMUNITY-BASED NURSING CARE GUIDELINES

Personal Safety Checklist for the Home Care Nurse

- Get to know the community, especially the differences between neighborhoods.
- Dress in sensible shoes and simple clothing, avoid long necklaces, expensive jewelry, or pins of political or religious nature.
- Get to know your client and family and determine if there is a history of violence.
- Know your agency policies and procedures and follow them.
- Keep your supervisor informed of any potential violent situations with your caseload.
- Have safety accessories in your car: a working cell phone, flashlight; and have a well-maintained car.
- Lock up equipment and your purse or valuables in the trunk of the car.
- Attend a course on safety, self-defense, or self-protection.

caregivers is on the rise. In fact, **lay caregiving** is one of the world's fastest growing unpaid professions. It is estimated that almost 75% of elderly persons with severe disabilities who receive home care services rely solely on family members or other unpaid assistance. Eight of 10 of these informal caregivers provide unpaid assistance for an average of 4 hours a day, 7 days a week. Three quarters of them are women, and one third are older than 65 years. A telephone survey in 1996 estimated that more than 22 million households in the United States had at least one member who provided some level of unpaid assistance to a spouse, relative, or other person older than 50 (NAHC, 2000). It is projected that by 2030, more than 12 million older adults will need either informal or formal long-term care (Blanchette, 1997).

Lay caregivers may have responsibilities for people at either end of the age spectrum: children and older people with chronic health problems. Usually the child's caregiver is a parent and the older client's caregiver is a spouse. The caregiver for an older person is often an older person with his or her own functional disabilities. However, lay caregivers may also be sons, daughters, in-laws, or friends. "Parentcaring" is the term used in the literature for sons and daughters caring for older parents. These caregivers are predominantly women, although recent research suggests that more men are becoming active in providing care in the home for an older spouse (Ruppert, 1996).

Caregiving includes providing emotional support, direct health services, and financial support; mediating with health and social service organizations; and sharing a household. It may include tasks such as bathing, toileting, shopping, preparing food, feeding, maintaining a household budget, and housekeeping. Family dynamics can be different from household to household. The nurse must be sensitive to this variety of family dynamics and work with the family and caregivers without being judgmental regarding their decisions.

Stress on the Caregiver

Caring for a client who has acute needs that are treated with complicated technologic devices can be difficult. Such care may weigh heavily on the family. The nurse may need to provide not only client care and treatment but also a great deal of support for the family. Studies have documented the strain of caregiving on the caregiver's physical and psychological health (Fisher & Eustis, 1994; Mastrian, Ritter, & Deimling, 1996). One study found that more than half of the parents caring for children with high-technology equipment in the home had psychological symptoms great enough to merit psychiatric intervention (Leonard et al., 1993). As family responsibility grows, parental distress increases. The nurse is in an important position to intervene.

The transition from visiting a family member in the hospital, where other people are responsible for care, to being a "paraprofessional" caregiver sometimes happens almost overnight. Suddenly the lay caregiver has 24-hour responsibility for tasks for which he or she has little or no knowledge and experience. The lay caregiver may have full- or part-time employment and have other family members to care for. The strain on caregivers can be great, and risks for depression and illness are high. Other psychosocial problems raise the risk. The family may already have mounting bills with a mortgage and utilities. Safety in the community may be an issue. Transportation may be a problem, especially if the person requiring care was the family's means of transportation. Drug abuse on the part of a family member may add to the burdens. The lay caregiver may have no support person or outlets on which to rely.

The 24-hour responsibility for the client's care means more than supplying physical care for the client. It means that the lay caregiver always has the client and his or her care in mind. The role is unrelenting. The day is organized around the care activities and needs of the client, and sometimes the client must be under observation all the time. Many times the client's personality, which may have changed with illness, places heavy demands on the caregiver's time and energy. The difficulty of the role has been associated with low levels of life satisfaction, high levels of depression, and symptoms of stress (Ruppert, 1996). If the care is to be provided temporarily, the stress may not be as great. If the length of time for care, however, is indefinite, as in chronic care, additional stress may be felt by the lay caregiver.

Because the stress on these lay caregivers is tremendous, and community-based nurses need to consider this fact as they plan care. Although their clients are their main concern, a holistic nursing style means that nurses also provide care for family and other support persons.

Interventions for Lay Caregivers

Nursing interventions may enhance quality of life for both the client and caregiver by ensuring that everyone has adequate preparation for ongoing care needs. Nursing interventions may also assist in planning with the client and family to meet those needs. The nurse must do ongoing assessment of the family's financial status, coping ability, and emotional adjustment to the demands of giving care in the home, including signs of depression. If the situation indicates that a referral should be made for emotional or psychological assistance, this must be done promptly.

The community-based nurse in any setting should be aware of the lay caregiver's circumstances and help the caregiver find solutions to problems. The nurse who initially establishes rapport and builds on that trust to work with both the client and caregivers is the most likely to successfully intervene. Sometimes working with the client to perform more self-care activities will take some of the responsibilities off the lay caregiver. Providing more teaching for the caregiver may help relieve the caregiver's feeling that the responsibilities are overwhelming. Other interventions include educational and support programs, burden-reducing programs, psychotherapeutic interventions, and self-help groups. Even a busy caregiver can find time in the schedule to attend a support group if it is deemed worthwhile. In these groups, people share their experiences and report on strategies that have or have not worked for them. Just knowing that other people are in the same situation or have the same feelings is helpful. Research pertaining to the development of a support group for caregivers is shown in Research Box 13–1.

RESEARCH RELATED TO COMMUNITY-BASED NURSING CARE

Research Box 13–1 ▶ Lives on Hold: Evaluation of a Caregiver's Support Program

This evaluation research of a caregiver support program found that the participants initially characterized their lives as being on hold. Socialization activities and learning to care for themselves helped them cope with feelings of being overwhelmed, isolated, and lacking personal time for themselves.

This caregiver support program was developed after a need assessment was completed by the Visiting Nurse Association (VNA) of East San Gabriel Valley of Los Angeles County, California. Using an interdisciplinary team, the VNA developed a 12-week program called the Comprehensive Caregiver Support Program (CSP), with three social support strategies. These included educational activities, emotional health activities, and directed activities.

The educational activities were led by a mental health nurse clinician and focused on provision of basic physical and mental health information, nurture and self-care, enhancement of self-esteem, stresses of caregiving, and the effects of chronic illness on family functioning. A medical social worker facilitated the emotional health activities, which involved group counseling support experiences and coping skills. An occupational therapist led the directed activities, which were intended to encourage, and stimulated leisure-time activities. Respite care was provided for all caregivers to allow them to attend the sessions.

Evaluation of the program revealed that all of the participants were committed to caring for their family member or friend. However, when they agreed to be a caregiver, few understood the major long-term changes which would follow. They described their lives as on hold because they were never free from caregiving responsibilities, fatigue, isolation, lack of personal time and space, loss of work, financial strain, and physical, emotional, and relational strain.

The aspects of the program the caregivers reported as most beneficial were the socialization and learning better self-care techniques.

The following suggestions for establishing a caregiver support group arose from this research:
- Encourage socialization and sharing at each session.
- Serve food and beverages at each session.
- Limit groups to 10 with diverse membership.
- Use a multidisciplinary approach choosing caring and supportive facilitators.
- Emphasize the importance of self-care without guilt.
- Provide continuing ongoing support and education including bereavement support if the care recipient dies.
- Provide qualified respite care for each participant for each session.

Kleffel, D. (1998). Lives on hold: Evaluation of a caregiver's support program. *Home Healthcare Nurse, 16*(7), 465–472.

Another method for structuring caregiver support is reported by Ruppert (1996), who writes about a series of classes used in helping lay caregivers understand and manage their caregiving experiences. The classes focus on wellness, stress management, psychological aspects of caregiving, communication techniques, nutritional aspects of wellness, and exercising for wellness.

Caregivers attending the classes begin with a self-inventory to examine their level of wellness. They are helped through feelings such as fatigue, exhaustion, denial, anger, frustration, hopelessness, powerlessness, guilt, and depression. Caregivers are encouraged to find their own support persons with whom they can share their emotions and concerns. Information about substance abuse is given because some caregivers may be tempted to rely on substances to help them cope. The caregiver learns how to communicate important information to the nurse or physician, how to discuss care with the client, and how to address legal issues such as power of attorney, advance directives, living wills, and organ donation. Proper nutrition, proper body mechanics, and exercise tips are some of the requirements for maintaining their energy levels.

The nurse helps caregivers cope by sharing realistic prognostic information, discussing alternative levels of care, and providing information regarding respite care. A community day care program may be available for the client to relieve the lay caregiver of constant responsibility. Some communities help with housekeeping provisions or meal programs. Churches may have volunteers who can provide respite care.

Respite care provides a temporary break for the caregiver. The care may include someone coming into the house for an hour or two so the caregiver can shop, go to a beautician or barber, or keep his or her own doctor's appointments. Respite care is an important aspect of hospice care. Another form of respite care is the client's temporary visit to a nursing home or other facility. While the client is cared for in other surroundings, the caregiver and family are free to vacation, perform household maintenance duties, or simply relax.

 ## HOSPICE CARE

Hospice care provides an essential alternative for the terminally ill client. "These agencies are committed to maintaining supportive social, emotional, and spiritual services to the terminally ill as well as support for the client's family" (NAHC, 1999. p. 1). Caring for the terminally ill includes caring for the family and caregivers. Care varies according to the client's and family's needs; however, the focus is always on the client and family as the unit of care. Hospice care is often interdisciplinary care that reaffirms the right of every individual and family to participate fully in the final stage of life.

Dr. Cecily Saunders founded the hospice movement in London in the late 1960s. Dr. Sylvia Lack established the first hospice in the United States based on the model developed in Great Britain. Since 1982, when the Medicare hospice program was established, the number of hospices has grown dramatically. According to the National Association of Home Care (1999), there were 31 Medicare-certified hospices in 1984. In 1985, there were 151. In 1991, there were 1011, and by September of 1998, the number had increased to 2287. In additional to all the other benefits to client and family provided by hospice care, the daily cost is substantially less than hospital and skilled nursing facilities.

When a client is diagnosed with a terminal illness and has 6 months or less to live, the client qualifies for hospice care through Medicare. Payment for hospice services under Medicare is based on four levels of care:

1. Routine care
2. Continuous home care (24 hours in a crisis situation)
3. Inpatient respite care not to exceed 5 days at a time
4. General inpatient care (Hamilton & Thomsen, 1998)

The focus of care shifts from aggressive, curative treatment to palliative care and to strengthening the client's and family's quality of life as the client faces death. The goal of hospice in the home is to maintain the client's quality of life, keep him or her as comfortable as possible in the home, and provide support and instruction to caregivers. The purpose of the care is to make the dying process as dignified as possible while keeping the client comfortable physically and providing emotional and spiritual support. Nursing care in this context also assists the client and family to define their needs at the end stages of life and to have the resources necessary to carry out their wishes. With hospice care, terminal illness no longer means dying alone in a hospital. People can remain in the comfort of their own home, surrounded by family and loved ones, and die peacefully without fear of major medical intervention and resuscitative measures. Death with dignity is the motto of hospice.

Hospice care is offered in a variety of settings. These include the free-standing hospice house where inpatient hospice services are provided at the end of life; hospital- and home-based services provided by free-standing hospice agencies; and home care-affiliated hospice agencies. Most of the programs in the United States are provided through autonomous, community-based, in-home hospice programs. Many hospice agencies are developed and supervised by nurses.

Intermittent hospice care is provided in the home by nurses; medical social workers; physical, occupational, and speech therapists; home health aides; and homemakers. Hospice programs provide short periods of continuous care in which a client is provided with shift nursing and aides for an acute episode and respite care for the family by placing the client in a nursing home for a few days. Hospice-trained volunteers provide a large amount of emotional and physical support for clients and families by assisting with transportation, household care, child care, errands, and companionship. Volunteers also provide a vital link between the client and health care providers.

At the time of death, bereavement counseling and support for the family continue for a year. Spiritual counseling is a common aspect of care. Spirituality expressed through the religious beliefs of the client and family can be a very useful tool in the care of people who are dying (Cairns, 1999).

 ## THE FUTURE OF HOME CARE AND HOSPICE CARE

Public and political consciousness and research allocation related to end-of-life issues, emphasis on personal choice, and increased public awareness of the limits of medical technology have all increased interest in hospice care. Recognition of the importance of pain management along with the joining of forces between palliative care and hospice have also contributed to increased availability and quality in hospice care (Head, 2000).

It is anticipated that both home care and hospice care will assume an increasingly important role in community-based care in the future. The client advocate role will continue to be a central element of both as complexity of health

COMMUNITY-BASED TEACHING

Community-Based Teaching for Hospice Clients and Their Families

Hospice realizes that this is a particularly difficult time. Your physical and emotional well-being is important, so although the following information may be disturbing, please know that the goal is to help prepare you for what to expect. Remember that a member of the hospice team is always available to you for emotional support or information. Be aware that a patient may exhibit many of these signs for several days.

Certain symptoms may appear as the body prepares itself for the final stage of life. Not all dying persons have all of these symptoms, but some common ones are presented below so that you will know when they occur that this is the natural process:

1. An individual may sleep most of the time and be difficult to wake up.
2. The person may be confused about where he or she is, what time it is, who people are. Speech may become difficult, confused, or unintelligible. (Talk calmly and assuredly.)
3. Sometimes the client may say things that seem to be in response to another reality. This may not be confusion; but they may be responding symbolically to another reality—preparing to die. Listen, talk to them.
4. Restlessness, pulling at linens, and seeing and hearing things you may not see or hear may occur.
5. They may not be able to see as well (keep a lot of light in the room).
6. Regardless of the person's condition, hearing is the last sense to leave. Do not assume the person cannot hear you. Always talk to the person even if he or she does not respond. It may bring comfort to reminisce or share your feelings.
7. There may be a decrease in amount of urine. The nurse can show you an appropriate bed padding or arrange for a urinary catheter.
8. Generally, breathing patterns will change. Breath will become irregular, cheeks may become limp, moving in and out with each breath. There may be 10- to 30-second periods of no breathing. This is called apnea.

Cheryl Skinner, RN, MPH. Based on National Hospice Organization information.

COMMUNITY-BASED NURSING GUIDELINES

Nursing Interventions Directed to the Needs of Grieving Partners

- Encourage the partner to be with and helpful to the dying loved one.
- Inform the partner of the loved one's condition.
- Ensure the comfort of the loved one.
- Inform the partner of the impending death
- Allow and encourage the expression of emotions.
- Accept, comfort, and support all family members.

Adapted from Hampe, S. (1979). Needs of the grieving spouse in a hospital setting. *Nursing Research, 24,* 113.

care delivery and concern for cost containment continue. Flexibility and accountability will remain fundamental as the pressure to meet professional practice standards intersects with pressure to contain costs. Challenges facing home care nurses will require that the nurse keep up with ever-changing regulations regarding coverage as well as the documentation requirements that will follow. In addition, nurses will be called on to counsel clients and families as they have increasing responsibility for acutely ill family members at home. As in all nursing specialties, it will be vital for home care and hospice nurses to welcome the increased use of technology (Harris, 2000).

 ## CONCLUSIONS

The setting for the provision of health care provision has shifted several times from the late 1800s to the present. Care of the ill in the home was at one point primarily physician care. The setting for care moved from the home to the hospital or acute care setting in the mid-1900s, but has now relocated back to the home and community. The major roles of home care are to educate, reinforce learning, and encourage clients and families to provide ongoing self-care. In home care the family and client experience a loss of privacy and an interruption in normal decision-making, but the advantages for the client and family outweigh the disadvantages when compared with inpatient care. Regardless of the client's diagnosis, the nurse in home care encourages self-care with a preventive focus, which is provided in the context of the client's family and community, and follows the principles of continuity of care.

What's On the Web

National Association for Home Care
Washington, DC 20003
Telephone: (202) 547-7424

Internet address: http://www.nahc.org

The National Association for Home Care is a professional organization that represents a variety of agencies providing home care services, including home health agencies, hospice programs, and homemaker/home health aide agencies. The Web site contains news and information about home care and hospice including publications, statistics about home care and hospice, job search, and hospice and home care locator and affiliates. It also has information about NAHC membership, meetings and conferences, grass roots activities, and state associations.

Canadian Home Care Association
17 York Street, Suite 401
Ottawa, Ontario, Canada K1N 9J6
Telephone: (613) 569-1585

Internet address: http://www.cdnhomecare.on.ca/index.html

The Canadian Home Care Association is dedicated to the accessibility, quality, and development of home care and community support services that permit people to stay in their homes and communities with safety and dignity. The Web site contains information on publications, related sites, employment opportunities, and education programs, as well as information related to the organization.

Last Acts
Robert Wood Johnson Foundation
P. O. Box 2316
College Road East and Route 1
Princeton, NJ 08543-2316
Telephone: (609) 452-8701

Internet address: http://www.lastacts.org

Last Acts is a call-to-action campaign dedicated to improving end-of-life care through sharing ideas and solutions by professional caregivers, institutions, and individuals. The Web site includes new updates, a resource center, and reports on palliative care, family needs, service providers, education and training, financing, and the workplace. This site is an outstanding resource for hospice issues.

References and Bibliography

Blanchette, D. (1997). *New directions for state long-term care system. Volume III: Supportive housing.* Washington, DC: American Association of Retired Persons.

Brady, M. (1999). Stories at the hour of our death. *Home Healthcare Nurse, 17*(3), 177–180.

Cairns, A. (1999). Spirituality and reigiousity in palliative care. *Home Healthcare Nurse, 17*(70), 450–455.

Capone, L. (1999). The twelve c's of clinical documentation. *Home Healthcare Nurse, 17*(6), 382–389.

Centers for Disease Control and Prevention. (2000). *Infections associated with home health care: Focus of health experts.* Available at: http://www.cdc.gov/od/oc/media.

Charkins-Drazin, R. & Drazin, S. (1992). A parent's perspective psychosocial clinical skills. *Children's Health Care, 21,* 116–117.

Clark, D. (2000). Old wine in new bottles: Delivering nursing in the 21st century. *Image: Journal of Nursing Scholarship, 32*(1), 11–15.

Cullen, J. (1998). How student nurses see home healthcare nurses today. *Home Healthcare Nurse, 16*(2), 75–79.

Documentation tips. (1999). *Home Healthcare Nurse, 17*(3), 193–194.

Durkin, N., & Wilson, C. (1999). Simple steps to keep yourself safe. *Home Healthcare Nurse, 17*(7), 430–435.

Fisch, N. (1993). Home care nursing and psychosocial emotional needs. *Home Healthcare Nurse, 11*(2), 64–65.

Fisher, L., & Eustis, N. (1994). Care at home: Family caregivers and home care workers. In E. Kahana, D. Biegel, & M. Wykle (Eds.), *Family caregiving across the lifespan.* Thousand Oaks, CA: Sage.

Forker, J., Gallagher, B., & Lewis, A. (1999). Care planning for the homebound elderly client. *Home Health Care Managed Practice, 11*(6), 42–48.

Frequently asked questions about OASIS. (2000). *Home Healthcare Nurse, 18*(4), 229–230.

Gropper, R., & Giovinco, G. (2000). Confidentiality in home and hospice nursing: Protecting vulnerable populations. *Home Healthcare Nurse, 18*(3), 161–163.

Hamilton, M., & Thomsen, R. (1998). Removing the label. *Continuing Care, 17*(9), 26–29, 40.

Hampe, S. (1979). Needs of the grieving spouse in a hospital setting. *Nursing Research, 24,* 113.

Harris, M. (2000). Challenges for home healthcare nurses in the 21st century. *Home Healthcare Nurse, 18*(1), 39–44.

Haynes, R., Montague, P., Oliver, T., McKibbon, D., Brouwers, M., & Kanani, R. (1999).

Interventions for helping patients to follow prescriptions for medications. *Cochrane Database System Review, 2,* CD000011.

Head, B. (2000). Home care in the new millennium. *Home Healthcare Nurse, 18*(1), 13–14.

Horton-Deutsch, S., Farran, C., Loukissa, D., & Fogg, L. (1997). Who are these patients and what services do they receive? *Home Healthcare Nurse, 15*(12), 847–853.

Kleffel, D. (1998). Lives on hold: Evaluation of a caregivers support program. *Home Healthcare Nurse, 16*(7), 465–472.

Layton, S. (1999). A patient's prayer. *Home Healthcare Nurse, 17*(5), 293.

Leonard, B., Brust, J., & Nelson, R. (1993). Parental distress: Caring for medically fragile children at home. *Journal of Pediatric Nursing: Nursing Care of Children & Families, 8*(1), 22–30.

Mastrian, K., Ritter, C., & Deimling, G. (1996). Predictors of caregiver health strain. *Home Healthcare Nurse, 14*(3), 209–217.

National Association for Home Care. (1999). *Basic statistics about hospice.* Washington, DC. Available at: http://www.nahc.org/Consumer/hpcstats.html.

National Association for Home Care. (2000). *Basic statistics about home health care 2000.* Washington, DC. Available at: http://www.nahc.org/Consumer/hcstats.html.

Pfaadt, M. (2000). A review of the basics—Understanding the categories of skilled nursing services. *Home Healthcare Nurse, 18*(5), 297–300.

Ruppert, R. A. (1996). Caring for the lay caregiver. *American Journal of Nursing, 96*(4), 40–45.

Russell, P., & Sander, R. (1998). Palliative care: Promoting the concept of a healthy death. *British Journal of Nursing, 7*(5), 256–261.

Schwarz, K., & Roberts, B. (2000). Social support and strain of family caregivers of older adults. *Holistic Nursing Practice, 14*(2), 77–90.

Scott, E. (1999). Hygiene issues in the home. *American Journal of Infection Control, 27*(6), s22–s25.

Shyu, Y. (2000). Patterns of caregiving face competing needs. *Journal of Advanced Nursing, 31*(1), 35–43.

Smith, B., Appleton, S., Adams, R., Southcott, A., & Ruffin, R. (2000). Home care by outreach nursing for chronic obstructive pulmonary disease. *Cochrane Database System Review, 2,* CD000994.

Smith-Stoner, M. (2000). Palliative care . . . 2000. *Home Healthcare Nurse, 18*(1),32.

Steven, R., & Katsekas, B. (1999). Nursing the terminally ill: Being with people in difficult times. *Home Healthcare Nurse, 17*(8), 504–509.

Stoker, J. (1999). Defining homebound status. *Home Healthcare Nurse, 17*(2), 119.

Stulginsky, M. (1993). Nurses' home health experience. *Nursing & Healthcare, 14*(8), 402–407.

Turkoski, B. (2000). Home care and hospice ethics: Using the code for nurses as a guide. *Home Healthcare Nurse, 18*(5), 309–317.

Watson, J. (1999). Becoming aware: Knowing yourself to care for others. *Home Healthcare Nurse, 17*(5), 317–322.

Weiss, R., & Milone-Nuzzo, P. (1999). A tool to assess homebound status. *Home Healthcare Nurse, 17*(8), 486–487.

LEARNING ACTIVITIES

LEARNING ACTIVITY 13-1

▶ **Client Care Study:** Home Care for an Older Client

The discharge planning nurse calls your home care agency with the following information on a referral.

Mrs. Gothie is an 87-year-old woman with severe congestive heart failure. She cared for her husband, who had dementia, for 7 years. He died 4 years ago. Mrs. Gothie has lived in the same third-floor apartment for 50 years. Although she has no children, she is close to her younger sister and brother and numerous nieces and nephews, who all live out of state. Her family is devoted to her, visiting her frequently, but most of her lifetime friends are no longer living. She has one friend who is able to help her on a limited basis, but most of her friends are aging.

When she came to the clinic 2 weeks ago, before being admitted to the hospital, her vital signs and laboratory values were:

Temperature: 98.6°F
Blood pressure: 128/88 mm Hg
Respirations: 26 breaths/min
Lung sounds: rales in all lung fields
Lab values: prothrombin time 4 × normal
Digoxin level: 0.1 ng/mL

Mrs. Gothie stated at the clinic visit:

I have had a terrible time getting my breath, especially at night. My ankles are three times as big as they used to be. I quit taking my water pill because it made me have to go to the bathroom all the time, and I couldn't sleep at night. I don't have any appetite but I do eat fruit. Most days, I don't even bother to get dressed or take a shower because I'm so tired. What's the use— I never go any where—I'm always too tired. I have had a lot of bruises on my arms and legs.

She was admitted to the hospital for acute congestive heart failure. After 3 days at the hospital she was discharged to Happy Day Extended Care Facility. After 1 week of physical therapy, she is scheduled to be discharged home. You are assigned to be the case manager for Mrs. Gothie. After reviewing the attached referral form, plan your first visit with Mrs. Gothie.

1. List the points you will cover when you telephone Mrs. Gothie to set up an appointment for the first visit.
2. Determine the primary purpose of the first visit.
3. Determine the focus of your physical assessment.
4. Identify your key areas of concern when you do your psychosocial assessment.
5. List the people who can provide support for Mrs. Gothie.
6. Identify learning needs you will assess in the first visit.
7. Discuss referrals you will make after the first visit.

LEARNING ACTIVITY 13-2

▶ **Practical Application:** Psychosocial Needs of Home Care Clients

Consider the psychosocial needs of home care clients in the following situations. Comment about the likelihood of their condition to produce anxiety or social isolation. Give a reason for your answer.

1. A 50-year-old retired government employee who is caring for his 50-year-old wife who has severe dementia
2. A 20-year-old woman caring for her 5-month-old baby, who has frequent episodes of apnea. The apnea has required frequent immediate action and on one occasion necessitated cardiopulmonary resuscitation to revive the baby.
3. A 70-year-old woman caring for her husband, who has terminal lung cancer
4. An 80-year-old woman with severe chronic obstructive pulmonary disease who lives alone and is homebound
5. A 60-year-old man with congestive heart failure who has frequent episodes of shortness of breath at night

LEARNING ACTIVITY 13-3

▶ **Critical Thinking Exercise:** Self-Evaluation and Reflection

THE HOME VISIT

1. In your clinical journal, reflect on a home visit you have made in clinical. Identify the nursing skills and competencies you used as you provided care.
2. What did you expect the visit to be like, and how did the actual visit compare?
3. How was caring for the client in the home different from an acute care setting? How was it similar? What did you do differently in the home setting?
4. What did you learn from this experience?
5. How will you use this information in your future practice?

LAY CAREGIVER

1. In your clinical journal, reflect on an experience you have observed or a client you have cared for in clinical who has been cared for by a lay caregiver for an expended period of time. Outline the case.
2. Discuss what you observed with this situation and how it applies to the theory in the text.
3. How did or would you support the caregiver based on what you learned reading the text?

Implications for Future Practice

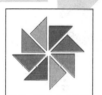

Any nurse, whether he or she has practiced for years or is just entering the profession, needs to think ahead. What are the implications for the future in community-based nursing care? How can you best prepare yourself to give quality care in your future practice?

Chapter 14 reviews current health care practice and anticipated future trends. The role of the nurse in the future, including educational preparation and advanced practice nursing, is discussed at length. Cost containment will remain a prominent deciding factor in health care delivery. It must also be weighed in relationship to the client's receiving quality care. The implications of technologic development and the information age, and their profound impact on everyday nursing care, are discussed. All of these trends are considered in light of the shift in demographics in the United States. Components of community-based care are discussed in light of the future.

With a knowledge base of basic concepts, development of your skills, and an understanding of how to apply this knowledge and skill to your community-based nursing care, you will be ready to practice as a nurse of the present and future.

Chapter 14 ▶ Trends in Community-Based Nursing

Trends in Community-Based Nursing

ROBERTA HUNT

▶ LEARNING OBJECTIVES ◀

- Discuss how current trends in community-based nursing will affect the role of the nurse in the future.
- Determine how market-driven economic policy affects the delivery of nursing care.
- Discuss the implications of technologic development on health care in general and on the nursing profession specifically.
- Identify trends in knowledge explosion related to alternative therapies, and relate the value of these therapies to client care.
- Outline how the shift in demographics affects the role of the nurse.
- Discuss the importance of the nursing competency of civic responsibility.
- Relate future trends in nursing to the components of community-based nursing.
- Develop a plan for your personal goals in your future in nursing in community-based care.

▶ KEY TERMS ◀

alternative therapies
health care organization
intergrated health care system
civic responsibility
knowledge explosion
market-driven economy

seamless care
service learning
pharmacogenomics
underserved populations
unlicensed assistive
    personnel

Trends in Heath Care

The Future of Nursing Care

Cost Containment

Technology and Information

Alternative Therapies

Shifting Demographics

Civic Responsibility

The Future of Community-Based Nursing Care

Conclusions

 TRENDS IN HEALTH CARE

Forces affecting health care in the future will also affect the role of the nurse. One can only speculate about what that future will be. According to Lindeman (2000), some broad changes can almost certainly be predicted in the future in health care, including the following:

► Emphasis on cost containment resulting from market-driven economic policy
► Advancements in technology
► Knowledge explosion
► Demographic shifts

Schools of nursing will have to revamp their curricula to meet these changing requirements. Content related to cost containment will be essential. It will be a given that nurses are technology competent. Not only does this mean computer competent, but able to constantly keep up with new ways of accessing and using information. The knowledge explosion requires that nurses develop skills in evaluating the legitimacy, efficacy, and importance of information and new treatments. All of these changes will occur within the context of changing demographics as nurses care for a population that is older, more diverse, and living with more chronic conditions.

This chapter discusses trends and concerns about current and future health care dealing with nursing care, cost containment, technologic development, the knowledge explosion, alternative therapies, and shifting demographics, and how they relate to components of community-based care. All these subjects have been discussed throughout the book, but here they are summarized with a look to the future.

 THE FUTURE OF NURSING CARE

Cost-containment concerns have resulted in several specific trends in nursing:

► A shift in the provision of nursing care from the acute care setting to the home and community
► Increased need for nurses to be technologically and transcultually competent
► Increased use of nonprofessional caregivers for roles and responsibilities formerly restricted to the practice of registered nurses (RNs)
► Increased use of advanced practice nurses (APNs) as primary care providers

Because community-based nursing practice will be central to the care of the large population of aging and chronically ill people, nurses will have to:

▶ Develop nurse-centered service models
▶ Consider going into independent practice
▶ Have competence in home care practices
▶ Be knowledgeable about client education techniques for every educational and socioeconomic level
▶ Have good organizational skills
▶ Be well versed in the aging process and have the skills necessary to care for the aged

Several broad general competencies will be demanded of nurses in practice in the 21st century. These include critical thinking and clinical judgment skills, effective organizational and teamwork skills, service orientation and cost awareness, accountability for clinical outcomes and quality of care, continuous improvement of health care, population-based approaches to care, an ethic of social responsibility, and commitment to continual learning and development (Bellack & O'Neil, 2000).

Nurses must be prepared to use critical thinking skills to solve problems and make decisions regarding care. They must also be able to make independent clinical judgments. They must be knowledgeable about making age-appropriate referrals to other disciplines and community agencies. Role responsibilities in community-based settings require a mutual decision-making model as nurses work with clients and families.

Because clients will be more ill when they are discharged home, nurses must be more technically advanced in their skills and adept at detailed documentation to ensure payment for services. The need to care for the acutely ill client in an isolated home environment creates an autonomous practice mode for home care nurses. The future will bring a need for competent, skilled nursing practitioners who are comfortable with practicing independently.

Flexibility will be important because cost-containment measures require decreased specialization. Some predict that current demands for care will lead to a decrease in specialization. Administrators are introducing multiskilled health care providers who are cross-trained to practice in a "seamless care" environment where practitioners provide care in different facilities or settings. With the trend away from specialization of health care personnel, nurses will be called on to perform more tasks and to cross discipline lines. In home care nursing, this is evidenced by nurses doing venipunctures (a laboratory technician's role) and teaching and monitoring administration of oxygen (a respiratory therapist's role). To prepare for the home care role, nurses must be competent as managers of care and teachers of self-care.

Nurses must become involved in the political, legislative, and regulatory processes of government. Nurses should not only know who their elected congressmen and senators are but also educate these officials about research findings so the officials can positively affect future legislation on health care reform (Fig. 14–1). Changes in professional licensing laws need to be made to reflect the realities of the 21st century. In 1994, one nursing futurist wrote that the RN of the future must maintain accountability when delegating duties to nonlicensed personnel; nurses, not physicians, should be ordering and directing paraprofessional services; and nurses should order nursing care that is recognized by third-party payers and is consequently reimbursed (Harris, 1994). Our profession has made major progress in two of these areas. The issue of delegating

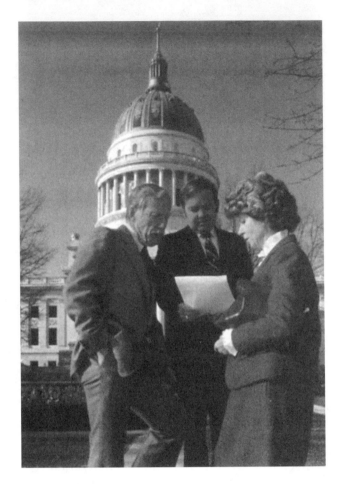

Figure 14–1. ▶ Nurses are an invaluable source of health care information for legislators.

duties to nonlicensed personnel has been and continues to be clarified. Today, APNs are able to bill directly through Medicare and in most states prescribe medication.

Unlicensed Assistive Personnel Performing Nursing Functions

Decreased specialization has resulted in the increased use of **unlicensed assistive personnel** (UAP) for some duties formerly assigned only to RNs. As a cost-containment strategy, many acute care settings are reducing the number of RNs and increasing the number of UAP (American Nurses Association, 1994). This change in the composition of the workforce, with employees crossing disciplines to deliver care, is a clearly emerging trend. However, the cost savings produced by using more nonprofessional employees and fewer professional staff is not well documented.

There is, and will be in the future, a danger of liability for the nurse supervising UAP. The importance of the nurse's following proper standards for delegation was covered in Chapter 7. Increasing use of UAP for nursing functions has caused a great deal of controversy. Nursing professionals may benefit from embracing a flexible position in regard to this issue, however. For instance, lay health care workers may be

> ... in some communities the critical link between the underserved or high-risk populations and the formal healthcare system. Nurses have partnered with community members to identify, support, and provide training and consultation to lay health workers, who are members of the community and committed to assisting themselves and their neighbors through outreach networks. In this way, nurses can significantly impact eliminating barriers to healthcare, increase accessibility of needed services, and thus improve the health status of the community. (Craven & Hirnle, 2000, p. 28)

Educational Preparation and Advanced Practice Nursing

If current trends continue, future nurses will perform a wider range of responsibilities. This will require both increased knowledge and skill. For example, community-based care demands a more proficient and autonomous practitioner. The current number of nurses educated at each level of preparation does not support this growing demand. Sixty percent of all new nurses graduate from an associate degree program; 36% receive baccalaureate degrees (National League for Nursing, 1994). The need for nurses with a baccalaureate degree will exceed the supply in the first 2 decades of the 21st century.

Nurse practitioners began to appear in the United States and Canada in the late 1960s, in response to a limited supply of physicians. Nurse practitioners most often provide primary care and diagnoses and treat common diseases and injuries. They prescribe medications in all states and Canada.

Currently, there is a great deal of support for APNs or RNs with specialty training at the master's degree level to provide primary care. During the early 1990s, state laws broadened the authority of nurse practitioners by allowing prescriptive authority and third-party billing. As a result, nurse practitioners can establish independent practices paralleling those of primary care physicians.

As early as the 1980s, studies have shown that when comparing the same type of clients, nurse practitioners have as good or better outcomes as physicians. An analysis of four random trials showed that the differences in outcomes between nurse practitioners and physicians was not significant (Ibrahim, 1986). The studies described the practice of nurse practitioners as safe, efficacious, and as effective as that of a physician, while being more cost-effective.

The Office of Technology Assessment, in a widely cited 1986 report, said that nurse practitioners are valuable in improving access to primary care and supplementary care in rural areas and in health programs for the poor, minorities, and people without health insurance. This report stated that the quality of care provided by nurse practitioners is as good as or better than care provided by physicians and that nurse practitioners' skills in communication, counseling, and interviewing are better than those of physicians (Congress of the United States Office of Technology Assessment, 1986). It is predicted that nurse practitioners will be used more extensively for primary care as a cost-effective alternative to physicians.

More recent studies show that nurse practitioners improve standards of care and increase efficiency and clinical effectiveness (Dawson & Benson, 1997). Nurse practitioners provide quality health care, but they also provide care at a fraction of the cost of physician care. It is estimated that nurse practitioner visits are 39% lower in cost than the average cost for comparable physician visits. Cost to society associated with not using nurse practitioners to their fullest potential is $6 to $9 billion a year, according to economist Nichols (1992).

Specialty areas of nurse practitioners include adult, gerontologic, neonatal, occupational, pediatric, psychiatric, school/college, and women's health. Nurse practitioners work in both rural and urban areas, from rural North Dakota to New York City. They practice in diverse settings such as community health centers, hospitals, college student health clinics, physician offices, nurse practitioner offices, nursing homes and hospices, home health care agencies, and nursing schools.

There is an established need for practitioners with an interest in research and advanced practice at the master's and doctoral levels. Nursing administrators must be educated and trained in management, finance, and the economic and social implications of our changing population as it affects the health care system.

Trends call for all nurses to be well prepared for the practice roles of today and tomorrow. Nurses must view education as an ongoing process and not limited to getting an entry degree. Continuing education is essential as the care delivery system demands more education, including baccalaureate, graduate, and postgraduate degrees. In most areas of the country, the curriculum at each level lays the groundwork for the next level of education, facilitating ongoing nursing education.

COST CONTAINMENT

The U.S. health care system is the most expensive in the world, using 14% of the gross national product (GNP), yet the country ranks 24th in terms of healthy life expectancy (Anderson & Poullier, 1999; World Health Organization, 2000). Every industrialized nation except the United States has a national health plan in place that covers all citizens (Anderson & Poullier, 1999). However, in the United States, health care is not a right but a commodity available to those who can purchase it, sold as a part of a **market-driven economy.** In a market-driven economy, consumer demand drives production regarding what services will be created and consumed and in what quantity. Keeping costs down and profits up is always a key aspect of a market-driven economy. Managed care has increasingly become an important provider of care because its central element is cost containment. Thus, cost containment as an important element of health care is here to stay. Consequently, nurses must continue to be aware of the financial aspects of the work they do, whatever the setting or position, now and in the future.

TECHNOLOGY AND INFORMATION

Technologic Development

The health care system of the future will be driven by technology and information. Technology is the tool to extend human abilities. Technology will be used to manage information and make decisions about care. Such technology may include medications, procedures, devices, and electronically based systems that support care delivery. Already clients are wearing programmable medication administration pumps. Nurses will need to program and troubleshoot such machines. These models will evolve constantly. The most promising advances are those related to high-speed telecommunications and portable computers. At present, it is possible to link a desktop computer to a modem and standard telephone line to transmit radiographs, computed tomography images, electrocardiograms, electroencephalograms, and health histories instantly. The potential for improving continuity is obvious. Some of the new technologies relevant to nursing care are described in Table 14–1.

TABLE 14–1 • Emerging Technologies for Nursing

Technology	Description	Nursing Applications	Implications
Internet	The vast collection of interconnected networks that all use the TCP/IP protocols and that evolved from the ARPANET of the late 1960s and early 1970s	Distance learning, research, clinical decision making, wellness models, telemedicine	Better information and much more of it can improve patient care Patient education can enhance wellness Degree of Internet access/experience is becoming a critical professional differentiator
Continuous speech recognition (CSR)	Natural or conversational speech is recorded, and phoneme recognition is used to recognize streams of sound	Charting	Reduces time spent on administration so that more time can be spent on patient care Lack of accepted nursing vocabulary limits data retrievability
Wireless computing	Any mobile terminal, mobile station, personal station, or personal terminal using nonfixed access to the network	Point-of-care data collection/retrieval	Improved patient care
Thin-client computing	A "stripped-down" personal computer designed specifically to be a client in a client/server network	Home care, ambulatory care, and nursing/ health care corporations	Cheaper technology; thin clients tend to cost less than fully-equipped models because they don't need full software or internal devices of their own Easier to learn/maintain
Data warehouses, data marts, and data mining	A data warehouse is a central repository for data collected by various business systems across the enterprise A data mart is a subset of the data warehouse, designed to serve a particular	Research, clinical decision making, and patient education	Improves clinical decision making by providing access to data from all parts of the enterprise and data that can be drilled down for nursing specificity Lack of defined nursing vocabulary

(continued)

TABLE 14–1 • Emerging Technologies for Nursing *(Continued)*			
Technology	**Description**	**Nursing Applications**	**Implications**
	community of knowledge workers (such as nurses) Data mining is the analysis of data for new relationships		limits data mart utility

Simpson, R. (1999). Toward a new millennium: Outlook and obligations for the 21st century. *Nursing Administration Quarterly, 24*(1), 94–97.

Several trends are shaping technology in health care. One trend is that of globalization. This began at the beginning of the 20th century with the invention of the telephone and was expanded at the end of the 20th century with the creation of the Internet. Gradually, the world's borders have dissolved as the world has become one. Thanks to telephones, telecommunications, and telehealth, nurses are now able to practice across geographic and national borders. Accelerated by the concerns for cost and profit, physicians and health care organizations are using globalization to export expertise (Simpson, 1999).

A second trend in technology is the culture of change. Society-wide change is evident in everyday life. In health care, change has been an unmistakable constant factor. Change requires ongoing adaptation and flexibility every day in every situation.

Clients are now aggressively treated for acute episodes of illness. This "recovery" from an acute situation may result in a long-term chronic condition and even technologic assistance for the rest of a client's life. What yesterday occurred in the intensive care unit may tomorrow occur at home. With the increase in available technology, care can be provided at an ever-higher level of sophistication in the home. If respirators, intravenous therapy (Fig. 14–2), and home dialysis are now common, what will technology allow in the future? It is anticipated that advancements in technology will improve the quality and efficiency of client care, raise the general health care status of the nation's population, and reduce the overall cost of health care. Box 14–1 reflects activities in which nurses can affect future home care through technology.

Knowledge Explosion

The **knowledge explosion** has produced what is often referred to as the information age. Major scientific developments have been occurring so quickly that knowledge overload is common. In the past, clients and families have consulted their nurse, nurse practitioner, or physician for information regarding health and illness. The health care provider has carried that information in their head or known where to go to explore the question. Now, an almost infinite amount of information is available to anyone who is computer literate.

Genetics is one area in which the information explosion is particularly evident. Because of the completion in 2000 of part of the Human Genome Project, which has mapped the human genetic code, treatments will be possible that were not even considered within the realm of possibility 10 years ago. For example, **pharmacogenomics** is the technology of developing and producing med-

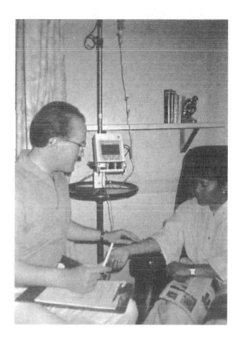

Figure 14–2. ▶ Intravenous therapy and other technologic treatments are performed in the home. Nurses are not always available to provide such services. More and more clients and families will need to be taught to perform highly specialized skills.

ications tailored to specific genetic profiles. What this means is that in the years to come, pharmacists will be able to provide a version of a blood pressure medication that is based on the individual client's specific genetic profile. Biotech companies are developing blood tests that reveal disease-gene mutations that forecast an individual's chances of developing a certain condition (Brown, 2000).

Nursing Implications

Rising health care costs and the need to enhance the quality of care are primary concerns for the nursing profession. In 1995, a study showed that approximately 55% of the overall cost in a home care agency is administrative, and up to 50% of the labor costs for nurses is dedicated to paperwork (Gogola, 1995). Computer technology frees the nurse from much paperwork so there is more time for teaching about self-care.

A significant change in nursing practice has resulted from the expanding

---

▶ **Box 14–1.** Ways for Nurses to Affect
Future Home Care Through Technology ◀

- Participate in national organizations and commissions on technology.
- Develop new computer technology.
- Stay current with emerging systems.
- Act as a client advocate in the development of computer-based educational programs.

Hales, G. D. (1995). Computers in nursing: The future revisited. *Gastroenterology Nursing, 18*(1), 30–32.

implementation of computer-based client records. With computerization, it is possible to retain the history of a client from birth to death. Automation in home care is viewed as a way to improve efficiency. Recent developments in information technology offer a variety of alternatives for documentation. For instance, the use of hand-held computers for field staff is a growing trend. Here the practitioner inputs clinical, financial, and administrative data and the system produces appropriate reports and forms. These systems are capable of redefining the data content, structure, and preconceptions about clinical information, patient assessment, care planning, and care delivery. Nurses chart information directly on a terminal or laptop computer with no need for copious written notes, charting from memory, or carrying around stacks of papers. Data entry is done through the keyboard, mouse, touch screen, voice activation, bar code, or pen touch. The system can alert nurses about inconsistencies in the data or the need to collect more information, generate a time-based report, or create a task list for each client. A growing number of manufacturers produce this developing technology that integrates data with a central system, facilitates the tracking of specific costs, and allows the client to interact with the system and retrieve information regarding care.

Imagine working as a home health care nurse, transmitting pertinent diagnostic data directly to the attending physician and having a three-way interaction with the client, physician, and nurse instantly. It has become common for nurses to electronically connect with client databases to obtain information from the client's complete nursing, medical, diagnostic, medication, and treatment history. Nurses are also able to order on-line prescriptions or home care equipment.

As a result of the explosion in information, people have access to near-infinite amounts of information. Many diagnostic kits will become available in the consumer market. The nurse may be called on to interpret or explain the results. Misinformation and misunderstanding by the consumer may be possible, which will require another service of the nurse (Hupfeld, 2000).

Are educational programs for nurses preparing students for this future? Are nurses comfortable moving into a present and future dominated by information systems? Educational institutions must have exit criteria that ensure basic computer knowledge. Faculty members must have computers to support their work. The profession of nursing has to have an impact on the future of home care.

The community-based nurse helps the client and the family by affirming that they do have choices. The nurse continues to reinforce this independence of action throughout the process of decision-making. Nurses are in a position to witness the impact of technology; they are the ones who help the client and the family to build their lives in a way that is meaningful to them in the face of a health care crisis. It is the responsibility of the nurse to recognize when technologic intervention is inappropriate and to help the family weigh the benefits and the burdens of their options.

 ## ALTERNATIVE THERAPIES

Twenty years ago, **alternative therapies** were considered fringe treatments by most Western health care practitioners. However, consumers wanted more choices for treatment and more control over their care. As a result of possible unpleasant side effects of conventional therapies and a growing skepticism about Western medicine, consumers have turned in larger numbers to alternative therapies. There is a basic distinction between alternative therapies and

Western medicine. Western medicine bases care on the disease model and the nature of pathology, whereas alternative therapies address holistic functioning within the social and environmental context, not focusing only on the function of the organs (Reed, Pettigrew, & King, 2000).

Today, alternative therapies are gaining respect and recognition from the general public and medical professionals as more people report positive results. Large numbers of individuals use alternative therapies, as seen in studies done in 1993 and 1998 by Eisenberg and colleagues. These studies reported that one third of persons contacted in a national survey had used unconventional therapy in the past year. Total out-of-pocket expenditure for alternative therapies was estimated at $10.3 billion in 1990, compared with $12.8 billion for all hospital care in the United States in that year. Estimates for growth by the year 2010 are 88% for certain alternative practitioners, compared with the estimate for growth for physicians of 16% (Cooper & Stoflet, 1996).

Alternative therapies are increasingly being valued and used by nurses and other health care providers. In the future, nurses will increasingly be called on to be knowledgeable about and use alternative therapies. Therefore, it is imperative that nurses build their knowledge and skills base about alternative therapies (Box 14–2).

For the person who feels intimidated and dehumanized by the sterility and business-like environment of most Western medical facilities, the warm, personal caring and concern of alternative practitioners may be therapeutic (Fig. 14–3). Because stress and anxiety are major factors in many illnesses, the soothing environment and supportive attitude of alternative practice have contributed to its appeal.

Research provides evidence that alternative therapies do enhance health and promote recovery from illness (Research Box 14–1). Those who support only Western methods of health care have ignored or repudiated the value of more traditional or alternative methods. These alternative therapies, however, have persisted and grown because people find them useful. Acknowledging the full breadth of services that individuals use, and working with them, is more productive than ignoring what the client chooses to do in the quest for wholeness and health.

Nursing Implications

To follow the holistic perspective, nurses must be knowledgeable about alternative therapies. With such knowledge they can monitor care and treatment and

---

▶ **Box 14–2.** Why Nurses Should Learn About Alternative Therapies ◀

- Large numbers of individuals are now using alternative therapies.
- As the population becomes more diverse ethnically, more methods of promoting health and treating illness are necessary.
- Alternative therapies have gained legitimacy with governmental agencies such as the National Institutes of Health, which has established an Office of Alternative Medicine.
- Medical education and physicians are integrating alternative therapies into their practice.

Adapted from Reed, F. C., Pettigrew, A., & King, M. O. (2000). Alternative and complemetary therapies in nursing curricula. *Journal of Nursing Education, 39*(3), 133–139.

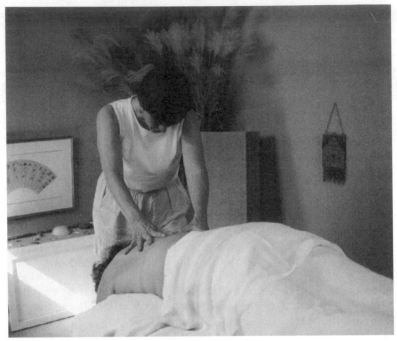

Figure 14–3. ► One complementary therapy is neuromuscular and therapeutic massage.

provide information about benefits for clients. The National Institute of Health has categorized alternative modalities and therapies into seven specific fields of practice, seen in Box 14–3. Nurses should attend training in multiple alternative therapies to provide expanded care to their clients.

Nurses can begin to broaden their perspectives about different health care therapies by addressing their own body, mind, and spirit issues. It is possible to work successfully with clients who use alternative approaches for their health care needs if nurses take an aggressive approach for a health care system defined by the needs of clients.

For example, Lisa is a 29-year-old woman who delivered a healthy, 9-lb, 10-oz baby boy 2 weeks ago. The home health care nurse makes a home visit. Lisa complains about continued perineal discomfort with no unusual discharge or odor. The nurse suggests hydrocortisone cream and suppositories. Lisa says that she wants to avoid steroid creams and asks if there is an alternative. The nurse is concerned but states that she cannot provide her with any other suggestions. The only things that work, she says, are hydrocortisone and time, and Lisa should adhere to the medications that are known to be effective. Lisa is left feeling insecure, unsatisfied, and without a remedy for her discomfort.

Aromatherapy, the use of essential oils with diverse medicinal qualities, has been shown to help in the treatment of a range of conditions, including perineal discomfort (Dale & Cornwell, 1994; Kuhn, 1999). If the home health care nurse had interest and training in alternative therapies, she may have been better equipped to care for her client. When the nurse is willing to acknowledge the client's philosophy and values, the client may be willing to consider what the nurse has to offer for the client's care.

RESEARCH RELATED TO COMMUNITY-BASED NURSING CARE

Research Box 14–1 ▶ Using Research to Evaluate the Effectiveness of Alternative Therapies

Because one in three individuals uses alternative therapies to manage health problems, it is imperative that the nurse develop skills to teach and counsel clients regarding the effectiveness of these interventions. "To offer the best possible advice on complementary therapy, the nurse needs to assess the scientific credibility of each treatment regimen." (Cerrato, p. 53)

This article recommends keeping an open but skeptical mind when assessing therapies and always considering the reliability of the evidence. The least reliable are client testimonials, with animal experience more reliable, and double-blind trials the most reliable form of research. In the double-blind study neither the clinicians nor the subjects know if they are getting the treatment or a placebo.

Some alternative therapies that have been shown to be effective treatments are chiropractic, massage, meditation, and nutrition therapy. A randomized open trial showed that chiropractic manipulation does relieve low back pain and has been shown to be more cost-effective than routine medical care.

Massage has been shown to reduce anxiety and pain and reduce lymphedema in clients with cancer. With postoperative clients who have undergone hysterectomy, massage lowers blood pressure, reduces the need for pain medication, and results in fewer visits to the physician after discharge.

Meditation has been shown to have measurable and profound physiologic effects with chronic pain and in lowering blood pressure in clients with hypertension. Meditation with relaxation training reduces nausea and vomiting with clients undergoing chemotherapy.

The value of nutrition therapy has been well documented in several instances. Two of the best known are the use of calcium supplements to prevent and treat osteoporosis in postmenopausal women and the use of folic acid in the prenatal period to prevent neural tube defects. One area that is less well documented as being effective is the use of vitamin E to protect against heart disease, but every year there is more new evidence to support this therapy.

More new data to support the value or lack of value of alternative therapies are available every day. To help evaluate alternative therapies for scientific credibility, use the MEDLINE database or consult the National Center for Complementary and Alternative Medicine (NCCAM).

Reliable information on alternative therapies is available from:

NCCAM Clearinghouse
P. O. Box 8218
Silver Spring, MD 20907-8218
Telephone: (888) 644-6226
TTY/TDT: (888) 644-6226
Fax: (301) 495-4957
Internet address: http://nccam.nih.gov/nccam
Cerrato, P. (1997). Use research to weigh the alternatives. *RN, 60*(2), 53–55.

SHIFTING DEMOGRAPHICS

The number and proportion of older people continues to increase. Since 1900, the percentage of the population older than 65 years has tripled, and growth is

> ▶ **Box 14–3.** Seven Fields of Practice of Alternative Therapies ◀

Herbal medicine encompasses herbal approaches for pharmacologic use and is derived from European, Asian, and Native American traditions.

Diet, nutrition, and lifestyle changes promote study of the effects of various food groups, vitamins, and minerals on acute and chronic disease as well as health promotion and disease prevention.

Mind/body or behavioral interventions include interventions such as biofeedback, relaxation, imagery, meditation, hypnosis, psychotherapy, prayer, mental healing, art, dance, music therapy, and yoga.

Alternative system of medical practice includes traditional Asian medicine, Ayuveda, homeopathy, naturopathic medicine, environmental medicine, and community-based health care practices.

Manual health methods use techniques such as osteopathy, massage therapy, chiropractic, physical therapy, and therapeutic touch as diagnostic and therapeutic tools.

Bioelectromagnetics explores how living organisms interact with electromagnetic fields for a variety for applications, including bone repair, wound healing, and immune system stimulation.

Pharmacologic and biologic treatments include drugs and vaccines not yet accepted by mainstream medicine.

Kuhn, M. (1999). *Complementary therapies for health care providers.* Philadelphia: Lippincott Williams & Wilkins.

expected to continue. By 2030, more than 20% of the U.S. population will be age 65 or older (National Center for Health Statistics, 1999). During the second decade of the 21st century, the postwar baby boom generation will move into the 65-and-older age group.

People living longer with more chronic conditions require an increased use of health care resources. It is estimated that nearly 20% of the population lives with disabilities, with this proportion on the rise. The number of people younger than 18 years with activity limitations increased by 33% for girls and 40% for boys between 1990 and 1994. Among adults ages 18 to 44, there was an increase of 16% in the number with activity limitations (U.S. Department of Health and Human Services, 2000).

In North America, cultural diversity continues to increase, with projections that 51.1% of the total U.S. population will be comprised of nonwhites by 2080 (U.S. Bureau of the Census, 1990). Immigrants and their children will reflect close to 50% of the growth in the U.S. population by 2020. By 2005, the Hispanic population will be the largest of the minority groups, and by 2025 their number will double (U.S. Immigration and Naturalization Service, 1997).

Nursing Implications

Providing nursing care to diverse populations has been discussed throughout this text and will increasingly be an issue for nurses. In the future, regardless of the nurse's own ethnic background, the nurse must be proficient at transcultural nursing to be effective in promoting self-care. Nurses will play a major role in addressing health promotion and disease prevention issues for elderly clients. A larger proportion of the nurse's caseload will include individuals with chronic, disabling conditions. Promoting self-care and health promotion and disease prevention with this population entails skills and knowledge that are different from those needed for clients in an acute episode of a resolvable condition.

Continuity is more difficult in cross-cultural nursing. Every decision hinges on the cultural context of the issue. Also, it is often more difficult to enhance continuity with an older client who has a weak support system or multiple chronic conditions that impair mobility or sensory perception than it is for a middle-aged client with a spouse.

Collaboration is even more important when working with diverse populations. Collaboration across disciplines is always challenging, but particularly so if the interdisciplinary team members are from several cultural backgrounds.

CIVIC RESPONSIBILITY

The Pew Commission's 21 competencies for the 21st century are shown in Box 1–2. It is easy to see how these competencies follow the trends discussed in this chapter. The first competency is "embrace a personal ethic of social responsibility and service." Cost containment has changed the delivery of nursing care and forced lay caregivers and clients themselves to be more responsible for self-care. Because health care is a commodity, many individuals (and often entire families) do not have access to care. Thus, a growing number of underserved individuals and families do not have access to health care but could benefit from nursing care. The competency of **civic responsibility** is intended to serve this growing **underserved population.**

One way to develop this competency is through volunteerism. Nurses, students, and nursing faculty must make a sustained commitment to community well-being through direct service. By carefully exploring options, students may find that by volunteering in a community-based setting, they learn more than they would in a traditional clinical setting.

A second way to develop the competency of social responsibility is through experiences that are structured to combine learning and volunteering. **Service learning** experience can be valuable for the nurse or student to develop empathy, social awareness, and social and cultural competence. Students and nurses can take the initiative to learn while volunteering by taking an internship or independent study in an area of community health that interests them.

THE FUTURE OF COMMUNITY-BASED NURSING CARE

Cost containment will continue to be a driving force for health care services, challenging nurses to be flexible, autonomous, and creative in their thinking. The current decrease in specialization calls for flexibility in the performance of roles across disciplines and the articulation of nursing as a profession. This requires the nurse to encourage clients and families to maximize their independence and follow through with self-care in all aspects of their lives. The educational preparation of the nurse will determine tasks; however, this may involve a broad range of activities from the simple to the complex. More education will be necessary for some who are required to perform, teach, and oversee complicated care.

Self-Care

In the future, the number of clients requiring assistance with self-care will grow as the percentage of the population with chronic disease increases. Self-care requires the nurse to recognize that assessment, planning, intervention, and evaluation revolve around the question, "How much care can the client and caregivers safely provide on their own?"

Self-care is especially challenging when the client is older or is from a different culture. The nurse of the future must be equipped to enhance the self-care skills of the client who is likely to be aging, from a different culture, and coping with several chronic conditions.

Self-care in the future will require mastery of an increasingly complex technology. To manage at home with a chronic health problem, the client and family caregiver will have to use complicated monitors and life-sustaining medical equipment, while the nurse uses sophisticated telecommunications devices to access information and transmit client data to the agency, attending physician, or nurse practitioner.

Preventive Care

The future focus of health care will be on treatment efficacy rather than technologic imperative. This promotes preventive nursing care, as discussed in Chapter 2. Community-based nursing considers all three levels of prevention. Focusing on prevention will be particularly challenging as the percentage of the aging and chronically ill increases. Growing trends in alternative health therapies allow more culturally sensitive options in preventive care.

Health care's focus on cost containment challenges the nurse to use prevention strategies to reduce costs. This is as true in the hospital as in other community-based settings. Rather than being seen as expensive baggage that can be eliminated, nurses need to be seen as keys to keeping beds empty by using their expertise in prevention. Dunham-Taylor, Marquette, and Pinczuk (1996) have developed creative ideas in using nurses in preventive care in the community-based hospital. A summary of their ideas follows:

Nurses can position themselves as the first link between clients and the hospital, thus developing long-term relationships. This involves periodically contacting clients with chronic problems.

Nurses can provide telephone triage services for the hospital by fielding calls, referring clients to more cost-effective services, and reducing the number of unnecessary visits to emergency departments.

Nurses can be proactive by contacting clients about immunizations and screening programs or fielding calls about medication administration, dressing changes, or proper diet. They can help correct problems before they become serious or identify already serious problems that need immediate care rather than postponed service.

Nurses can conduct educational programs on drug counseling, substance abuse, birth control, diet, and prenatal and well-baby care.

Nurses can contact aging clients routinely to identify health problems at early stages and to eliminate some physician visits that are motivated by loneliness and boredom. Nurses can lead self-help groups for this population.

Care Within the Context of Community

Earlier chapters explained the value of the community in providing health care, and Chapter 3 discussed the cultural aspects of community-based nursing. Nursing care must be provided within this cultural context, taking into consideration the strengths and resources of the client, family, and community. Considering affordable health care, the nurse will provide care in the home within the parameters of the family, community, and client. As the population ages, this challenge will be further complicated by the demands of high technology. Acceptance of alternative methods of care will allow care within the context of the client's family and community, including, in many cases, popular and folk healers. Because the racial and ethnic face of the nation is changing, nurses will be required to speak languages other than English or to be knowledgeable about using interpreters. An example of a card the nurse may need to carry is shown in Box 14–4. Nurses should also encourage representatives of minority groups to enter the profession of nursing.

► **Box 14–4.** Home Care Interpretation Services ◄

If you do not speak English, or if you have a hearing or speech impairment, you can have interpretation services provided for you at no charge. Tell the person helping you that you need an interpreter.

SPANISH SI NO HABLA INGLÉS, O NO OYE BIEN, O TIENE ALGÚN IMPEDIMENTO AL HABLAR, USTED PUEDE CONSEGUIR SERVICOS GRATIS DE INTERPRETATIÓN. DÍGALE A LA PERSONA QUE LE ESTÁ ATENDIENDO QUE USTED NECESITA UN INTÉRPRETE.

VIETNAMESE NẾU BẠN KHÔNG THÔNG THẠO ANH-NGỮ HOẶC BỊ LẶNG TAI HAY BỊ BỆNH TẬT VỀ BỘ PHẬN NGÔN NGỮ, BẠN CẦN NHỜ CƠ QUAN THÔNG DỊCH GIÚP ĐỠ MIỄN PHÍ CHO BẠN. NÓI VỚI NGƯỜI GIÚP ĐỠ BẠN RẰNG BẠN CẦN THÔNG DỊCH VIÊN.

LAOTIAN ຖ້າວ່າເຈົ້າເວົ້າພາສາອັງກິດບໍ່ໄດ້ຫລືວ່າເຈົ້າບໍ່ໄດ້ຍິນ ຫລືເຈົ້າເວົ້າບໍ່ໄດ້, ທາງພະແນກແປພາສາຈະຈັດຫາ ຜູ້ແປພາສາໃຫ້ເຈົ້າໂດຍບໍ່ໄດ້ຄິດຄ່າ. ບອກຜູ້ທີ່ຊ່ວຍເຈົ້ານັ້ນວ່າເຈົ້າຕ້ອງ ການຜູ້ແປພາສາ.

KHMER (CAMBODIAN) បើលោកអ្នកមិនសូវចេះភាសាអង់គ្លេស ឬ ខ្វះត្រចៀកស្តាប់មិនសូវបានឬក្រញ្ញ ។ សូមលោកទាក់ទងនិងបុគ្គលិកក្នុងការព្យាបាលយើងឲ្យរកអ្នក បកប្រែភាសារដោយឥតគិតកំរៃ ។

Please notify your nurse if another language is used, other languages are available.

Continuity of Care and Collaborative Care

The hospital of the future may be known as a **health care organization** or an **integrated health care system.** These systems already exist in many parts of the country. More community-based care programs will come from these integrated systems. Another term used is **seamless care**, in which all levels of care are available in an integrated form. Continuity allows quality care to be preserved in a changing health care delivery system. It is an essential component of cost containment and prevents duplication of services, rehospitalization, and inappropriate use of services. An older, more diverse population will provide challenges to the nurse as continuous care becomes the expected norm.

As a result of increased use of alternative therapies, the importance of continuity is evident. It will be essential for traditional and nontraditional providers to respect one another's contributions to the client's care and to communicate and coordinate care effectively.

 CONCLUSIONS

Cost-effective and quality health care accessible to everyone remains at the forefront of health care goals for the 21st century. In addition, flexibility will be an important aspect of community-based care. Trends demand nurses to be flexible when performing roles across disciplines while simultaneously articulating nursing as a profession. Ongoing professional development will be imperative to keep pace with professional demands of community-based nursing.

The nurse of the future must be equipped to care for the client who is likely to be aging, from a different culture, and coping with several chronic conditions. It will be essential for traditional and nontraditional providers to respect one another's contributions to the client's care and to communicate effectively. Trends in alternative methods of healing allow more culturally sensitive options. The nature and scope of nursing are broader than any one setting in which care is offered. Nursing care has remained constant in its philosophy over the decades. However, nurses must now adapt their care delivery models to include clients in acute care settings, long-term care, ambulatory settings, and the home. Nurses follow the standards of nursing care in all settings. In the future, this will require a more educated and proficient nurse.

What's on the Web

Alternative Medicine Homepage

Internet address: http://www.pitt.edu/~cbw/altm.html

This site, maintained by the Falk Library of the Health Sciences at the University of Pittsburgh, is a starting point for sources of information on alternative therapies.

American Medical Informatics Association
Nursing Informatics Work Group

Internet address: http://www.amia-niwg.org

This organization's goal is to promote the advancement of nursing informatics within an interdisciplinary context. This goal is pursued in professional practice, education, research, and governmental and other service.

Online Journal of Issues in Nursing

Internet address: http://www.nursingworld.org/ojin

This on-line publication provides a forum for discussion of current issues in nursing.

National Center for Complementary and Alternative Medicine (NCCAM)

Internet address: http://www.nccam.nih.gov

The NCCAM at the National Institutes of Health (NIH) conducts and supports basic and applied research on complementary and alternative therapies. This site disseminates information on complementary and alternative interventions to practitioners and the public. This is an excellent site for current, reliable information based on research.

GENERAL WEB RESOURCES
adam.com

Internet address: http://www.adam.com

This is a commercial site that provides health and wellness information.

American Heart Association

Internet address: http://www.americanheart.org

This Web page contains information related to patient information, support groups links, licensed products and services, and science and research. There is an excellent patient and caregiver education area, Living with Heart Failure, at http://www.american-heart.org/chf.

American Lung Association

Internet address: http://www.lungusa.org

This site contains information on lung disease in all forms, with special emphasis on asthma, tobacco control and environmental health

The Body: An AIDS and HIV Information Resource

Internet address: http://www.thebody.com

A comprehensive resource with information on the disease process, safe sex, support groups treatment, mental health, and legal and financial issues from a variety of sites and links.

CancerNet

Internet address: http://www.cancernet.nci.nih.gov

Maintained by the National Cancer Institute, this site has extensive credible information on cancer, reviewed by oncology experts and based on research.

drkoop.com

Internet address: http://www.drkoop.com

This is a commercial site that offers news, feature articles, and links to on-line support communities. C. Everett Koop, MD, former U.S. Surgeon General, heads it.

Health on the Net Foundation

Internet address: http://www.hon.ch

This international initiative has a multilingual search engine for information on health and health care.

Health Promotion Online

Internet address: http://www.hc-sc.gc.ca/hppb/hpo/index.html

This Canadian site addresses a wide range of health promotion and disease prevention programs. Offers content in French.

Health Resources on IHP Net

Internet address: http://www.ihpnet.org/4health.html

Designed to save time, this site provides direct routes to health information.

Healthfinder

Internet address: http://www.healthfinder.gov

This site from the U.S. Department of Health and Human Services leads to publication, clearinghouses, databases, Web sites, and support and self-help groups as well as reliable information.

Healthy People 2010

Internet address: http://web.health.gov/healthypeople

This site provides access to all of the *Healthy People 2010* documents and initiatives.

InteliHealth

Internet address: http://www.intelihealth.com

This site provides physician-reviewed consumer-friendly articles, on-line communities, and a medical dictionary. The "Ask the Doc" feature is very popular.

Internet Mental Health

Internet address: http://www.mentalhealth.com

This encyclopedia of mental health information is designed to promote understanding, diagnosis, and treatment of mental health.

Lippincott Williams & Wilkins

Internet address: http://www.lww.com

Lippincott leads in the world of information resources for nursing, medical, and allied health professionals and students.

March of Dimes

Internet address: http://www.modimes.org

This organization focuses on issues related to prenatal care and preventing birth defects, infant mortality, and low-birth weight infants. The Web site includes information on research, programs, and public affairs.

Mayo Clinic Health Oasis

Internet address: http://www.mayohealth.org

Sponsored by the Mayo Clinic, this site features reliable information on a variety of health issues with resources for each.

Medscape

Internet address: http://www.medscape.com

This commercial site is a professional site built around practice-oriented information.

Mental Health InfoSource

Internet address: http://www.mhsource.com

Included in this site are lay and professional information, news, continuing education, and consultation related to issues of mental health.

Mental Health Net

Internet address: http://www.mentalhelp.net

This free service includes thousands of resources and information for lay and professional consumers.

McGill Medical Informatics

Internet address: http://www.mmi.mcgill.ca

This Canada-wide database for medical teaching and learning has a wide variety of medical information.

National Institutes of Health (NIH)

Internet address: http://www.nih.gov

The NIH Web site is an excellent all-around resource for nurses from all specialties. It contains news and events, health information, grants, scientific resources and links to other sites including National Institute of Nursing Research and the W.G. Magnuson Clinical Center Nursing Department.

National Institutes of Health
Warren Grant Magnuson Clinical Center Nursing Department

Internet address: http://www.cc.nih.gov/nursing

This site provides links to federal resources, Internet search engines, and other useful resources. This nursing-specific site provides information from universities, the Centers for Disease Control and Prevention, and the National Institute of Nursing Research.

National League for Nursing

Internet address: http://www.nln.org

A resource for nursing education, practice, and research, this site has the latest information about the organization and nursing in general.

National Women's Health Information Center (NWHIC)

Internet address: http://www.4woman.gov

The NWHIC is a free information and resource service on women's health issues for consumers, health care professionals, researchers, educators, and students. This bilingual site (English and Spanish) contains a wealth of information on health issues that is free of copyright restrictions and may be copied.

NursingNet

Internet address: http://www.nursingnet.org

Created to further the knowledge and understanding for student nursing, specialty nursing, health care issues, and links to other nursing-specific sites.

Nursing Student WWW page

Internet address: http://www.csn.net/~tbracket/htm.htm

This site contains information and resources for nursing students.

OncoLink

Internet address: http://www.oncolink.upenn.edu

This site is maintained by the University of Pennsylvania Cancer Center. It contains news, education on treatment options, reporting on clinical trials, psychosocial support through an active on-line community, and resources such as associations, support groups, on-line journals, and book reviews.

Parent's Page

Internet address: http://www.efn.org/~djz/birth/babylist.html

An outstanding place to start to link to organizations, multimedia, and health resources that specialize in pregnancy and birth, this site also has information about and connections to midwifery resources, adoption, family planning, infertility, and grief and loss.

PharmInfoNet; Pharmaceutical Information Network

Internet address: http://www.pharminfo.com

This comprehensive site for pharmaceutical information provides articles, drug information, disease information, discussion groups, and a glossary.

Planned Parenthood

Internet address: http://www.plannedparenthood.org

In both Spanish and English, this Web site includes legislative updates, statistics, newsletters, and a library with information on family planning.

PubMed

Internet address: http://www.ncbi.nlm.nih.gov/entrez/query.fcgi

This search service of the National Library of Medicine provides access to over 10 million citations.

RealAge

Internet address: http://www.realage.com

This commercial site provides news, an on-line support community, and interactive health assessment tools.

Resources for Nurses and Families

Internet address: http://pegasus.cc.ucf.edu/-wink/home.html

This site contains resources for families, nurses, and nurse educators.

Stanford Health Pages

Internet address: http://stanford.thehealthpages.com

This site publishes information on general health care topics and community-specific comparative information with a library of articles on a variety of health topics.

Sudden Infant Death Syndrome and Other Infant Death (SIDS/OID) Information Web Site

Internet address: http://sids-network.org

At this site you will find up-to-date information about SIDS.

Transcultural Nursing

Internet address: http://www.megalink.net/~vic/index.html

This site's goal is to provide information about transcultural nursing to help other nurses understand behavior and its cultural basis.

U.S. Department of Health and Human Services

Internet address: http://www.dhhs.gov

This site provides links to numerous health resources from the federal government.

U.S. National Library of Medicine

Internet address: http://www.nlm.nih.gov

The U.S. National Library of Medicine is the largest medical library.

World Health Organization

Internet address: http://www.who.int

This is the Web site of the international World Health Organization, which is committed to the attainment of the highest possible level of health for everyone worldwide.

Source: Nicoll, L. (2000). *Nurses' guide to the Internet* (3rd ed). Philadelphia: Lippincott Williams & Wilkins.

References and Bibliography

American Academy of Nurse Practitioners. (1997). *The nurse practitioner: A primary health care professional* [Brochure]. Austin, TX.

American Nurses Association. (1995). *The report of survey results: The 1994 ANA layoffs survey.* Washington, DC: Author.

Anderson, M., & Poullier, J.(1999). Health spending, access, and outcomes: Trends in industrialized countries. *Health Affairs, 18*(3), 178–193.

Bellack, J., & O'Neil, E. (2000). Recreating nursing practice for a new century: Recommendations and implications of the pew health professions commission final report. *Nursing and Health Care Perspectives, 21*(1), 15–19.

Brown, K. (2000). The human genome business today. *Scientific America, 283*(1), 50–55.

Chang, E., Daly, J. H., Hawkins, A., McGirr, J., Fielding, K., Hemmings, L., et al. (1999). An evaluation of the nurse practitioner role in major rural emergency department. *Journal of Advanced Nursing, 30*(1), 260–268.

Ciaccio, J., & Walker, G. (1998). Nursing and service learning: The Kibyshi Maur. *Nursing and Health Care Perspectives, 19*(4), 175–177.

Clark, D. (2000). Old wine in new bottles: Delivering nursing in the 21st century. *Journal of Nursing Scholarship, 32*(1), 11–15.

Congress of the United States Office of Technology Assessment. (1986). *Nurse practitioners, physicians' assistants and certified nurse midwives: A policy analysis.* HCS 37.

Cooper, R., & Stoflet, S. (1996). Trends in the education and practice of alternative medicine clinicians. *Health Affairs, 15*(3), 226–238.

Craven, R. F., & Hirnle, C. J. (2000). *Fundamentals of nursing: Human health and function* (3rd ed.). Philadelphia: Lippincott Williams & Wilkins.

Dale, A., & Cornwell, S. (1994). The role of lavender oil in relieving perineal discomfort following childbirth: A blind randomized clinical trial. *Journal of Advanced Nursing, 19*(1), 89–96.

Dawson, A., & Benson, S. (1997). Clinical nurse consultant: Defining the role. *Clinical Nurse Specialist, 11*(6),250–254.

Dunham-Taylor, J., Marquette, R. P., & Pinczuk, J. Z. (1996). Surviving capitation. *American Journal of Nursing, 96*(3), 26–29.

Eisenberg, D., Kessler, R., Foster, D., Norlock, F., Calhins, D., & Delbanco, J. (1993). Unconventional medicine in the United States. *New England Journal of Medicine, 328,* 246–252.

Eisenberg, D., Davis, R., Ettner, S. L., Appel, S., Wikey, S., Van Rompay, M., & Kessler, R. C. (1998). Trends in alternative medicine use in the United States, 1990–1997: Results of a follow-up national survey. *Journal of the American Medical Association, 280*(18), 1569–1575.

Ellis, J. R., & Hartley, C. L. (1995). *Nursing in today's world: Challenges, issues, and trends.* Philadelphia: Lippincott.

FITNE launches advanced communication system for community based nursing education. (1999). *Computers in Nursing, 16*(3), 140.

Gogola, M. (1995). A joint hospital/vendor project brings CQI and point-of-care technology to home care. *Computers in Nursing, 13*(4), 143–150.

Grandinetti, D. (1999). NP progress report: How is this practice doing? *RN, 62*(7), 36–38.

Hales, G. D. (1995). Computers in nursing: The future revisited. *Gastroenterology Nursing, 18*(1), 30–32.

Harris, M. D. (1994). Home healthcare nursing is alive, well, and thriving. *Home Healthcare Nurse, 12*(3), 17–20.

Health Partners Today, Alternative Health Services, April 1999, 3. Minneapolis: Health Partners.

Heller, B., Oros, M. T., & Durney-Crowley, J. (2000). The future of nursing education: 10 trends to watch. *Nursing and Health Care Perspectives, 21*(1), 9–13.

Hupfeld, S. (2000) Through the looking glass: Tomorrow's hospital. *RN, 63*(6), 52–65.

Ibrahim, M. (1986). *Epidemiology and health policy* (pp. 133–135). Rockville, MD. Aspen.

Integrating alternatives into managed care. (1999). *RN, 62*(3), 30bb–30dd.

Kirk, S., & Glendinning, C. (1998). Trends in community care and patient participation: Implications for the roles of informal carers and community nurses in the United Kingdom. *Journal of Advanced Nursing, 28*(2), 370–381.

Kuhn, M. (1999). *Complementary therapies for health care providers.* Philadelphia: Lippincott Williams & Wilkins

Larsen, P. D. (2000). Community-based curricula: New issues to address. *Journal of Nursing Education, 39*(3), 140–141.

Lindeman, C. A. (2000). The future of nursing education. *Journal of Nursing Education, 39*(1), 5–12.

Lo-Mon, B. (2000). The role of the nurse practitioner. *Nursing Standard, 14*(21), 49–51.

Martin, S., & Hutchinson ,S. (1999). Nurse practitioners and the problem of discounting. *Journal of Advanced Nursing, 29*(1), 9–17.

Mawn, B., & Reece, S. (2000). Reconfiguring a curriculum for the new millennium: The process of change. *Journal of Nursing Education, 39*(3), 101–107.

National Center for Health Statistics, United States. (1999). *Health and aging chartbook.* Hyattsville, MD: Author.

Nichols, L. M. (1992). Estimating costs of under using advanced practice nurses. *Nursing Economics, 10,* 343–351.

Reed, F. C., Pettigrew, A., & King, M. O. (2000). Alternative and complementary therapies in nursing curricula. *Journal of Nursing Education, 39*(3), 133–139.

Simpson, R. (1999). Toward a new millennium: Outlook and obligations for 21st century health care technology. *Nursing Administration Quarterly, 24*(1), 94–97.

Tagliareni, M., Pollok, C., Horns, P., & LeDane, S. (1999). The Councils respond: What will nursing be like when the towers come down? *Nursing and Health Care Perspectives, 20*(1), 15–16.

U.S. Bureau of the Census. (1999). *General population characteristics.* Washington, DC: U.S. Government Printing Office.

U.S. Department of Health and Human Services. (2000). *Healthy people 2010* (Conference edition I & II). Washington, DC: U.S. Government Printing Office.

U.S. Immigration and Naturalization Service. (1997). *Statistical abstracts of the United States 1996.* Washington, DC: U.S. Government Printing Office.

White, S., & Henry, J. (1999). Incorporation of service learning into a baccalaureate nursing education curriculum. *Nursing Outlook, 47*(6), 257–261.

World Health Organization. (2000). *WHO issues new health live expectancy rankings.* Press release. Available at: http://www.who.int/inf-pr-2000/en/pr2000-life.html

LEARNING ACTIVITIES

LEARNING ACTIVITY 14-1

▶ **Client Care Study:** Case Manager in the Clinic of the Future

The year is 2015—the future is here. You are a case manager in a busy, urban nursing clinic. You have a caseload of clients who live in the community where your center is located. You either see your clients in the ambulatory clinic or you communicate with them by computer. Today, one of your clients, Alfred Martinez, 64-years-old, is having a sigmoid bowel resection with a temporary colostomy by laparoscopic laser surgery at the day surgery center. Home care will be provided by his wife, who will be assisted by their three adult sons on a rotating basis. It is your responsibility to coordinate the disciplines involved in his health care and manage his nursing care.

1. Identify risk factors that must be addressed when you plan for Mr. Martinez's postoperative recovery at home.
2. List five questions you will ask Mr. Martinez when you assess his care needs. Review the questions.

   Do these questions view the client holistically?
   Are they indicative of a contextual approach to identifying the client's needs?

3. Organize topics you will include when you teach Mrs. Martinez and sons about his postoperative care. Compare and contrast current care from the care provided in 1987.
4. State alternative treatments or nursing interventions you included in the plan of care. Determine if they are paid for by a third-party payer.
5. Analyze how technology will assist you in Mr. Martinez's care (eg, in making the assessment, communicating, and implementing the plan of care).

LEARNING ACTIVITY 14-2

▶ **Critical Thinking Exercise:** Self-Evaluation and Reflection

NURSING IN THE FUTURE

1. In your clinical journal, identify a future trend in health care. Find at least two articles about this trend and summarize each.
2. Follow the summary with two paragraphs in which you discuss how this trend could change or affect nursing.

Glossary

acculturation: individuals or groups from one culture learning the ways to exist in a new culture

activities of daily living (ADL): normal tasks of daily life

acute care: short-term medical or nursing care

advance directives: written guide that allows people to state in advance what their choices for health care would be if certain circumstances should develop

adult foster care homes: small residential sites that provide housing and protective oversight; also known as board and care homes or family care homes

advanced practice nurse: registered nurse who has completed graduate study in a specialty area according to specific academic requirements

advocacy: protection and support of another's rights

affective interventions: those teaching and nursing interventions that facilitate changes in attitudes, values, and feelings

affective learning: changes in attitudes, values, and feelings

alternative therapies: interventions that focus on body, mind, and spirit integration; may be used in addition to conventional treatments. Examples include relaxation, imagery, prayer.

ambulatory care center: any health care setting that provides a wide variety of services, including those related to medical, surgical, mental health, or substance abuse

assessment: a dynamic, ongoing process that uses observations and interactions to collect information, recognize changes, analyze needs, and plan care

assimilation: individuals or groups from one culture identifying more strongly with the dominant culture in values, activities, and daily living

assisted-living facilities: multiple dwellings that provide help with activities of daily living, such as being reminded to take medication, assistance with dressing and bathing, and meal preparation

barriers: factors that may adversely affect a process, (eg, referral process)

behavioral interventions: teaching or nursing interventions that assist clients to change their own behavior

boarding care homes: homes for the disabled or older person who needs meal service and housekeeping only and can manage most personal care

brokerage model: a model of case management that defines the role of the case manager as a coordinator of care mediating between all parties

care of the caregiver: nursing interventions intended to assist the individual providing care for the client

care manager: individual who manages the care of the client

case finding: a set of activities used by the nurse working in community settings that identifies clients who are not currently receiving health care, but who could benefit from such care

case management: a systematic process used by nurses to ensure that clients' multiple health and service needs are met. These include assessing client needs, planning and coordinating services, referring to other appropriate providers, and monitoring and evaluating progress.

civic responsibility: a personal ethic of social responsibility and service

client advocacy: intervening or acting on behalf of the client to provide the highest quality health care obtainable.

clinical nurse specialist: a registered nurse with a graduate degree in a specialty or subspecialty area of nursing who usually practices in acute care settings, providing direct or indirect client care

cognitive interventions: teaching or nursing actions that enhance the client's ability to intellectually process information

cognitive learning: the ability to intellectually process information including remembering, perceiving, abstracting, and generalizing

collaboration: purposeful interaction between nurse, clients, and other professional and community members based on mutual participation and joint effort

community: people, location, and social systems

community assessment: the process of determining the real or perceived needs of a defined community of people

community-based nursing: nursing care within the context of the client's family and community with a prevention focus that enhances the client's ability for self-care; a collaborative effort to maintain continuity of care

community health problem: the health need identified in community assessment

community resources: a collection of health care providers or supportive care providers who share common interests or a sense of unity

complementary therapies: interventions that focus on body, mind, and spirit integration; may be used in addition to conventional therapies. (Examples: relaxation, imagery, prayer.)

constructed survey: a time-consuming and expensive method of collecting information about a community with a valid and reliable survey, using a random sample of a targeted population where the data collected are analyzed for patterns and trends

consultation: an interactive problem-solving process between the nurse and the client

continuity of care: coordination of services provided to clients before they enter a health care setting, during the time they are in the setting, and after they leave the setting

coordinated care: the coordination of interdisciplinary sources of care and support to provide successful continuity of care

coordination: harmonious adjustment or working together

cultural awareness: self-awareness of one's own cultural background, influences, and biases

cultural blindness: lack of recognition of one's own beliefs and practices or of the beliefs and practices of others

cultural care: health care in a cultural context, acknowledging the client's cultural beliefs about disease and treatment

cultural encounter: direct contact with members of cultural communities

cultural knowledge: familiarity with a culturally or ethnically diverse group's world view, beliefs, values, practices, lifestyles, and problem-solving strategies

cultural sensitivity: the considerate, respectful, compassionate, empathic, and sensible response to a person or situation

cultural skill: the ability to collect relevant cultural data regarding the client's health history

culture: a set of values, beliefs, and attitudes that characterizes a group and provides guidance in determining one's behavior

cultural assessment: considers the cultural beliefs, values, and practices of an individual, group, or community to determine needs and interventions within a specific cultural context

day surgery centers: ambulatory services that provide preoperative, operative, and postoperative care on an outpatient basis

delegation: a management principle used to obtain desired results through the work of others, and a legal concept used to empower one person to act for another

demographics: the statistics of birth, deaths, and diseases of a community

detoxification center: facility that provides individuals safe detoxification of chemicals. The focus is on immediate health care needs and discharge planning

developmental family assessment: determination of family developmental stage and ability to meet the developmental tasks of that stage

developmental task: the usual and expected psychosocial, cognitive, or psychomotor skills at certain periods in life; failure to master the developmental task can lead to unhappiness and difficulty with later tasks

diagnosis-related groups (DRGs): classification of clients by major medical diagnosis for the purpose of standardizing health care costs

discharge planning: coordinating, planning, and arranging for the transition from one health care setting to another

diversity: the condition of being different

documentation: the process of obtaining and recording information used for communication, reference, and legal issues

emic care: care determined by the local or insider's views and values

employee assistance programs: provision of assistance to an employee when emotional or physical illness threatens to interfere with the employee's health

employee wellness programs: plans that focus on keeping employees healthy and preventing illness and accidents

environmental assessment: evaluation of the client's home and neighborhood environment

epidemic: disease occurrence that exceeds normal or expected frequency in a community or region

ethnicity: cultural differences based on heritage

ethnocentrism: belief that one's own cultural beliefs and values are best for all

etic care: care determined by the professional's or outsider's views and values

extended care facilities: synonymous with nursing homes; provide care for individuals who need daily care generally for the rest of their lives

extended family: nuclear family and other related people

family developmental tasks: the usual and expected family psychosocial, cognitive, or psychomotor skills at certain periods in life; failure to master a developmental task can lead to unhappiness and difficulty with later tasks

family functions: activities or behaviors of family members that maintain the unity of the family and meet the family's needs

family health: how well the family functions together as a unit; the family's ability to carry out usual and desired daily activities

family roles: expected set of behaviors associated with a particular family position

family structure: the characteristics of individuals (age, gender, number) who make up the family unit

family systems theory: a theory that says the family is a collection of people who are integrated, interacting, and independent, and that the actions of one member impact the actions of other members

fee-for-service: retrospective method of reimbursing medical care where each service requires payment

financial assessment: evaluation of a client's ability to pay for service

function: subjective and objective evidence of ability to perform activities of daily living

functional assessment: determination of level of health defined by one's ability to carry out usual and desired daily activities

genogram: an assessment to show family structure

gerontology nursing: the nursing care of older adults, particularly those older than 65 years

health: state of physical, mental, and social well-being and not merely the absence of disease or infirmity

health disparity: differences in health by gender, race, or ethnicity, education or income, disability, living in rural localities, or sexual orientation

health indicator: reflects the major public health concerns and illuminates factors that affect the health of individuals and communities

health maintenance organizations (HMOs): health care systems that provide comprehensive health service delivered by a defined network of providers to their members, who pay a fixed premium

health promotion: activities that enhance the well-being of an already healthy individual

health protection: environmental or regulatory measures that confer protection on large population groups

health-illness continuum: health described in a range of degrees from optimal health at one end to total disability or death at the other

healthy family functioning: optimal level of family health as defined by the family's ability to carry out usual and de-sired daily activities

holism: a way of viewing the person as an integrated whole of mind, body, and spirit; reflects the interactive process that occurs in all of us

holistic assessment: considers not only physical and psychosocial factors, but also cultural, functional, nutritional, en-vironmental, and spiritual aspects of the client

home care agencies: official, hospital-based, or proprietary organizations that provide health care in the client's resi-dence

home health care: component of compre-hensive health care whereby health ser-vices are provided to individuals and families in their places of residence for the purpose of promoting, maintaining, or restoring health

home visit: assessment, diagnosis, plan-ning, and evaluation of nursing care in the client's home

homeless shelter: facility that provides food and shelter for individuals without homes

hospice care: holistic services provided to dying persons and their loved ones to provide a more dignified and comfort-able death

hospital-based home care agency: an op-erating department of a hospital that has no mandates and no tax support to determine which services to provide

infant mortality rate: rate of death per 1,000 infants defined as 1 month to 1 year of age

informant interviews: asking community residents who are either key informants or members of the general public about their observations and concerns re-garding their community

instrumental activities of daily living (IADL): abilities to plan and prepare meals, travel, do laundry, do house-keeping, shop, and use the telephone

interdisciplinary team model: a model of case management built on the concept of collaboration that allows each pro-fessional on the team to offer his or her particular specialty

lay caregiving: care provided by families, friends, or other nonprofessionals in the home

learning domains: three areas (cognitive, affective, and psychomotor) in which teaching and learning occur

learning need: a deficit in knowledge, skills, or attitude that interrupts func-tioning

learning objectives: expected outcome for the client, including a subject, action verb, performance criteria, target time, and special conditions

lifeways: beliefs about dress, diet, and other activities of daily living

living will: written advance directive specifying the medical care a person de-sires to refuse should he or she lack the capacity to consent or refuse treatment at some point

managed care: health care systems that coordinate medical care for specific groups to promote provider efficiency and control costs

market-driven economy: a system in which consumer demand drives produc-tion regarding what services will be cre-ated and consumed and in what quantity

medication safety: concern with taking medication the correct way and avoid-ing taking medication with other drugs and substances that cause harmful in-teractions

minority: race, ethnic, or cultural group that does not belong to the dominant group

morbidity rates: rates of illness or injury

mortality rates: rates of causes of death

need to learn: perception that informa-tion or skill is relevant or necessary for immediate or delayed application

nuclear family: mother, father, and chil-dren living together

nurse midwife: a nurse who provides in-dependent care for women during nor-mal pregnancy, labor, and delivery

nurse practitioner: see advance practice nursing

nursing centers: clinics that deliver pri-mary health care, managed and served by nurses, practitioners, and other ad-vanced practice nurses

nursing functions: those activities that enable the nurse to fulfill the roles of caregiver, manager, educator, planner, and advocate

occupational health nurse: registered nurse employed in a work setting who focuses on the health and well-being of people in the workplace

official home care agency: mandated to offer a particular group of services and supported by tax dollars

outpatient services: also called ambulatory care centers or clinics; provide a broad range of health care services for the client who does not require inpatient care

parish nurse: registered nurse employed by a religious organization to provide nursing care to members of the congregation

participant observations: examination of formal and informal social systems at work for the purpose of community assessment

pharmacogenomics: the technology of developing and producing medications tailored to specific genetic profiles

polypharmacy: the prescription of more than one medication

power system: a group of people who determine how control is distributed throughout a community or social system

preferred provider organizations (PPOs): a network of physicians, hospitals, and other health-related services that contract with a third-party payer organization to provide comprehensive health services to subscribers on a fee-for-service basis

preventive services: services attempting to avoid disease or injury or minimize the consequences

primary prevention: actions that avoid the initial occurrence of disease or injury

proprietary home care agency: a free-standing for-profit home care agency; services are provided based on third-party reimbursement schedules or by self-pay

prospective payment: payment for health care services in advance based on rate derived from predictions of annual service costs

psychomotor learning: physical skills that can be demonstrated

race: to characterize a distinct human type by traits that are transmitted by descent

readiness to learn: emotional state, abilities, and potential that allow learning to occur

referral process: a dynamic process between community resources that ensures continuity of care for the well-being of a client

rehabilitation centers: either residential or outpatient facilities providing services to those requiring either physical or emotional rehabilitation. Residence is generally limited to the achievement of goals

reimbursement requirements: governmental or proprietary requirements that must be met before a service is paid for

residential centers: supervised group facilities with various levels of independence, including, among other levels, retirement communities, assisted living facilities, board and care, skilled nursing facilities, and subacute rehabilitation centers

respite care: services to a family or caregivers to temporarily relieve caregiving demands

retirement communities: homes or apartments with supportive services provided by the retirement community, providing a community living style for individuals who choose to live with other seniors

school nurse: a registered nurse charged with the health care of school-age children and school personnel in an educational setting

secondary data: records, documents, or any previously collected information

secondary prevention: actions providing early identification and treatment of disease or injury with the purpose of limiting disability

self-care: the actions of individuals, families, and communities to preserve and promote their own health, life, and sense of well-being

skilled nursing facilities: provision of nursing, medical, and therapy services for the individual who does not require acute care, but requires ongoing care. Generally transferred to extended care or to home

sliding fee scale: payment schedule based on the client's ability to pay for service

social system: the various components of a community, including economic, educational, religious, political, legal, and methods of communication

specialized care centers: facilities that provide health care for a specific population group

spiritual assessment: allows the nurse to determine the presence of spiritual distress or identify other spiritual needs and incorporate them into the plan of care

spirituality: a flowing, healing, dynamic balance that allows and creates health and well-being; sometimes involves organized religion

stereotyping: a mental picture or an assumption about a person based on a characteristic that comes from myths or generalizations based on the perceived membership in a group

structural family assessment: family assessment that maps out the composition of the family, such as a genogram

subacute rehabilitation centers: limited time residence; discharge usually occurs when the client has met certain goals

support services: services that help people avoid problems or solve problems that interfere with their well-being

technology: a tool to extend human abilities

tertiary prevention: actions to maximize recovery and potential after an injury or illness

transcultural nursing: a body of knowledge and practice for caring for people from other cultures

transferring: moving from one tertiary care setting to another

transitional housing: temporary service often used between acute illness episodes or a personal housing crisis and permanent housing

underserved populations: individuals and families who do not have access to health care

unlicensed assistive personnel (UAP): persons without a professional license

vital statistics: information related to on-going registration of births, deaths, adoptions, divorces, marriages, causes of death, and other statistics that reflect the vital signs of a community

wellness promotion: to encourage or promote a healthy state

windshield survey: motorized equivalent of a simple observation where the observer drives through a chosen neighborhood and uses the power of observation to conduct a general assessment of that neighborhood

work site health promotion: programs that focus on the health of employees within business and industry

INDEX

References with "t" denote tables; "f" denote figures, "b" denote boxes.